THE SCIENCE OF YOGA

cover art by JANE EVANS

THE SCIENCE OF YOGA

THE **YOGA-SŪTRAS** OF PATAÑJALI IN SANSKRIT
WITH TRANSLITERATION IN ROMAN, TRANSLATION
IN ENGLISH AND COMMENTARY

BY
I. K. TAIMNI

A QUEST BOOK
Published under a grant from The Kern Foundation

THE THEOSOPHICAL PUBLISHING HOUSE
Wheaton, Ill., U.S.A.
Madras, India / London, England

Fourth Quest Book edition 1975 published by The Theosophical Publishing House, Wheaton, Ill., a department of The Theosophical Society in America.

ISBN: 0-8356-0023-8
Library of Congress Catalog Card number 67-4112

PRINTED IN THE UNITED STATES OF AMERICA

PREFACE

A LARGE number of thoughtful people, both in the East and the West, are genuinely interested in the subject of *Yoga*. This is natural because a man who has begun to question life and its deeper problems wants something more definite and vital for his spiritual needs than a mere promise of heavenly joys or 'eternal life' when he passes out of his brief and feverish life on this planet. Those who have lost faith in the ideals of orthodox religions and yet feel that their life is not a meaningless and passing phenomenon of Nature naturally turn to the philosophy of *Yoga* for the solution of problems connected with their 'inner' life.

People who take up the study of *Yoga* with the object of finding a more satisfactory solution of these problems are likely to meet with one serious difficulty. They may find the philosophy interesting, even fascinating, but too much enveloped in mystery and rigmarole to be of much practical value in their life. For there is no subject which is so much wrapped up in mystery and on which one can write whatever one likes without any risk of being proved wrong. To a certain extent this atmosphere of mystery and obscurity which surrounds *Yoga* is due to the very nature of the subject itself. The philosophy of *Yoga* deals with some of the greatest mysteries of life and the Universe and so it must inevitably be associated with an atmosphere of profound mystery. But much of the obscurity of *Yogic* literature is due, not to the intrinsic profundity of the subject, but to the lack of correlation between its teachings and the facts with which an ordinary educated man is expected to be familiar. If the doctrines of *Yoga* are studied in the light of both ancient and modern thought it is much easier for the student to understand and appreciate them. The discoveries made in the field of Science are especially helpful in enabling the student to understand certain facts of *Yogic* life, for there is a certain analogous relationship between the laws of higher life and life as it exists on the physical plane, a relationship which is hinted at in the well-known Occult maxim ' As above, so below '.

Some teachers of *Yoga* have attempted to meet this difficulty by taking out of the philosophy and technique of *Yoga* those particular practices which are easy to understand and practise, placing these before the general public as *Yogic* teachings. Many of these practices like *Āsana*, *Prāṇāyāma* etc. are of a purely physical nature and when divorced from the higher and essential teachings of *Yoga* reduce their systems to a science of physical culture on a par with other systems of a similar nature. This over-simplification of the problem of *Yogic* life, though it has done some good and helped some people to live a saner and healthier physical life, has greatly vulgarized the movement for *Yogic* culture and produced a wrong impression, especially in the West, about the real purpose and technique of *Yoga*.

What is needed, therefore, for the average student of *Yoga* is a clear, intelligible presentation of its philosophy and technique which gives a correct and balanced idea of all its aspects in terms of modern thought. For, while it is true that many aspects of *Yogic* life are beyond the comprehension of those confined within the realms of the intellect, still, the general philosophy and the broader aspects of its technique can be understood by the serious student who is familiar with the main trends of philosophical and religious thought and is prepared to bring to his study an open and eager mind.

He can, at least, understand this philosophy sufficiently to be able to decide whether it is worth his while to undertake a deeper study of the subject and later, to enter the path of *Yoga* as a *Sādhaka*. For, it is only when he enters the path of practical *Yoga* and begins to bring about fundamental changes in his nature that he can hope to gain real insight into the problems of *Yoga* and their solution.

This book is meant to give to the serious student of *Yoga* a clear idea with regard to the fundamental teachings of *Yoga* in a language which he can understand. It does not present *Yoga* from any particular angle or on the basis of any particular school of philosophy. Those who study the book will see for themselves that this Science of sciences is too comprehensive in its nature and too profound in its doctrines to be fitted into the framework of any particular philosophy, ancient or modern. It stands in its own right as a Science based upon the eternal laws of the higher life and does not require the support of any science or philosophical system to uphold its claims. Its truths are based on the experiences and experiments of an unbroken line of mystics, occultists, saints and sages who have realized and borne witness to them throughout the ages. Although an attempt has been made to explain the teachings of *Yoga* on a rational basis so that the student may be able to grasp them easily nothing is sought to be proved in the ordinary sense. The facts of higher *Yoga* can neither be proved nor demonstrated. Their appeal is to the intuition and not to the intellect.

There is a vast literature dealing with all aspects and types of *Yoga*. But the beginner who attempts to dive into this chaotic mass is likely to feel repulsed by the confusion and exaggerated statements which he is likely to find everywhere. Round a small nucleus of fundamental and genuine teachings of *Yoga* has grown up during the course of thousands of years a volume of spurious literature composed of commentaries, expositions of minor systems of *Yogic* culture and *Tāntric* practices. Any inexperienced student who enters this jungle is likely to feel bewildered and to come out of it with a feeling that his pursuit of the *Yogic* ideal might prove a waste of time. The student would, therefore, do well to confine himself to the basic literature to avoid confusion and frustration.

In this basic literature of *Yoga*, the *Yoga-Sūtras* of Patañjali stand out as the most authoritative and useful book. In its 196 *Sūtras* the author has condensed the essential philosophy and technique of *Yoga* in a manner which is a marvel of condensed and systematic exposition. The student who studies the book for the first time or superficially may find the treatment rather strange and haphazard, but a more careful and deeper study will reveal the rational basis of the treatment. The following synopsis will show how rational the whole treatment is.

The first Section deals with the general nature of *Yoga* and its technique. It is meant really to answer the question 'What is *Yoga*?' Since *Samādhi* is the essential technique of *Yoga*, naturally, it occupies the most important position among the various topics dealt with in the Section. This Section is, therefore, called *Samādhi Pāda*.

The first part of the second Section deals with the philosophy of *Kleśas* and is meant to provide an answer to the question 'Why should anyone practise *Yoga*?' It gives a masterly analysis of the conditions of human life and the misery and suffering which are inherent in these conditions. The philosophy of *Kleśas* must be thoroughly understood by any person who is to take to the path of *Yoga* with the unalterable determination to persevere, life after life, until he has reached the End. The second part of Section II deals with the first five practices of *Yogic* technique which are referred to as *Bahiraṅga* or external. These practices are of a preparatory nature and are meant to make the *Sādhaka* fit for the practice of *Samādhi*. As this Section is meant to fit the aspirant physically, mentally, emotionally and morally for the practice of Higher *Yoga* it is called *Sādhana Pāda*.

The first part of the third Section deals with the three remaining practices of *Yogic* technique which are referred to as *Antaraṅga* or internal. It is through these practices which culminate in *Samādhi* that all the mysteries of *Yogic* life are unravelled and the powers or *Siddhis* are acquired. In the second part of this Section these accomplishments are discussed in detail and the Section is, therefore, called *Vibhūti Pāda*.

In the fourth and the last Section are expounded all those essential philosophical problems which are involved in the study and practice of *Yoga*. The nature of the mind and mental perception, of desire and its binding effect, of Liberation and the results which follow it, are all dealt with briefly but systematically to enable the student to have an adequate background of theoretical knowledge. Since all these topics are connected in one way or another with the attainment of *Kaivalya*, the Section is called *Kaivalya Pāda*.

On account of its comprehensive and systematic treatment of the subject the *Yoga-Sūtras* is the most suitable book for deep and systematic study of *Yoga*. In the olden days all students of *Yoga* were made to commit it to memory and meditate regularly and deeply on the *Sūtras* for bringing out their hidden meanings. But the modern student, who has to be convinced first that the study and practice of *Yoga* is worthwhile, needs a more detailed and elaborate treatment of the subject to enable him to understand its philosophy as a whole. Even for this purpose the *Yoga-Sūtras* is the most suitable basis, not only because it gives all the essential information about *Yoga* in a masterly manner but also because it is recognized as a masterpiece in the literature of *Yoga* and has stood the test of time and experience. It is for this reason that it has been made the basis of the present book.

The task of an author who undertakes to write a commentary on a book like the *Yoga-Sūtras* is not an easy one. He is dealing with a subject of the most profound nature. The ideas which he has to interpret are given in the form of *Sūtras* which embody the art of condensation to the utmost limit. The language with which the *Sūtras* are constructed is an ancient one which, though extraordinarily effective in the expression of philosophical ideas, can lend itself to an extraordinary variety of interpretations. And what is most important, he is dealing with a Science which is related to facts which come within the range of human experience. He cannot like the academic philosopher give free rein to his imagination and put forward merely an ideal interpretation. He has to show things, to the best of his ability, as they actually are and not as they should be or might be. Keeping in view the possibility of the changes which are always brought about in the connotations of words with lapse of time it is extremely hazardous to interpret the *Sūtras* rigidly according to their literal meaning. Of course, one cannot take liberties with a book like the *Yoga-Sūtras* which has been written by a master mind in a language which is considered almost perfect. But it is one thing to interpret a *Sūtra* in a loose and careless manner and another to bring out its meaning with due regard to facts of experience and recognized traditions of ages. The sensible way, of course, is to take into consideration all the factors which are involved, avoiding especially explanations which explain nothing.

Another difficulty in writing a commentary in English is the impossibility of finding exact equivalents for many *Saṃskṛta* words. Since the Science of *Yoga* has flourished mainly in the East and the interest in *Yoga* in the West is of recent origin there are no equivalents in the English language corresponding to many *Saṃskṛta* words which stand for well-defined philosophical concepts. And in many cases the available English words with approximate meanings are liable to give a totally wrong impression. To avoid this danger *Saṃskṛta* words have been used freely in the commentary if an exact equivalent in English is not available. But to facilitate careful study of the subject, not only is the original *Saṃskṛta* text given in the case of each *Sūtra* but also the meanings of the *Saṃskṛta* words used in the *Sūtra*. Of course, as pointed out above, the exact English equivalents of many *Saṃskṛta* words are not available. In such cases only approximate meanings have been given and the student is expected to find the exact significance of the words from the following commentary. The above procedure will enable the student to judge for himself how far the interpretation is in accordance with the literal meanings of the words used in the *Sūtra*, and if there is a divergence, how far the divergence is justified. But, of course, the final justification for any interpretation is its conformity with the facts of experience and if this kind of verification is not possible, commonsense and reason should be the guide. The seeker after Truth should concern himself especially with facts and the truth underlying the various *Sūtras* and should not allow himself to get involved in controversies about the meanings of words. This pastime he can leave to the mere scholar.

A careful study of the *Yoga-Sūtras* and the kind of preparation and effort which is needed for attaining the objective of *Yogic* endeavour might give to the student the impression that it is an extremely difficult, if not impossible undertaking, beyond the capacity of the ordinary aspirant. This impression is certain to dishearten him, and if he does not think deeply over the problems of life and clarify his ideas about them, it might lead him to abandon the idea of embarking on this Divine adventure or to postpone it to a future life. There can be no doubt that the serious pursuit of the *Yogic* ideal is a difficult task and cannot be undertaken as a mere hobby or to find an escape from the stress and strain of ordinary life. It can be undertaken only on understanding fully the nature of human life and the misery and suffering which are inherent in it and the further realization that the only way to end this misery and suffering permanently is to find the Truth which is enshrined within ourselves, by the only method which is available, namely, *Yogic* discipline. It is also true that the attainment of this objective is a long-term affair and the aspirant should be prepared to spend a number of lives—as many lives as may be required—in its whole-hearted and single-minded pursuit. No one can know in the beginning his potentialities and how much time will be needed. He can hope for the best but must be prepared for the worst.

Those who do not feel themselves equal to this task are not under any compulsion to attempt it immediately. They can continue the theoretical study of *Yoga*, think constantly over life's deeper problems, try to purify their minds and strengthen their characters, until their power of discrimination becomes sufficiently strong to enable them to pierce through ordinary illusions and see life in its naked reality. In fact, this is the purpose of *Kriyā Yoga* to which Patañjali has referred in the beginning of Section II. When the inner eyes of true discrimination begin to open as a result of the practice of *Kriyā Yoga* they will cease to wonder whether they are strong enough to undertake this long and difficult journey to their true homes. Then nothing will be able to stop them, and they will naturally and whole-heartedly devote themselves to this difficult but sacred task.

The important point is to make a definite beginning somewhere and as soon as possible—Now. The moment such a serious beginning is made forces begin to gather round the centre of endeavour and take the aspirant forward towards his goal, slowly at first, but with increasing speed until he becomes so absorbed in the pursuit of his ideal that time and distance cease to matter for him. And one day he finds that he has reached his goal and looks back with a kind of wonder at the long and tedious journey which he has completed in the realm of Time while all the time he was living in the Eternal.

I. K. Taimni

CONTENTS

	PAGE
PREFACE	.. v
SECTION I	
Samādhi Pāda	.. 1
SECTION II	
Sādhana Pāda	.. 125
SECTION III	
Vibhūti Pāda	.. 273
SECTION IV	
Kaivalya Pāda	.. 375
INDEX	.. 447

SECTION I

SAMĀDHI PĀDA

SAMĀDHI PĀDA

१. अथ योगानुशासनम् ।

Atha Yogānuśāsanam.

अथ now; herewith योग (of) Yoga अनुशासनम् expounding; exposition (teaching).

1. Now, an exposition of *Yoga* (is to be made).

Generally, a treatise of this nature in *Saṃskṛta* begins with a *Sūtra* which gives an idea with regard to the nature of the undertaking. The present treatise is an 'exposition' of *Yoga*. The author does not claim to be the discoverer of this Science but merely an expounder who has tried to condense in a few *Sūtras* all the essential knowledge concerning the Science which a student or aspirant ought to possess. Very little is known about Patañjali. Although we have no information about him which can be called definitely historical, still according to occult tradition he was the same person who was known as Govinda Yogi and who initiated Śaṃkarācārya in the Science of *Yoga*. From the masterly manner in which he has expounded the subject of *Yoga* in the *Yoga-Sūtras* it is obvious that he was a *Yogi* of a very high order who had personal knowledge of all aspects of *Yoga* including its practical technique.

As the method of expounding a subject in the form of *Sūtras* is peculiar and generally unfamiliar to Western students having no knowledge of the *Saṃskṛta* language, it would perhaps not be out of place to say here a few words on this classical method which was adopted by the ancient Sages and scholars in their exposition of some of the most important subjects. The word *Sūtram* in *Saṃskṛta* means a thread and this primary meaning has given rise to the secondary meaning of *Sūtram* as an aphorism. Just as a thread binds together a number of beads in a rosary, in the same way the underlying continuity of idea binds together in outline the essential aspects of a subject. The most important characteristics of this method are utmost condensation consistent with clear exposition of all essential aspects and continuity of the underlying theme in spite of the apparent discontinuity of the ideas presented. The latter characteristic is worth noting because the effort to discover the hidden 'thread' of reasoning beneath the apparently unconnected ideas very often provides the clue to the meaning of many *Sūtras*. It should be remembered that this method of exposition was prevalent at a time when printing was unknown and most of the important treatises had to be memorized by the student. Hence the necessity of condensation to the utmost limit. Nothing essential was, of course, left out but everything with which the student was expected to be familiar or which he could easily infer from the context was ruthlessly cut out.

The student will find on careful study what a tremendous amount of theoretical and practical knowledge the author has managed to incorporate in this very small treatise. Everything necessary for the proper understanding of the subject has been given at one place or another in a skeleton form. But the body of the requisite knowledge has to be dug out, prepared properly, chewed and digested before the subject can be understood thoroughly in its entirety. The *Sūtra* method of exposition may appear to the modern student needlessly obscure and difficult but if he goes through the labour required for the mastery of the subject he will realize its superiority to the all too easy modern methods of presentation. The necessity of struggling with the words and ideas and digging out their hidden meanings ensures a very thorough assimilation of knowledge and develops simultaneously the powers and faculties of the mind, especially that important and indispensable capacity of digging out of one's own mind the knowledge which lies buried in its deeper recesses.

But while this method of exposition is very effective it has its drawbacks also. The chief disadvantage is the difficulty which the ordinary student who is not thoroughly conversant with the subject has in finding the correct meaning. Not only is he likely to find many *Sūtras* difficult to understand on account of their brevity but he may completely misunderstand some of them and be led astray in a hopeless manner. We have to remember that in a treatise like the *Yoga-Sūtras*, behind many a word there is a whole pattern of thought of which the word is a mere symbol. To understand the true significance of the *Sūtras* we must be thoroughly familiar with these patterns. The difficulty is increased still further when the words have to be translated into another language which does not contain exactly equivalent words.

Those who wrote these treatises were master-minds, masters of the subject and language they dealt with. There could be no fault in their method of presentation. But in the course of time fundamental changes can sometimes be brought about in the meaning of words and the thought patterns of those who study these treatises. And this fact introduces endless possibilities of misunderstanding and misinterpretation of some of the *Sūtras*. In treatises of a purely philosophical or religious nature such a misunderstanding would perhaps not matter so much, but in one of a highly technical and practical nature like the *Yoga-Sūtras* it can lead to great complications and even to dangers of a serious nature.

Luckily for the earnest student, *Yoga* has always been a living Science in the East and it has had an unbroken succession of living experts who continually verify by their own experiments and experiences the basic truths of this Science. This has helped not only to keep the traditions of *Yogic* culture alive and pure but to maintain the meanings of the technical words used in this Science in a fairly exact and clearly defined form. It is only when a Science is divorced completely from its practical application that it tends to lose itself in a morass of words which have lost their meaning and relation with the actual facts.

While the method of presenting a subject in the form of *Sūtras* is eminently suited for the practical and advanced student it can hardly be denied that it does not quite fit in with our modern conditions. In the olden days those who studied these *Sūtras* had easy access to the teachers of the Science who elaborated the knowledge embodied in a condensed form, filled up the gaps and gave practical guidance. And these students had leisure in which to think, meditate and dig out the meanings for themselves. The modern student who is interested merely in the theoretical study of the *Yogic* philosophy and is not practising it under an expert teacher has none of these facilities and needs an elaborate and clear exposition for an adequate understanding of the subject. He needs a commentary which not only aims at explaining the obvious meaning but also the hidden significance of the words and phrases used in terms of the concepts with which he is familiar and can easily understand. He wants his food not in ' tabloid ' form but in bulk, and if possible, in a palatable form.

२. योगश्चित्तवृत्तिनिरोधः ।

Yogaś citta-vṛtti-nirodhaḥ.

योगः (the essential technique of) yoga चित्त (of) mind वृत्ति (of) modifications निरोधः inhibition; suppression; stoppage; restraint.

2. Yoga is the inhibition of the modifications of the mind.

This is one of the most important and well-known *Sūtras* of this treatise not because it deals with some important principle or technique of practical value but because it defines with the help of only four words the essential nature of *Yoga*. There are certain concepts in every science which are of a basic nature and which must be understood aright if the student is to get a satisfactory grasp of the subject as a whole. The ideas underlying all the four words in this *Sūtra* are of such a fundamental nature and the student should try to grasp through study and reflection their real meaning. Of course, the significance of these words will become sufficiently clear only when the book has been studied thoroughly, and the various aspects of the subject considered in their relation to one another. It might be expected that words of such fundamental importance will be carefully defined and such definitions inserted wherever they are needed. But in the case of the present

Sūtra no such definitions have been given and we can therefore conclude that the author expected the student to acquire a clear idea with regard to the import of the words from his study of the whole book. But as it is necessary for the student not to start his study with wrong or confused ideas it will perhaps be worthwhile considering at this initial stage the import of the words and the *Sūtra* in a general way.

Let us begin with the word *Yoga*. The word *Yoga* in *Saṃskṛta* has a very large number of meanings. It is derived from the root *Yuj* which means 'to join' and the idea of joining runs through all the meanings. What are the two things which are sought to be joined by the practice of *Yoga*? According to the highest conceptions of Hindu philosophy of which the Science of *Yoga* is an integral part, the human soul or the *Jīvātmā* is a facet or partial expression of the Over-Soul or *Paramātmā*, the Divine Reality which is the source or substratum of the manifested Universe. Although in essence the two are the same and are indivisible, still, the *Jīvātmā* has become subjectively separated from *Paramātmā* and is destined, after going through an evolutionary cycle in the manifested Universe, to become united with Him again in consciousness. This state of unification of the two in consciousness as well as the mental process and discipline through which this union is attained are both called *Yoga*. This conception is formulated in a different way in the *Sāṃkhya* philosophy but on close analysis the fundamental idea will be found to be essentially the same.

Then we come to the word *Citta*. This word is derived from the *Cit* or *Citi* (IV-34) one of the three aspects of *Paramātmā* called *Sat-Cit-Ānanda* in *Vedānta*. It is this aspect which is at the basis of the form side of the Universe and through which it is created. The reflection of this aspect in the individual soul which is a microcosm is called *Citta*. *Citta* is thus that instrument or medium through which the *Jīvātmā* materializes his individual world, lives and evolves in the world until he has become perfected and united with the *Paramātmā*. Broadly, therefore, *Citta* corresponds to 'mind' of modern psychology but it has a more comprehensive import and field for functioning. While *Citta* may be considered as a universal medium through which consciousness functions on all the planes of the manifested Universe, the 'mind' of modern psychology is confined to the expression of only thought, volition and feeling.

We should not, however, make the mistake of imagining *Citta* as a sort of material medium which is moulded into different forms when mental images of different kinds are produced. It is fundamentally of the nature of consciousness which is immaterial but affected by matter. In fact, it may be called a product of both, consciousness and matter, or *Puruṣa* and *Prakṛti*, the presence of both being necessary for its functioning. It is like an intangible screen which enables the Light of consciousness to be projected in the manifested world. But the real secret of its essential nature lies buried in the origin of the manifested Universe and can be known only on attaining Enlightenment. It is true that the theory of perception which is developed in Section IV gives some general indication with regard to the nature of *Citta* but it does not say what *Citta* essentially is.

The third word we have to consider in this *Sūtra* is *Vṛtti*. It is derived from the root *Vṛt* which means ' to exist '. So *Vṛtti* is a way of existing. In considering the ways in which a thing exists we may consider its modifications, states, activities or its functions. All these connotations are present in the meaning of *Vṛtti* but in the present context this word is best translated by the words ' modifications ' or 'functionings '. Sometimes the word is translated as ' transformations '. This does not seem to be justified because in transformation the emphasis is on the change and not on the condition. The transformations of *Citta* may be stopped and it may still remain in one particular modification as happens in *Sabīja Samādhi*. As the ultimate aim of *Yoga* is inhibition of all modifications in *Nirbīja Samādhi* it will be seen that the word ' transformation ' will not adequately express the meaning of the word *Vṛtti*. Besides, the word ' transformation ' has to be used for the three *Pariṇāmas* dealt with in the first part of Section III. Since *Citta* has a functional existence and comes into being only when consciousness is affected by matter, the word ' functionings ' perhaps expresses to the maximum degree the significance of *Vṛtti* in the present context, but the word ' modifications ' is also used generally and understood more easily and may therefore pass.

In trying to understand the nature of *Citta-Vṛttis* we have to guard against a few misconceptions which are sometimes prevalent among those who have not studied the subject deeply. The first thing to note is that *Citta-Vṛtti* is not a vibration. We have seen above that *Citta* is not material and therefore there can be no question of any vibration in it. Vibrations can take place only in a vehicle and these vibrations may produce a *Citta-Vṛtti*. The two are different though related. The second point to be noted in this connection is that a *Citta-Vṛtti* is not a mental image though it may be and is generally associated with mental images. The five-fold classification of *Citta-Vṛttis* in I-5 definitely shows this. Mental images may be of innumerable kinds but the author has classified *Citta-Vṛttis* under five heads only. This shows that *Citta-Vṛttis* have a more fundamental and comprehensive character than the mere mental images with which they are associated. This is not the place to enter into a detailed discussion of the essential nature of *Citta-Vṛttis* because the question involves the essential nature of *Citta*. But if the student studies carefully the six *Sūtras* (I-6-11) dealing with the five kinds of *Vṛttis* he will see that they are the fundamental states or types of modifications in which the mind can exist. The author has given five types for the modifications of the lower concrete mind with which the ordinary man is familiar. But the number and nature of these different types are bound to be different in the higher realms of *Citta*.

The last word to be considered is *Nirodha*. This word is derived from the word *Niruddham* which means 'restrained', 'controlled', 'inhibited'. All these meanings are applicable in the different stages of *Yoga*. Restraint is involved in the initial stages, control in the more advanced stages and inhibition or complete suppression in the last stage. The subject of *Nirodha* has been dealt with in considering III-9 and the student should read carefully what is written in that connection.

If the student has understood the meaning of the four words in this *Sūtra* he will see that it defines in a masterly manner the essential nature of *Yoga*. The effectiveness of the definition lies in the fact that it covers all stages of progress through which the *Yogi* passes and all stages of unfoldment of consciousness which are the result of this progress. It is equally applicable to the stage of *Kriyā-Yoga* in which he learns the preliminary lessons, to the stages of *Dhāraṇā* and *Dhyāna* in which he brings the mind under his complete control, to the stage of *Sabīja Samādhi* in which he has to suppress the 'seeds' of *Saṃprajñāta-Samādhi* and to the last stage of *Nirbīja Samādhi* in which he inhibits all modifications of *Citta* and passes beyond the realm of *Prakṛti* into the world of Reality. The full significance of the *Sūtra* can be understood only when the subject of *Yoga* has been studied thoroughly in all its aspects and so it is useless to say anything further at this stage.

३. तदा द्रष्टुः स्वरूपेऽवस्थानम् ।

Tadā draṣṭuḥ svarūpe 'vasthānam.

तदा then द्रष्टुः (of) Seer स्वरूपे in his 'own form' or essential and fundamental nature अवस्थानम् establishment.

3. Then the Seer is established in his own essential and fundamental nature.

This *Sūtra* points out in a general way what happens when all the modifications of the mind at all levels have been completely inhibited. The Seer is established in his *Svarūpa* or in other words attains Self-realization. We cannot know what this state of Self-realization is as long as we are involved in the play of *Citta-Vṛttis*. It can only be realized from within and not comprehended from without. Even the partial and superficial comprehension which we can obtain under our present limitations by means of study and reflection is possible only after we have mastered the whole theory and technique of *Yoga* outlined in this treatise. The higher stages of consciousness which unfold in the state of *Samādhi* and which are referred to in I-44 and 45 are called *Ṛtaṃbharā* or truth-right-bearing. In their light the *Yogi* can know the truth underlying all things in manifestation. But he can know the truth in this way of only those things which are part of *Dṛśyam*, the Seen, not of the *Draṣṭā*, the Seer. For this he has to practise *Nirbīja Samādhi* (I-51).

४. वृत्तिसारूप्यमितरत्र ।

Vṛtti-sārūpyam itaratra.

वृत्ति (with) modifications (of the mind) सारूप्यम् identification; assimilation इतरत्र elsewhere, in other states.

4. In other states there is assimilation (of the Seer) with the modifications (of the mind).

When the *Citta-Vṛttis* are not in the state of *Nirodha* and the *Draṣṭā* is not established in his *Svarūpa* he is assimilated with the particular *Vṛtti* which happens to occupy the field of his consciousness for the moment. A simile will perhaps help the student to understand this assimilation of consciousness with the transformation of the mind. Let him imagine a lighted electric bulb suspended in a tank full of limpid water. If the water is churned violently by some mechanical contrivance it will make all kinds of patterns in three dimensions round the bulb, these patterns being illuminated by the light from the bulb and changing from moment to moment. But what about the bulb itself? It will disappear from view, all the light emanating from it being assimilated with or lost in the surrounding water. Now, let him imagine the churning of water slowed down gradually until the water becomes perfectly still. As the three dimensional patterns begin to subside gradually the electric bulb gradually emerges into view and when the water is quite at rest the bulb alone is seen. This simile illustrates in a rather crude way both the assimilation of the consciousness of the *Puruṣa* with the modification of the mind and its reversion to its own unmodified state when the mind comes to rest. The mind may come to rest either through *Para-Vairāgya* developed by *Īśvara-pra.idhāna* or through the practice of *Samādhi*, the result in both cases is the same—Enlightenment—and Liberation.

This *Sūtra*, like the previous one, is meant to answer only in a general way the question 'what happens to the *Puruṣa* when he is not established in his *Svarūpa*?' Its full significance can be understood only after the whole book has been studied thoroughly, and the various aspects of the subject understood adequately.

५. वृत्तयः पञ्चतय्यः क्लिष्टाक्लिष्टाः ।

Vṛttayaḥ pañcatayyaḥ kliṣṭākliṣṭāḥ.

वृत्तयः (plural of वृत्तिः) modes, modifications or functionings of the mind पञ्चतय्यः fivefold; of five kinds क्लिष्टा painful अक्लिष्टाः (and) not-painful.

5. The modifications of the mind are five-fold and are painful or not-painful.

After indicating the essential nature of *Yogic* technique the author then proceeds to classify the *Vṛttis*. He classifies them in two ways. Firstly, in relation to our feelings whether they are painful, pleasurable or neutral in their character. And secondly, according to the nature of the *Pratyaya* which is produced in our consciousness.

Let us consider first the reaction of these *Vṛttis* on our feelings. This reaction according to Patañjali is either painful or not-painful. This will appear to a superficial student a rather strange way of classifying the mental modifications. Of course, there are certain modifications which are of a neutral character, i.e., they do not produce any pleasurable or painful reaction in our mind. When, for example, we notice a tree while walking it is a mere sensuous perception which does not arouse any pleasurable or painful feeling within us. The vast majority of our sensuous perceptions which result in the modification of the mind are of this neutral character. They have been classed as 'not-painful'.

But there are other modifications of the mind which do arouse a pleasurable or painful feeling within us. For example, when we taste some palatable article of food, or see a beautiful sunset or smell a rose there is a distinct feeling of pleasure. On the other hand, when we see a horrible sight or hear a cry of anguish the resulting transformation of the mind is definitely painful. Why has then Patañjali classified all such modifications of the mind which arouse some feeling within us as painful? The reason for this is given in II-15 in connection with the philosophy of *Kleśas*. It will suffice to mention here that according to the theory of *Kleśas* upon which the *Yogic* philosophy is based, all pleasurable and painful experiences are really painful to the people who have developed the faculty of discrimination and are not blinded by the illusions of the lower life. It is our ignorance, caused by these illusions, which makes us see pleasure in experiences which are a potential source of pain and therefore makes us run after those pleasures. If our inner eyes were open we would see the 'potential' pain hidden within these pleasures and not only when the pain is present in an 'active' form. We would then see the justification for classifying all experiences which involve our feelings and thus give rise to *Rāga* and *Dveṣa* as painful. This may appear to the student a rather pessimistic view of life but let him withhold his judgment until he has studied the philosophy of *Kleśas* in Section II.

If all experiences involving our feelings are painful then it is logical to classify the remaining experiences which are of a neutral character and do not affect our feelings as not-painful. It will be seen, therefore, that the primary classification of *Citta-Vṛttis* as painful and not-painful is not without reason and from the *Yogic* point of view perfectly logical and reasonable.

The other point of view from which the *Citta-Vṛttis* have been classified is the nature of the *Pratyaya* produced in the *Citta*. The object of classifying them in this manner is to show that all our experiences in the realm of the mind consist of mental modifications and nothing else. The control and complete suppression of these modifications, therefore, extinguishes our lower life completely and leads inevitably to the dawning of the higher consciousness. When classified in this manner the *Vṛttis* or modifications are stated to be of five kinds as shown in the next *Sūtra*.

६. प्रमाणविपर्ययविकल्पनिद्रास्मृतयः ।

Pramāṇa-viparyaya-vikalpa-nidrā-smṛtayaḥ.

प्रमाण right knowledge विपर्यय wrong knowledge विकल्प fancy; imagination निद्रा sleep स्मृतयः (and) memory.

6. (They are) right knowledge, wrong knowledge, fancy, sleep, and memory.

Here again, on a cursory examination, the five-fold classification may appear rather odd but a deeper study will show that it is perfectly scientific. If we analyse our mental life, as far as its content is concerned, we shall find it to consist of a great variety and number of images, but a closer study of these images will show that they can all be classified under the five broad sub-heads enumerated in this *Sūtra*. Before we deal with each of these separately in the subsequent five *Sūtras* let us try to understand the underlying system of classification in a general way.

Pramāṇa and *Viparyaya* comprise all those images which are formed by some kind of direct contact through the sense organs with the outer world of objects. *Vikalpa* and *Smṛti* comprise all those images or modifications of the mind which are produced without any kind of direct contact with the outer world. They are the result of the independent activity of the lower mind using the sensuous perceptions which have been gathered before and stored in the mind. In the case of *Smṛti* or memory these sensuous perceptions are reproduced in the mind faithfully, i.e., in the form and order in which they were obtained through the sense-organs previously. In the case of *Vikalpa* or imagination they are reproduced in any form and order from the sensuous material present in the mind. The imagination can combine these sensuous perceptions in any form or order, congruous or incongruous, but the power of combining the sensuous perceptions is under the control of the will. In the dream state the will has no control over these combinations and they appear before consciousness in haphazard, fantastic and frequently absurd combinations influenced to a certain extent by the desires present in the sub-conscious mind. The higher Self with its will and reason has, as it were, withdrawn beyond the threshold of consciousness, leaving the lower mind partly entangled with the brain deprived of the rationalizing influence of reason and the controlling influence of will.

When even this remnant of the lower mind also withdraws beyond the threshold of brain consciousness we have dreamless sleep or *Nidrā*. In this state there are no mental images in the brain. The mind continues to be active on its own plane but its images are not reflected on the screen of the physical brain.

Now, let the student examine his mental activity in the light of what has been said above. Let him take any modification of the lower concrete mind which works with names and forms and see whether he cannot put it under one or the other of these five groups. He will find to his surprise that all modifications of the lower mind can be classed under one or the other of these sub-heads and therefore the system of classification is quite rational. It is true that many modifications on analysis will be found to be complex and to come under two or more groups but the various ingredients will all be found to fit under one or another of the five groups. That is why the *Vṛttis* are called *Pañcatayyaḥ*, five-fold.

It may be asked why only the modifications of the lower concrete mind have been taken into account in this classification of the *Citta-Vṛttis*. *Citta* comprises all the levels of the mind, the lowest of which is called the lower *Manas* functioning through the *Manomaya Kośa* and dealing with concrete mental images with names and forms. The answer to this question is obvious. The ordinary man whose consciousness is confined to the lower mind can conceive of only these concrete images which are derived from perceptions through the physical sense-organs. The *Citta-Vṛttis* corresponding to the higher levels of the mind though more definite and vivid and capable of being expressed indirectly through the lower mind are beyond his comprehension and can be perceived on their own planes in the state of *Samādhi* when consciousness transcends the lower mind. *Yoga* starts with the control and suppression of the lowest kind of *Citta-Vṛttis* with which the *Sādhaka* is familiar and which he can understand. No useful purpose could be served by dealing with the *Citta-Vṛttis* corresponding with the higher levels of the mind even if these *Citta-Vṛttis* were amenable to ordinary classification. The *Sādhaka* has to wait till he learns the technique of *Samādhi*.

Let us now consider the five kinds of modifications individually, one by one.

७. प्रत्यक्षानुमानागमाः प्रमाणानि ।

Pratyakṣānumānāgamāḥ pramāṇāni.

प्रत्यक्ष direct cognition; sense-evidence अनुमान inference आगम (and) testimony; revelation प्रमाणानि tested and attested facts.

7. (Facts of) right knowledge (are based on) direct cognition, inference or testimony.

Pramāṇā which may be translated approximately as right knowledge or knowledge related to facts, comprises all those experiences in which the mind is in direct or indirect contact with the object of the senses at the time and the mental perception corresponds with the objects. Although three sources of right knowledge are mentioned in the *Sūtra* and only in one (*Pratyakṣa*) there is direct contact with the object, this does not mean that there is no contact with the object in the other two. The contact in these two cases is indirect, through some other object or person. A simple illustration will make this point clear. Suppose you see your car coming to your door. You recognize it at once. This knowledge is, of course, *Pratyakṣa*. Now, if you are sitting in your room and hear the familiar sound of your car in front of your house you recognize it at once as your car. Here your knowledge is based on contact with the object but the contact is indirect and involves the element of inference. Now suppose again you neither see nor hear the car but your servant comes and says that your car is at the door. Here again the contact with the object is indirect but your knowledge is based on testimony. In all these three cases since the image which springs up in your brain corresponds with a fact, the *Citta-Vṛtti* comes under the category of *Pramāṇa* or right knowledge. If it does not, for example, if your inference with regard to the presence of your car is wrong or the servant makes an incorrect report, then your knowledge is wrong and belongs to the second category i.e., *Viparyaya*. Knowledge of the *Pramāṇa* type may be based partly on one and partly on another of these three sources but if it corresponds with facts, it belongs to this type.

८. विपर्ययो मिथ्याज्ञानमतद्रूपप्रतिष्ठम् ।

Viparyayo mithyā-jñānam atad-rūpa-pratiṣṭham.

विपर्ययः wrong knowledge; erroneous impression; mistake; delusion मिथ्या false; illusory ज्ञानम् knowledge; conception अतद् (of) not its own रूप (real) form प्रतिष्ठम् possessing; occupying; based.

8. Wrong knowledge is a false conception of a thing whose real form does not correspond to such a mistaken conception.

The second type of *Vṛtti* called *Viparyaya* is also based on some kind of contact with an external object but the mental image does not correspond with the object. The examples usually given to illustrate this kind of *Vṛtti* such as a mirage in a desert may give the impression that it is very rare but this is not a fact. Cases of *Viparyaya* are very frequent. Wherever there is lack of correspondence between our conception of a thing and the thing itself we have really an instance of *Viparyaya*. But it should be remembered that in *Viparyaya* we are not concerned with the correctness or definiteness of our mental impressions but only with the correspondence between the object and the mental image formed in our mind. In partial darkness our impression of an object may be blurred but if it corresponds with the object it is not a case of *Viparyaya*.

९. शब्दज्ञानानुपाती वस्तुशून्यो विकल्पः ।

Sabda-jñānānupātī-vastu-śūnyo vikalpaḥ.

शब्द word ज्ञान cognizance अनुपाती following upon वस्तुशून्यः empty of substance; devoid of objectivity विकल्पः fancy.

9. An image conjured up by words without any substance behind it is fancy.

The first two categories of mental modifications exhaust all kinds of experiences in which there is some kind of contact with an object outside the mind. These may therefore be called ' objective ' in their nature. Now we come to the other two kinds of *Vṛttis* in which there is no such contact and the mental image is a pure creation of the mind. Here again we have two subdivisions. If the mental modification is based upon a previous experience and merely reproduces it we have a case of memory. If it is not based upon an actual experience in the past or has nothing to correspond to in the field of actual experience but is a pure creation of the mind then it is fancy or imagination. When we mentally review the events of our past life such mental modifications belong to the realm of memory. When we read a novel our *Vṛttis* belong to the realm of fancy. Of course, even in the case of fancy the mental images will be found on analysis to be derived ultimately from the sensuous perceptions which we have actually experienced sometime or other, but the combinations are novel and these do not correspond to any actual experience. We may imagine a horse with the head of a man. Here the head of a man and the body of a horse have been perceived separately and belong to the realm of memory but the combination of the two in one composite image which does not correspond to an actual experience makes the mental image a case of *Vikalpa*. The two categories of memory and fancy on account of the absence of any contact with an external object which stimulates the mental image may be called ' subjective ' in their nature.

१०. अभावप्रत्ययालम्बना वृत्तिर्निद्रा ।

Abhāva-pratyayālambanā vṛttir nidrā.

अभाव absence; nothingness प्रत्यय content of mind आलम्बना support; basis object वृत्तिः modification निद्रा sleep.

10. That modification of the mind which is based on the absence of any content in it is sleep.

This is an important *Sūtra* and should be studied carefully. Of course, the literal meaning of the *Sūtra* is obvious. Even that modification of the mind in which there is no content in the mind is classed as *Vṛtti* which is called *Nidrā*. And for a very good reason. During the time a person is in this state his mind is, as it were, a blank or a void. There is no *Pratyaya* in the field of consciousness. This state outwardly appears to be the same as that of *Citta-Vṛtti-Nirodha* in which also there is complete suppression of mental modifications. How does this state then differ from the condition of *Nirbīja-Samādhi* for the two are poles apart. The difference lies in the fact that in the state of *Nidrā* or deep sleep the mental activity does not stop at all, only the brain is disconnected from the mind and so does not record the activities which are going on in the mind. When the person wakes up and the contact is established again, the brain again becomes the seat of mental activity as before. When a car is put out of gear the engine does not stop, only the effect of the running of the engine on the car disappears and so there is no motion of the car. In the same way, in deep sleep although there is no *Pratyaya* in the brain the mental activity is transferred to a subtler vehicle and goes on as before. Only the brain has been put out of gear. Experiments in hypnotism and mesmerism partly corroborate this view.

Now, in *Yoga* it is the activity of the mind or *Citta* which is suppressed and for this it is necessary to stop the vibrations of the lower mental body *while in the waking state*. In the waking state the brain is connected with the lower mind and by controlling the activity of the mind *in the brain* we can control its own activity. When the engine of a car is in gear, by regulating or stopping the motion of the car we can regulate or stop the movement of the engine itself. It will be seen therefore that the state of deep sleep and the state of *Citta-Vṛtti-Nirodha* though superficially they may appear similar are quite different.

११. अनुभूतविषयासंप्रमोषः स्मृतिः ।

Anubhūta-viṣayāsaṃpramoṣaḥ smṛtiḥ.

अनुभूत (of) experienced विषय object; subject-matter असंप्रमोषः (non-theft); not letting go or allowing to escape स्मृतिः memory.

11. Memory is not allowing an object which has been experienced to escape.

The mental process involved in recalling a past experience is a peculiar one and the reason why memory is considered as a type of *Citta-Vṛtti* has already been discussed in dealing with I-9. Memory is here defined as the retention of past experiences in the mind. But it is to be noted that these experiences are retained in the mind as mere impressions (*Saṃskāra*) and as long as they are present in their potential form, as mere impressions, they cannot be considered as a *Citta-Vṛtti*. It is only when the potential impressions are converted into their active state in the form of mental images that they can properly be considered as a *Citta-Vṛtti*.

१२. अभ्यासवैराग्याभ्यां तन्निरोधः ।

Abhyāsa-vairāgyābhyāṃ tan-nirodhaḥ.

अभ्यास (by) persistent practice वैराग्याभ्यां (and) non-attachment or absence of desire or detachment (तत्+निरोधः) तन्निरोधः control or suppression or inhibition of that (*Citta-Vṛttis*).

12. Their suppression (is brought about) by persistent practice and non-attachment.

After classifying and explaining the different forms which modifications of the mind may assume, the author gives in this *Sūtra* the two general means of bringing about the suppression of these modifications. These are practice and non-attachment. Two apparently simple words, but what a tremendous effort of the human will and variety of practices they stand for. Both these words have been defined in the subsequent *Sūtras* but their full significance can be understood only after the study of the book has been completed.

१३. तत्र स्थितौ यत्नोऽभ्यासः ।

Tatra sthitau yatno'bhyāsaḥ.

तत्र of those (two) स्थितौ for being firmly established or fixed यत्नः effort; endeavour अभ्यासः practice.

13. *Abhyāsa* is the effort for being firmly established in that state (of *Citta-Vṛtti-Nirodha*).

What is *Abhyāsa*? All effort directed towards the attainment of that transcendent state in which all *Citta-Vṛttis* have been suppressed and the light of Reality shines uninterruptedly in its fullest splendour. The means of attaining this objective are many and various and all these may be included in *Abhyāsa*. It is true that in the particular system of *Yoga* put forward by Patañjali only eight kinds of practices have been included and hence it is called *Āṣṭāṅga-Yoga*, i.e. *Yoga* with eight component parts. But there are other systems of *Yoga* prevalent in the East and each has its own particular technique. Many practices are common but there are some which are peculiar to each system. Patañjali has included in his system practically all those which are essential or important. The *Yogi* can adopt any of these according to his needs or temperament though he is generally advised to confine himself to those practices which are prescribed in the particular school to which he belongs.

It need hardly be pointed out that *Yoga* is an experimental science and as in all sciences new techniques are being constantly discovered by individual teachers and taught to their disciples. Thus each advanced teacher, though he follows the broad principles of *Yoga* and techniques of his particular school, imparts a personal touch to his teachings by introducing certain minor practices of his own. These are generally continued in a more or less modified form as long as the school lasts. But in most cases such schools quickly degenerate into mere academic bodies carrying on a dead tradition.

१४. स तु दीर्घकालनैरन्तर्यसत्कारासेवितो दृढभूमिः ।

Sa tu dīrgha-kāla-nairantarya-satkārāsevito dṛḍha-bhūmiḥ.

सः that तु indeed; दीर्घ (for) long काल time नैरन्तर्य (with) uninterrupted continuance; (incessantly) सत्कार (and) reverent devotion; earnestness आसेवितः pursued; practised; followed; continued दृढ firm भूमिः ground.

14. It (*Abhyāsa*) becomes firmly grounded on being continued for a long time, without interruption and with reverent devotion.

In order that the practice of *Yoga* may bear fruit and may enable the *Sādhaka* to be firmly established on the path there are three conditions which must be fulfilled. These conditions as defined in this *Sūtra* are (1) These practices must be continued for a long time. (2) There should be no interruptions. (3) The path must be trodden with devotion and in a spirit of reverence. The necessity for pointing out these conditions will be seen if one takes into account the enormous number of failures on this path. The path of *Yoga* appears very fascinating in the beginning and many are the people who are caught by its glamour and make a start in the hope of plucking its fruit in a very short time. But alas! Of those who enter the path, only a microscopical minority are able to make good progress. Even those who have the courage and perseverance to continue are very few in number. The vast majority of aspirants drop out sooner or later, giving up the practice completely or keeping up a semblance of mere external forms as soon as the glamour wears out. They either come to believe that it is all 'moonshine' or manage to convince themselves that conditions in the present life are not favourable and they had better postpone the effort to the next life when they vainly hope to be placed in better circumstances. Leaving out a few cases where *Karma* interposes a real obstacle in the path of the aspirant the real cause of discontinuing the practice is, in the vast majority of cases, the lack of spiritual maturity without which no success on this path is possible. The world and its pursuits have still a great deal of attraction for such people and they are not prepared to make the sacrifices which are demanded on this path.

Coming back to the essential conditions of success the necessity for continuing the practices for a long time is obvious. The nature of the changes which have to be brought about in our character, mind and vehicles is such that unless the practices are continued for a long time no appreciable improvement can be expected. Our nature has to be completely changed and the change is so fundamental that we must be prepared to continue the work until it is finished. How long this will take will depend upon many factors: our evolutionary stage, the time we have already given to the work in previous lives and the effort that we make in this life. Theoretically, if a man is able to surrender himself *completely* to *Īśvara* he can pass into *Samādhi* immediately, but it is a very big 'if' and the *Saṃskāras* of the past will not in actual life allow him to accomplish suddenly what can be done only after a long and strenuous course of discipline. In a few rare cases where the progress is extremely rapid there is always the momentum of the past, due generally to a number of successive lives devoted to the practice of *Yoga*. So, no one can predict when the final goal will be reached and he who enters the path seriously must make up his mind to continue not only for a long time but through many lives until the goal is reached. He who is ready for treading this path is so much absorbed in the fascinating work and has so much to do that he has no time to worry as to when he will reach the goal. If time hangs heavy on our hands and we are continually worrying when success will be ours it shows lack of real interest and is a danger signal.

To appreciate the requirement of not allowing any interruptions we have to remember that much of the work in *Yoga* involves bringing about very deep-seated and fundamental changes in the various vehicles through which consciousness functions on the different planes. And success in bringing about the desired changes depends upon continuity of practice. Interruption means not only waste of so much time but a considerable sliding back and retraversing the same ground which has already been covered. An example will make this clear. Suppose a *Sādhaka* is trying to purify his mind. He has to exclude rigidly from his mind all impure thoughts and emotions and to make his mental vehicle or *Manomaya Kośa* vibrate to the highest and purest thoughts until the ordinary coarse material of the vehicle has been completely replaced by the finest and subtlest matter which can respond to only pure and lofty thoughts and emotions. If this is accomplished the very vibratory capacity of the vehicle is completely changed and it becomes very difficult for the *Sādhaka* to entertain any impure thoughts in the same way as it is difficult for a licentious person to entertain pure thoughts. But suppose he gives up the effort after making some progress then the original conditions tend to reassert themselves gradually, and if he resumes the practice after considerable time the process of purification has to start *ab initio*.

Most of the required changes in our mind and character involve some changes in various vehicles and these latter processes which are really material must be almost completed if they are to be made practically irreversible. Even in ordinary life this continuity of practice is of importance for most undertakings. A boy who wants to make himself strong and muscular must take exercise regularly. If he does strenuous exercise but gives it up from time to time he does not make much progress. Prolonged and steady practice is the secret of success in all such undertakings. Even interrupted practice gives some advantage and is better than no practice at all because it creates favourable *Saṃskāras* and thus strengthens tendencies in the desired direction but when *Yoga* is taken up seriously uninterrupted practice is essential and every new technique which is initiated must be practised continuously until it is sufficiently mastered.

The third condition requiring an attitude of devotion and earnestness is equally important. *Yoga* is a serious business and requires intense and whole-hearted application. It cannot be pursued as a hobby, one of a number of pursuits in which we are equally interested. If a person desires success even in a worldly pursuit like science or art he has to give himself completely to his work, the more difficult the undertaking the greater the devotion it demands. Now, the objective of *Yoga* is the highest prize of human achievement and its pursuit must necessarily be very exacting in its demand on the time and energy of the *Sādhaka.* That is why in the olden days people who wanted to practise *Yoga* retired into forests so that they could devote themselves completely to this task. Complete retirement may not be possible or necessary but a whole-hearted devotion to this holy task is absolutely necessary. Many people think that they can combine the pursuit of worldly ambitions with *Yogic* discipline and glibly cite the example of Janaka. But Janaka had already attained the ideal of *Yoga* before he undertook the worldly duties. The ordinary *Sādhaka* especially the beginner who tries to combine the two ideals is sure to be swamped by his worldly desires and activities and to pursue the path of *Yoga* merely in name. Circumstances and habits of past lives may not allow the *Sādhaka* to adopt this one-pointed attitude all at once but he must work steadily and deliberately towards this end, eliminating one by one all the activities and interests which either interfere with his main work or uselessly consume his time and energy. This capacity to throw oneself whole-heartedly and persistently into the task which the *Sādhaka* has placed before himself is a necessary qualification and shows the readiness of the soul to embark on the Divine Adventure.

The word *Satkāra* also implies an attitude of reverence towards his task. In pursuing his ideal the *Sādhaka* is trying to find that Ultimate Reality which is the basis and the cause of the whole Universe, manifest and unmanifest. This very fact that he is trying to unravel the greatest mystery of life should fill him with a sense of awe and reverence provided he is conscious of the nature of his high purpose and the tremendous nature of the Reality which he is approaching.

When the three conditions mentioned in the *Sūtra* are present progress on the path of *Yoga* is assured. It may be slow owing to inadequate momentum from past lives but the *Sādhaka* is at least firmly established on the path and the attainment of the final goal becomes only a question of time.

१५. दृष्टानुश्रविकविषयवितृष्णस्य वशीकारसंज्ञा वैराग्यम् ।

Dṛṣṭānuśravika-viṣaya-vitṛṣṇasya vaśīkāra-
saṃjñā vairāgyam.

दृष्ट (for) seen (here in this world); visible; physical आनुश्रविक (and) heard; promised in the scriptures; revealed विषय objects वितृष्णस्य of him who has ceased to thirst वशीकारसंज्ञा conciousness of perfect mastery (of desires) वैराग्यम् non-attachment; detachment.

15. The consciousness of perfect mastery (of desires) in the case of one who has ceased to crave for objects, seen or unseen, is *Vairāgya*.

This *Sūtra* defines *Vairāgya* the second general means of bringing about the suppression of *Citta-Vṛttis*. The full significance of *Vairāgya* and its role in bringing the mind to a condition of rest will be fully understood only after the study of the philosophy of *Kleśas* outlined in Section II. Here we shall discuss only certain general principles. The word *Vairāgya* is derived from the word *Rāga* which has been defined in II-7 as the attraction which arises due to pleasure derived from any object. *Vairāgya* therefore means the absence of any attraction towards objects which give pleasure. The question may be asked: why absence of attraction only, why not absence of repulsion also, because attraction and repulsion are a pair of opposites and repulsion binds the soul to the objects as much as attraction. The reason why *Dveṣa* has been left out in the etymological expression of the idea as *Vairāgya* is not oversight but the fact that *Dveṣa* is really included in *Rāga* and forms with it a pair of opposites. The alternation of attraction and repulsion between two individuals who are attached to each other shows the underlying relation of attraction and repulsion and their common derivation from attachment. So, non-attachment which means freedom from both attraction and repulsion correctly expresses the underlying meaning of *Vairāgya*.

The reason why *Vairāgya* plays such an important part in restraining and then eliminating *Citta-Vṛttis* lies in the fact that desire in its two expressions of *Rāga* and *Dveṣa* is a tremendous driving and disturbing force which is incessantly producing *Vṛttis* in the mind. In fact, in the earlier stages of evolutionary progress, desire is the sole driving force and the development of the mind takes place almost solely as a result of the constant driving to which it is subjected by desire. In the later stages other factors also come in and as desire gradually changes into will the latter more and more becomes the driving force behind the evolutionary development.

All aspirants who are treading the path of *Yoga* must therefore try to understand clearly the role which desire plays in our life and the manner in which it keeps the mind in a constant state of agitation. Many *Sādhakas* not realizing sufficiently the disturbing influence of desire try to practise meditation without giving sufficient attention to the problem of controlling desires with the result that they do not succeed to any considerable extent in freeing the mind from disturbances at the time of meditation. Trying to render the mind calm without eliminating desire is like trying to stop the movement of a boat on a surface of water which is being violently agitated by a strong wind. However much we may try to hold it down in one position by external force it will continue to move as a result of the impulses imparted to it by the waves. But if the wind dies down and the waves subside competely the boat will come to rest—in time—even without the application of an external force. So is the case with the mind. If the driving force of desire is eliminated completely the mind comes to rest (*Niruddha* state) naturally and automatically. The practice of *Vairāgya* is the elimination of the driving force of desire using the word desire in its widest sense of *Vāsanā* as explained in Section IV. But the elimination of *Citta-Vṛttis* by practising *Vairāgya* alone, though theoretically possible, is neither feasible nor advisable. It is like trying to stop a car by merely shutting off the supply of gas. Why not also apply the brakes and make the car stop more rapidly and effectively. Herein comes the role of *Abhyāsa*. *Abhyāsa* and *Vairāgya* are therefore jointly utilized for *Citta-Vṛtti-Nirodha*. After this general consideration of the role of *Vairāgya* let us now take note of some of the phrases used in I-15 with a view to understand the full implication of the definition given therein.

Viṣaya are the objects which produce the attraction and consequent attachment. They have been divided under two heads, those which are seen and those about which we merely hear, i.e. those which are mentioned in scriptures. *Ānuśravika*, of course, refers to the enjoyments which the followers of orthodox religions expect to gain in the life after death. The practice of *Vairāgya* seeks to destroy the thirst for both kinds of enjoyments.

It will be seen from what has been stated above that the *Yogic* ideal is entirely different from the orthodox religious ideal. In the latter, a particular kind of life and conduct are prescribed and if the votary of the particular religion conforms to that code of conduct he expects to live after the dissolution of the physical body in a superphysical world with all kinds of enjoyments and means of happiness. The heavens of different religions may differ with regard to the amenities which they provide but the underlying idea is the same, i.e. a particular kind of life which consists in following certain observances and moral code ensures a happy life in the hereafter.

The *Yogic* philosophy does not deny the existence of heaven and hell but it places before the *Yogi* an ideal of achievement in which the enjoyments and pleasures of heaven life have no place because these also are temporary and subject to illusion. The enjoyments of the heaven world are nothing as compared with the bliss and powers which the *Yogi* acquires when his consciousness passes into the still higher planes of existence. Even these transcendent states have to be renounced by him in his progress towards his ultimate goal. Every power and pleasure which is 'born' out of contact with *Prakṛti* and which is not contained in the Self and therefore does not make the *Yogi* self-contained is to be included in *Ānuśravika Viṣaya*.

It may be pointed out here that it is not the feeling of enjoyment on coming in contact with those *Viṣayas* which constitutes *Tṛṣṇa*. In our contact with objects of senses some must necessarily produce a sensation of pleasure. When consciousness functions on the higher planes through the subtler vehicles bliss is the natural inevitable accompaniment but it is not this feeling of pleasure or bliss which constitutes *Rāga*. It is the attraction and consequent attachment which is the cause of bondage and must be destroyed by the practice of *Vairāgya*.

It is also necessary to remember that mere absence of attraction due to the inactivity of the body or satiety or preoccupation with other things does not constitute *Vairāgya*. A man who becomes old may lose his sex-desire for the time being. A politician engaged in the pursuit of his ambitions may for the time being become indifferent to sensuous enjoyments. But this temporary indifference towards objects has nothing to do with *Vairāgya*. The attraction is merely in abeyance ready to come to the surface as soon as the necessary conditions are present. What is needed for true *Vairāgya* is the deliberate destruction of all attractions and the consequent attachments and conscious mastery over the desires. This is the meaning of the phrase *Vaśīkāra-Saṃjñā*. Control over the vehicles through which the desires are felt and the consciousness of mastery which comes from such control are the essential elements of *Vairāgya*. For gaining this kind of mastery one should have come in contact with temptations of every kind and should have passed through ordeals of every description and come out not only triumphant but even without feeling the slightest attraction. For, if the attraction is felt, even though we may not succumb to the temptation, we have not completely mastered the desire.

It will be seen, therefore, that isolation from the world or running away from temptations does not help us in acquiring true *Vairāgya* though this may be necessary in the very early stages of acquiring self-control. We have to learn the lesson and test ourselves in the midst of pleasures and temptations—of course not by yielding to temptations and indulging in pleasures, but by trying to pierce through the glamorous illusions which surround such pleasures while we are under their domination. Real *Vairāgya* is not characterized by a violent struggle with our desires. It comes naturally and in its most effective form by the exercise of our discriminative faculty which is called *Viveka*. Glamour plays a very great part in producing *Rāga* or attachment and even ordinary intellectual analysis combined with reason and commonsense, can free us from many unreasonable habits and attachments. But the real weapon to be used in acquiring true *Vairāgya* is the more penetrating light of *Buddhi* which expresses itself as *Viveka*. As our bodies are purified and our mind becomes free from the cruder desires this light shines with increasing brightness and destroys our attachments by exposing the illusions which underlie them. In fact

Viveka and *Vairāgya* may be considered as two aspects of the same process of dissipation of illusion through the exercise of discrimination on the one hand and renunciation on the other. As the process reaches a deeper level it merges more and more in *Jñāna* and becomes almost indistinguishable from it.

१६. तत् परं पुरुषख्यातेर्गुणवैतृष्ण्यम् ।

Tat paraṃ puruṣa-khyāter guṇavaitṛṣṇyam.

तत् that परम् highest; ultimate पुरुषख्यातेः by or from awareness of the Puruṣa or the Self गुणवैतृष्ण्यम् freedom from the least desire for the *Guṇas*.

16. That is the highest Vairāgya in which, on account of the awareness of the *Puruṣa*, there is cessation of the least desire for the *Guṇas*.

It has been pointed out in connection with the previous *Sūtrā* that discrimination and renunciation mutually strengthen each other and bring about progressively the destruction of illusions and attachments which are the root cause of bondage. This results in the release of consciousness from fetters which bind it to the lower worlds and the whole process culminates as we shall see later in *Kaivalya*, the final objective of *Yoga*. In that state the *Puruṣa* having realized his true nature and having shaken off the yoke of matter has no attraction left even for the subtlest kinds of bliss experienced on the highest planes of existence. He is completely self-sufficient and above all such attractions which are based on the play of the *Guṇas*. This *Vairāgya* which is based upon the destruction of *Avidyā* and the realization that everything is contained in the *Puruṣa* himself or the *Puruṣa* is the source of everything is the highest kind of *Vairāgya* and is called *Para-Vairāgya*. It will be seen that this *Para-Vairāgya* which is a characteristic of the *Puruṣic* consciousness—if this word can be used—can appear only on the attainment of *Kaivalya*.

The fact that complete *Vairāgya* develops only on the attainment of *Puruṣa-Khyāti* means that though there may be no active attachment in the lower stages, still, the seeds of attachment remain. This means that while there is the possibility of attachment developing again before *Puruṣa-Khyāti* is attained no such possibility exists after this stage is reached. This fact has also been expressed very well in the Bhagavad-Gītā in the well-known *Śloka* (II-59). "The objects of sense, but not the relish for them turn away from an abstemious dweller in the body; and even relish turneth away from him after the Supreme is seen".

१७. वितर्कविचारानन्दास्मितानुगमात् संप्रज्ञातः ।

Vitarka-vicārānandāsmitānugamāt saṃprajñātaḥ.

वितर्क (of) reasoning; argumentation विचार deliberation; reflection आनन्द bliss; joy अस्मिता (and; or) I-am-ness; sense of individuality; sense of pure being अनुगमात् by accompaniment; with association संप्रज्ञातः *Samādhi* with *Prajñā* or consciousness.

17. *Saṃprajñāta Samādhi* is that which is accompanied by reasoning, reflection, bliss and sense of pure being.

I-17 and I-18 deal with the two varieties of *Samādhi* called *Saṃprajñāta* and *Asaṃprajñāta*. Before we take up for discussion these two important *Sūtras* it is desirable that we deal in a general way with the nature of *Samādhi* and the mutual relationship of the different kinds and stages of *Samādhi* which are mentioned in the *Yoga-Sūtras*. This will make it easier for the student to tackle this very difficult though fascinating subject and enable him to see its different aspects in their true relationship. The subject of *Samādhi* is too often studied in a haphazard and disjointed manner without making any effort to view its different parts in their correct perspective.

As the *Sūtras* bearing on the different aspects of *Samādhi* are scattered in the *Yoga-Sūtras* at different places it will help the student if a brief analysis of these *Sūtras* is given here and the order in which they should be studied by the beginner pointed out. The manner in which the subject of *Samādhi* is treated in the *Yoga-Sūtras* may appear rather strange to the student. He should remember, however, that these *Sūtras* are meant to provide in a very condensed form all the essential knowledge for the advanced student of *Yoga* and not to serve as an introduction for the beginner who has yet to learn the A.B.C. of the subject. That is why Patañjali allows himself to plunge into a discussion of the more abstruse aspects of *Samādhi* in Section I and deals with the different stages of concentration leading upto *Samādhi* in Section III. This manner of treating a difficult subject must appear very confusing to the modern student for whom the conditions for understanding any subject are made as easy as possible. If, therefore, the student is new to the subject and his ideas about *Samādhi* and related subjects are not quite clear it would perhaps be better for him to take up the *Sūtras* bearing on *Samādhi* in the following order:

SAMĀDHI

(1) The three stages of meditation leading upto *Samādhi*	III-1, 2, 3, 4
(2) *Saṃprajñāta* and *Asaṃprajñāta Samādhi*	I-17, 18
(3) The essential process involved in *Sabīja Samādhi*	I-41
(4) The different phases of *Sabīja Samādhi*	I-42, 43, 44, 45, 46, 47, 48, 49, 50
(5) The technique of *Nirbīja Samādhi*	I-51, III-8, IV-26, 27, 28, 29
(6) The three kinds of transformations involved in *Samādhi*	III-9, 10, 11, 12

Samādhi may be defined generally as a process of diving into the deeper layers of one's consciousness which functions through different grades of the mind. Consciousness is an aspect of the Ultimate Reality in manifestation and its expression depends upon the particular grade of the mind through which it is functioning, the coarser the medium the more limited the expression. As the progressive involution of consciousness in matter for the purpose of its unfoldment imposes upon it increasing limitations, so the reverse process of evolution progressively releases consciousness from these limitations. The different stages of *Samādhi* represent this progressive release of consciousness from the limitations in which it is involved and *Kaivalya* is that state in which it can again function in perfect freedom.

As consciousness functions at different levels in different grades of the mind through different mechanisms which are called vehicles or *Kośas* its progressive release from limitations may be looked at from another point of view. It may be considered as its withdrawal from one vehicle into a subtler vehicle. Each vehicle has its own functions and limitations but the functions become more inclusive and the limitations more tenuous as the matter of which it is composed becomes more refined. This progressive withdrawal of consciousness in *Samādhi* into increasingly subtler vehicles is represented in the diagram showing ' Stages of *Samādhi* '. The diagram is self-explanatory but can be understood fully only when the different aspects of *Samādhi* have been studied in detail.

The first aspect of *Samādhi* with which Patañjali deals in the first Section is the distinction between *Saṃprajñāta* and *Asaṃprajñāta Samādhi*. There is a lot of misunderstanding with regard to the nature of these two kinds of *Samādhi* and many students confuse them with *Sabīja* and *Nirbīja Samādhis*. In fact the words used for different kinds of *Samādhis* are generally used by commentators in a haphazard manner and the subtler distinctions which characterize the different kinds and phases of *Samādhi* are frequently overlooked. A student of the *Yoga-Sūtras* should bear in mind that this is a scientific treatise in which each word has a specific and definite meaning and there is no possibility of looseness of expression or the use of alternate words for the same idea. When Patañjali uses two pairs of words—*Saṃprajñāta* and *Asaṃprajñāta* on the one hand and *Sabīja* and *Nirbīja* on the other—in entirely different contexts it is because he is dealing with two entirely different ideas or subjects and to take these two pairs of words as if they mean the same thing shows lack of comprehension of the whole subject. We shall discuss later the significance of *Sabīja* and *Nirbīja Samādhis*. Let us first try to understand what *Saṃprajñāta* and *Asaṃprajñāta Samādhis* mean.

As frequently happens in the use of *Saṃskṛta* words the clue to the meaning of a particular word is given by the etymological structure of the word. *Saṃprajñāta Samādhi* means '*Samādhi with Prajñā*'. The prefix *A* in *Saṃskṛta* means 'not' and therefore *Asaṃprajñāta Samādhi* means '*not the Samādhi with Prajñā*'. *Asaṃprajñāta Samādhi* is therefore not the *Samādhi* without *Prajñā*, which would be the opposite of *Saṃprajñāta Samādhi*. It is a state of *Samādhi* which, though associated with *Prajñā*, is yet different from *Saṃprajñāta Samādhi*. It may therefore be considered a correlative of *Saṃprajñāta Samādhi*. The word *Prajñā* in *Saṃskṛta* stands for the higher consciousness working through the mind in all its stages. It is derived from *Pra* which means high and *Jñā* which means to 'know'. The distinctive characteristic of this higher consciousness which unfolds in *Samādhi* is that the mind is cut off completely from the physical world and the consciousness is centred in one or the other of the set of vehicles beginning with the lower mental body and ending with the *Ātmic* vehicle. The consciousness is thus free from the burden and interference of the physical brain.

If both *Saṃprajñāta* and *Asaṃprajñāta Samādhis* are associated with *Prajña* (*Saṃprajña*) where lies the difference between the two? The difference lies in the presence or absence of a *Pratyaya* in the field of consciousness. *Pratyaya* is a technical word used in *Yoga* to denote the total content of the mind at any moment using the word mind in its widest sense and not merely the intellect. This *Pratyaya* may be of any kind and may exist on any plane of the mind. A mental image of a child, a concept of a mathematical principle, an all-embracing vision of the Unity of life are all *Pratyayas* of different kinds and belonging to different planes.

Now, in *Saṃprajñāta Samādhi* there is a *Pratyaya* (which is called a 'seed') in the field of consciousness and the consciousness is fully directed to it. So the direction of consciousness is from the centre outwards. In *Asaṃprajñāta Samādhi* there is no *Pratyaya* and therefore there is nothing to draw the consciousness outwards and hold it there. So as soon as the *Pratyaya* (P) is dropped or suppressed the consciousness begins to recede automatically to its centre O and after passing momentarily through this *Laya* centre, tends to emerge into the next subtler vehicle. When this process has been completed the *Pratyaya* (P′) of the next higher plane appears and the direction of consciousness again becomes from the centre outwards. The progressive stages of the recession of consciousness to its centre and its emergence into the next higher plane may be illustrated by the following diagram:

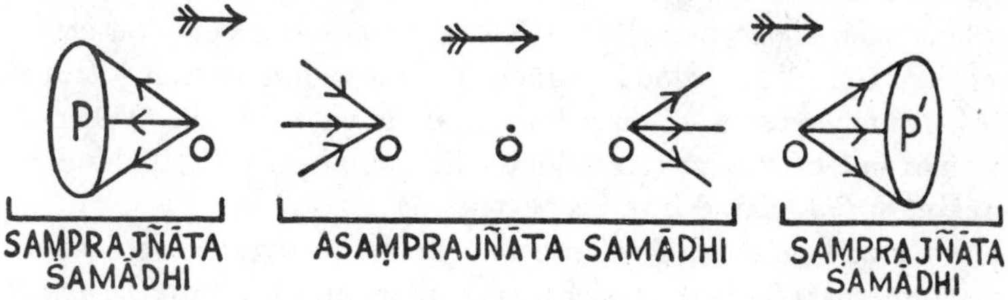

FIG. 1

From the time the *Pratyaya* P is suppressed to the time when the *Pratyaya* P′ of the next plane appears the *Yogi* is in the stage of *Asaṃprajñāta Samādhi.* During all this time he is fully conscious and his will is directing this delicate mental operation in a very subtle manner. The mind is no doubt blank but it is the blankness of *Samādhi* and not the blankness of an ordinary kind such as is present in deep sleep or coma. The mind is still completely cut off from the outer world, is still perfectly concentrated, is still under complete control of the will. *Asaṃprajñāta Samādhi* therefore represents a very dynamic condition of the mind and differs from *Saṃprajñāta Samādhi* only in the absence of *Pratyaya* in the field of consciousness. In intensity of concentration and alertness of the mind it is on a par with *Saṃprajñāta Samādhi.* That is why it is denoted by merely adding the prefix *A* to *Saṃprajñāta Samādhi.*

The void of *Asaṃprajñāta Samādhi* is sometimes called a 'cloud' in *Yogic* terminology and the experience may be compared to that of a pilot whose aeroplane passes through a cloud bank. The clear landscape is blotted out suddenly, the ordinary sense of direction disappears and he flies on in the certainty that if he holds on he is bound to come out again into the clear sky. When the consciousness of the *Yogi* leaves one plane and the *Pratyaya* of that plane disappears he finds himself in a void and must remain in that void until his consciousness automatically emerges into the next plane with its new and characteristic *Pratyaya.* He cannot do anything but wait patiently, with mind concentrated and alert, for the darkness to disperse and the light of the higher plane to dawn in his mind. In the case of the advanced *Yogi* this experience can be repeated over and over again and he passes from one plane to another until he takes the final plunge from the subtlest plane (the *Ātmic* plane) into Reality itself—the consciousness of the *Puruṣa.* The 'cloud' which he now enters is called *Dharma Megha* for reasons discussed in dealing with IV-29. When he comes out of this sacred 'cloud' he has already left behind the realm of *Prakṛti* and is in his own *Svarūpa.*

It will be seen, therefore, that in the progressive recession of consciousness from the lower mental plane to its origin *Saṃprajñāta Samādhi* with its characteristic *Pratyaya* and *Asaṃprajñāta Samādhi* with its void follow each other in succession until the last hurdle has been crossed and the *Yogi* is established in his *Svarūpa* and his consciousness has become one with the consciousness of the *Puruṣa.* The recession of consciousness towards its centre is thus not a steady and uninterrupted sinking into greater and greater depths but consists in this alternate outward and inward movement of consciousness at each barrier separating two planes.

The time taken for passage through the different planes and the intervening voids depends upon the advancement of the *Yogi.* While the beginner may remain entangled on the lower planes for a considerable time extending to years, the advanced *Yogi* can transfer his consciousness from one plane to another with lightning rapidity, and in the case of the Adept who has attained *Kaivalya* all the planes really merge into one because the passage up or down is so swift and easy that it is merely a question of focussing consciousness in one vehicle or another. As a rule, when the *Yogi* is still learning the technique of *Samādhi* he has to spend considerable time on a particular plane in studying its phenomena and laws before he is in a position to attempt passage into the next higher plane. His progress depends not only on his present effort but also on the momentum of the past and the *Saṃskāras* which he brings from his previous lives. The Science of *Yoga* cannot be mastered in one life but only in a succession of strenuous lives devoted exclusively to the *Yogic* ideal. And those who are impatient and cannot adopt this long term view are not yet qualified to enter this path and make steady progress towards their goal.

After dealing with the nature of *Saṃprajñāta* and *Asaṃprajñāta Samādhis* in a general way let us now consider the two *Sūtras* in which Patañjali has referred to these aspects of *Samādhi*. In I-17 he hints at the characteristics of the consciousness which unfolds in the four stages of *Saṃprajñāta Samādhi* which correspond to the four stages of the *Guṇas* mentioned in II-19. The word *Anugamāt* means 'associated with' or 'accompanied by' and the *Sūtra* therefore broadly means that the four successive phases or stages of *Saṃprajñāta Samādhi* are accompanied by the activities or states of the mind which are denoted by *Vitarka*, *Vicāra*, *Ānanda* and *Asmitā* respectively. Anyone who is familiar with the old *Vedāntic* classification or the modern Theosophical classification of the planes of manifestation and the functions of vehicles on those planes will easily see how closely this progressive unfoldment of consciousness through the four stages mentioned in the *Sūtra* corresponds with this classification. The classification of the elements which constitute the phenomenal side of the Universe according to *Sāṃkhya* and *Yogic* philosophies is functional and not structural and that is obviously the reason why Patañjali in denoting the successive stages of *Saṃprajñāta Samādhi* has given only the essential and dominant functions of the mind and not the names of the vehicles through which these functions are exercised. There is something to be said in favour of this functional representation of these stages as compared with the structural. While it certainly appears vague and difficult to understand it has the advantage of being independent of any particular mode of classifying the planes and the terminology adopted for denoting them. Besides, the *Yogi* who is following the path of mysticism and is bent on finding his Beloved may not be interested in the constitution and phenomena of the different planes and may not like to study these planes objectively. A simple functional treatment of the different stages of *Saṃprajñāta Samādhi* should therefore meet the needs of most people who are practising *Yoga*. But as a constitutional treatment has the great advantage of clarifying in a remarkable manner the whole technique of *Yoga* there is no reason why we should not take advantage of the knowledge which is available to us.

In the following diagram are shown the different stages of

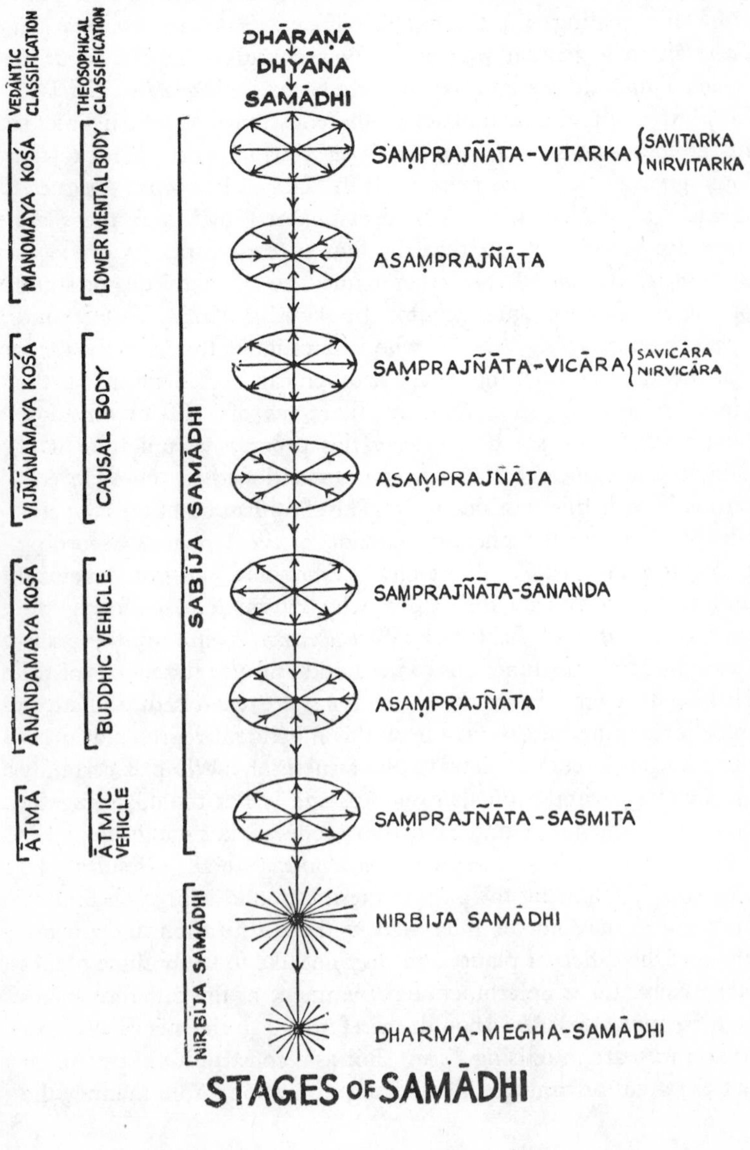

STAGES OF SAMĀDHI

Saṃprajñāta and *Asaṃprajñāta Samādhi* as well as their correspondences to the different vehicles and other aspects of the question involved in our study. It will be seen that *Saṃprajñāta Samādhi* begins when the consciousness is completely cut off from the outer world after passing through the two preliminary stages of *Dhāraṇa* and *Dhyāna*. In the first stage of *Saṃprajñāta Samādhi* the consciousness is therefore centred in the lower mental world and functions through the *Manomaya Kośa*. The essential function of the mind in this stage is denoted by the word *Vitarka*. It should be noted that when a person can leave the physical body and function in the two subtler vehicles called astral or lower mental body he is not necessarily in a state of *Samādhi* though his physical body is in an inert condition. He may be merely functioning in these subtler bodies in the ordinary manner exercising his clairvoyant powers and bringing down the knowledge he has gained into the physical brain when he returns to the physical body. This state in which clairvoyance, etc. can be exercised is quite different from the state of *Samādhi* because the peculiar condition of the mind described in III-3 is not present. The mind is directed to different objects in succession and is not concentrated upon one object.

After mastering the technique of *Savitarka* and *Nirvitarka* phases in the first stage the *Yogi* practises *Asaṃprajñāta Samādhi* and withdraws his consciousness into the next higher plane, passing through the 'cloud' which accompanies *Asaṃprajñāta Samādhi*. The consciousness of the *Yogi* then emerges into the higher mental world and functions through the *Vijñānamaya Kośa* or the causal body. The essential function of the mind working through this vehicle is called *Vicāra*. The *Yogi* now starts practising *Samādhi* on this plane, slowly masters the technique of the *Savicāra* and *Nirvicāra* phases and again practises *Asaṃprajñāta Samādhi* to free his consciousness from the higher mental plane. The whole cyclic process has to be repeated twice again during the last two stages of *Saṃprajñāta Samādhi* in order to release the consciousness of the *Yogi* from the extremely subtle and hardly comprehensible vehicles which are called the *Ānandamaya Kośa* and *Ātmā* and whose essential functions are called *Ānanda* and *Asmitā*. The significance of the words *Vitarka*, *Vicāra*, *Ānanda* and *Asmitā* is explained in dealing with the four stages of the *Guṇas* in II-19 and the student should refer to that *Sūtra* in this connection.

The student should also note that throughout the recession of consciousness in the four stages there is always something in the field of consciousness. It is true that during the period of *Asaṃprajñāta Samādhi* there is no *Pratyaya* but only a 'cloud' or void but a 'cloud' or void is also a cover on pure consciousness. It is only the blurred impression produced in consciousness when it passes through the critical phase between the *Pratyaya* of two successive planes. This phase is like the critical state between two states of matter, liquid and gaseous, when it can be called neither liquid nor gaseous. So this presence of a *Pratyaya* which is characteristic of all stages of *Saṃprajñāta Samādhi* means that in *Saṃprajñāta Samādhi* consciousness can only know the nature of something which is placed within its field of illumination. It cannot know its own nature. If we pass a beam of light through a dark chamber and then place in the path of the beam different kinds of objects the light will immediately illuminate those objects and enable us to see them. The objects are seen with the help of the light but we cannot see the light itself, for if all the objects are removed from the path of the beam of light the chamber will become quite dark although the beam of light is still there. Is there a means of seeing the light itself? There is no means of seeing physical light apart from the objects which it illuminates. But the light of consciousness can be seen as it really is after all the stages of *Saṃprajñāta Samādhi* have been passed and *Nirbīja Samādhi* is practised to remove the final and the subtlest veil covering Reality, the consciousness of the *Puruṣa*.

We have been referring to the *Pratyayas* of the different planes and the student might like to know what these *Pratyayas* are like. Although efforts have been made to describe the glorious and vivid *Pratyayas* of the higher planes by mystics and occultists in all ages those who read these descriptions can see that these efforts are a failure, the higher the plane which is sought to be depicted the more complete the failure. The fact is that it is impossible to have any idea of these higher planes except in the most general and vaguest manner. Each world can be known only through the vehicle which consciousness uses in that world.

The successive descent of consciousness into the lower worlds is not like a progressive and general dimming of a brilliant light by a number of covers. Each successive descent involves a decrease in the number of dimensions of space and time and this imposes at each step additional limitations on consciousness which are inherent in the working of that plane.

In some of the subsequent *Sūtras* the nature of the different kinds of *Samādhis* is further elaborated. But it will be seen that no attempt is made anywhere to describe the experiences of the higher planes. The knowledge which these *Sūtras* give is like the knowledge derived from the study of the map of a country. A map does not give us any idea regarding the landscapes, scenery, etc. of a country. It can merely give us information regarding the relative positions and contour of different parts of the country. If we want really to know the country we must go and see it ourselves. So if we want to know what these higher planes are like we must practise *Samādhi* and come into direct touch with them through their respective vehicles. And even when we have seen those planes ourselves we are unable to give to others any idea about them. Such knowledge is always direct and incommunicable.

१८. विरामप्रत्ययाभ्यासपूर्वः संस्कारशेषोऽन्यः ।

Virāma-pratyayābhyāsa-pūrvaḥ saṃskāra-śeṣo'nyaḥ.

विराम cessation; dropping प्रत्यय content of the mind (the 'seed' of *Saṃprajñāta Samādhi*) अभ्यास practice -पूर्वः preceded by संस्कार impressions शेषः remnant अन्यः the other.

18. The remnant impression left in the mind on the dropping of the *Pratyaya* after previous practice is the other (i.e. *Asaṃprajñāta Samādhi*).

The nature of *Asaṃprajñāta Samādhi* is defined in this *Sūtra*. The meaning of the *Sūtra* should be clear to some extent in the light of what has been said already in connection with the previous *Sūtra*. Let us dwell for a while on the various phrases used in this *Sūtra*. *Virāma-Pratyaya* means ' the cessation of *Pratyaya* '. This of course refers to the ' seed ' of *Saṃprajñāta Samādhi* which is dropped and disappears from the field of consciousness in the practice of *Asaṃprajñāta Samādhi*. Some commentators interpret this phrase as ' the idea of cessation ' or ' the cause of cessation '. This would mean that the *Yogi* meditates on the idea of cessation of *Pratyaya* or on *Para-Vairāgya*. This interpretation does not seem to be justified in the present context and if analysed carefully will be seen to mean nothing but the dropping of the ' seed ' held in the preceding *Saṃprajñāta Samādhi*. A *Yogi* who is meditating on a ' seed ' can drop it with the production of a void state of the mind but he cannot leave the ' seed ' of *Saṃprajñāta Samādhi* and start meditating on the idea of cessation. Anyone can see that such a switch over from one idea to another of an entirely different nature in the state of *Samādhi* is impossible.

Abhyāsa Pūrvaḥ means ' preceded by practice '. Practice of what? Practice of holding in the mind the ' seed ' of *Saṃprajñāta Samādhi*. This phrase therefore serves to emphasize the fact that *Asaṃprajñāta Samādhi* can be practised only after the prolonged practice of *Saṃprajñāta Samādhi*. It is, as has been pointed out already, an intensely active and not a passive condition. In fact the recession of consciousness in *Asaṃprajñāta Samādhi* and its passage through the *Laya* centre depends upon the continuance of the constant pressure of the will which is at the back of the effort to keep the mind in the state of *Saṃprajnāta Samādhi*. There is no change in this condition of the mind except the disappearance of the *Pratyaya*. The pressure must be built up in *Saṃprajñāta Samādhi* before it can be utilized in *Asaṃprajñāta Samādhi*. The bow must be drawn before the arrow is released to pierce through the target.

Saṃskāra Śeṣaḥ means ' the remnant impression '. The impression which is left in the mind after the *Pratyaya* of one plane has been dropped, and before the *Pratyaya* of the next plane appears can under normal conditions only be void. But this void is not a static state although it may be felt to be so by the *Yogi* when he is passing through it. It is a dynamic condition because consciousness is being slowly or quickly transferred from one plane to another as shown in Fig. 1. Consciousness cannot remain suspended indefinitely in a void. It must emerge on one of the two sides of the *Laya* centre. If the technique of *Nirodha Pariṇāma* has not been mastered sufficiently it may spring back into the plane which it has just left and the ' seeds ' which had been dropped will then reappear. But if the mind can remain in the *Niruddha* state for a sufficiently long time as indicated in III-10, consciousness will emerge sooner or later into the next higher plane.

There are two other interesting points which may be discussed briefly before we leave the subject of *Asaṃprajñāta Samādhi.* One is the nature of the point O (Figure No. 1) through which consciousness passes from one plane to another. This point which has been called the *Laya* centre is the common centre in which all the vehicles of the *Jīvātmā* may be said to be centred. It is only through such a centre which is called a *Bindu* in *Saṃskṛta* that transference of consciousness from one plane to another can take place.

As a matter of fact there is only the centre of Reality surrounded by a number of concentric vehicles and whichever vehicle is illuminated by consciousness derives its illumination from that centre. But the concentration of consciousness in a particular vehicle makes it appear as if the consciousness is moving up and down along the line or point which connects all the vehicles. An Adept whose consciousness is permanently centred on the *Ātmic* plane focusses his attention temporarily in any particular vehicle and for the time being the objects connected with that vehicle come within the field of his consciousness. The centre of his consciousness thus appears to have moved into one vehicle or another but in reality it has not moved at all. Consciousness which is all the time centred in Reality has merely been focussed in one vehicle or another. It is in this particular sense that the transference of consciousness from one vehicle to another in *Samādhi* must be understood if we are not to become involved in the philosophical absurdity of imagining consciousness which transcends Time and Space moving from one place to another.

The second point which the student may note in this connection is that the common centre of all vehicles being the meeting point of all the planes, consciousness must always be withdrawn to this before it can be transferred to another vehicle, just as a person going along one road must return to the crossing before he can take to another road. *Asamprajñāta Samādhi* will be thus seen to be nothing but this withdrawal of consciousness to its *Laya* centre before it can begin to function on another plane. If the consciousness remains permanently established in the centre of Reality as it is in the case of a highly advanced Adept the question of withdrawing it to the centre does not arise. From this vantage-ground he commands an all-embracing view of all the lower planes and can instantaneously begin to function on any plane he likes.

The question may be asked why if this common centre of all vehicles is also the centre of Reality within each *Yogi*, he does not get a glimpse of Reality in passing through it from one plane to another. The possibility of such a glimpse certainly exists on account of the unique nature of this point. What then prevents the *Yogi* from touching Reality every time he practises *Asamprajñāta Samādhi*? The answer to this question is contained in some of the *Sūtras* occurring in the latter portion of Section IV. It is the *Saṃskāras* still burdening the *Yogi's* mind which obscure his vision and prevent him from obtaining a glimpse of Reality. These *Saṃskāras* must be destroyed completely before he is free to pass into the realm of Reality from whatever point he wills. But though the *Yogi*, still burdened with *Saṃskāras*, cannot gain a clear glimpse of Reality, he can sense, as it were, the Reality more and more as he makes progress towards his goal and the burden of his *Saṃskāras* becomes lighter. Viewed in this manner every successive *Asamprajñāta Samādhi* is a precursor of *Nirbīja Samādhi* which alone gives an unobstructed vision of Reality.

१९. भवप्रत्ययो विदेहप्रकृतिलयानाम्

Bhava-pratyayo videha-prakṛtilayānām.

भव (by) birth; objective existence -प्रत्ययः caused विदेह the 'bodiless' प्रकृतिलयानाम् of the 'merged-in-Prakṛti'; of the absorbed in Prakṛti.

19. Of those who are *Videhas* and *Prakṛtilayas* birth is the cause.

This *Sūtra* and the next are meant to differentiate between two kinds of *Yogis*. The first kind of *Yogis* referred to in II-19 are called *Videhas* and *Prakṛtilayas* and their trance is not the result of the regular self-discipline outlined in the *Yoga-Sūtras*. It depends upon their 'birth', that is, they possess the capacity to pass into trance naturally without any effort as a result of their peculiar physical and mental constitution. In the case of the second kind of *Yogis* their *Samādhi* is the result of regular practice of *Yoga* which requires certain high traits of character like faith, energy, etc. mentioned in I-20. While the meaning of I-20 is quite clear and obvious the interpretation of I-19 has become involved in confusion on account of the different meanings associated with the words *Bhava*, *Videha* and *Prakṛtilaya* by different commentators. Let us, therefore, see whether it is not possible to find a reasonable interpretation of this *Sūtra* based on experience and commonsense rather than on far-fetched meanings which merely cause confusion.

The first point to note in the interpretation of this *Sūtra* is that it points out a class of *Yogis* in contra-distinction to the class of *Yogis* referred to in I-20. What are the characteristics of the *Yogis* described in I-20? In their case the state of *Samādhi* or enlightenment is preceded by faith, energy, memory, high intelligence, in other words, it is the result of the possession by the *Yogi* of those essential traits of character which are needed in any high endeavour. The true *Yogis* of this class achieve their objective in the normal manner by adopting the usual means outlined in the *Yoga-Sūtras*. It follows therefore that the *Yogis* of the other class mentioned in I-19 do not owe their *Yogic* faculties and powers, whatever they may be, to the adoption of the usual means. Their faculties and powers come to them in an abnormal manner. This is the important point which gives a clue to the meaning of the *Sūtra*.

Who are the *Yogīs* who happen to possess *Yogic* faculties and powers without adopting the usual means? Anyone who moves among people possessing these faculties or powers is likely to come across some cases in which these powers and faculties are not at all the result of *Yogic* practice in this life but appear during the course of their life naturally without any considerable effort on their part. Such people are born with such faculties or powers, a fact which is also corroborated by IV-1, ' birth ' being mentioned in that *Sūtra* as one of the means of acquiring *Siddhis*. The *Saṃskṛta* word *Bhava* has also the connotation of ' to happen ' which further strengthens the idea of the accidental nature of the presence of these faculties. Of course, there is nothing really accidental in the Universe which is governed by natural laws in every sphere. Everything that happens is the result of causes known or unknown, and the fortuitous appearance of psychic powers is no exception to this Law (see IV-1).

The question now arises who are the *Videhas* and *Prakṛtilayas*, the two classes of people in whom these psychic powers appear without any apparent cause. The word *Videha* literally means the ' bodiless ' and *Prakṛtilaya* means ' merged-in-*Prakṛti* '. Some commentators have given meanings to these words which appear to be far-fetched and unjustifiable in the context in which the *Sūtra* is placed. *Videhas* most probably refers to the large number of psychics scattered throughout the world who are mediumistic by nature. A medium is a person with a peculiar physical constitution, the peculiarity consisting in the ease with which the dense physical body can be partially separated from the etheric double or the *Prāṇamaya Kośa*. It is this peculiarity which enables the medium to pass into trance and to exercise some psychic powers. The word *Videha* probably owes its origin to this peculiarity of being capable of becoming partially ' disembodied ', the peculiarity which is generally accompanied by the capacity to exercise psychic faculties of a spurious kind.

In the same way *Prakṛtilayas* are not high class *Yogis* who have obtained some kind of *Mokṣa* as suggested by some commentators. On the other hand they are pseudo-*Yogis* who have the capacity to pass into a kind of passive state or trance which outwardly resembles *Samādhi* but is not real *Samādhi*. Such a *Samādhi* is called *Jaḍa-Samādhi*. In real *Samādhi* the *Yogi's* consciousness becomes merged more and more first in the Universal Mind and then in the Universal Consciousness which is *Caitanya*. How can those who are merged in *Prakṛti* which is *Jaḍa* be considered high class *Yogis*! Such pseudo-*Yogis* are found in large numbers and undoubtedly possess some capacity to reflect the higher consciousness in their vehicles. But such powers as they possess are not under their control and the consciousness which they bring down is blurred giving them at best a sense of peace and strength and a vague realization of the Great Mystery hidden within them. These powers are undoubtedly due to *Saṃskāras* brought forward from previous lives in which they have practised *Yoga* but also done something to forfeit the right to make further progress for the time being. These *Saṃskāras* give them a peculiar constitution of the lower vehicles but not the will and capacity to tread the regular path of *Yoga*. It is only in the case of the true *Yogis* referred to in the next *Sūtra* that these qualifications are present.

The interpretation of the *Sūtra* as given above is at complete variance with those given by the well-known orthodox commentators. If it has no authority to back it, it has at least the advantage of being based on commonsense and facts of experience. If we take into account the context of the *Sūtra* it is apparent that the *Yogis* referred to in this *Sūtra* are of the pseudo variety and inferior to those who tread the normal path of *Yoga* outlined in the *Yoga-Sūtras*. In fact, it is probably to help the neophyte to avoid confusion on this subject that Patañjali has pointed out this distinction. Whether Patañjali actually meant the class of pseudo-*Yogīs* mentioned above, when he used the words *Videhas* and *Prakṛtilayas* it is difficult to say with certainty and in view of the theoretical nature of the question is not of much consequence.

२०. श्रद्धावीर्यस्मृतिसमाधिप्रज्ञापूर्वक इतरेषाम् ।

Śraddhā-vīrya-smṛti-samādhi-prajñāpūrvaka itareṣām.

श्रद्धा faith वीर्य indomitable energy or will स्मृति memory समाधिप्रज्ञा (and) intelligence or 'high knowledge' or keen intellect essential for *Samādhi* -पूर्वकः preceded by इतरेषाम् for others; of others.

20. (In the case) of others (*Upāya-Pratyaya Yogis*) it is preceded by faith, energy, memory and high intelligence necessary for *Samādhi*.

In the case of the true *Yogis*, in contra-distinction to pseudo-*Yogis* referred to in the previous *Sūtra* the attainment of various progressive states of consciousness in *Samādhi* is preceded by the presence in the *Sādhaka* of certain traits of character which are essential for the attainment of a high spiritual ideal. Patañjali has mentioned only four such traits in the *Sūtra* but the list is not necessarily meant to be exhaustive and each trait which has been mentioned implies far more than the literal meaning of the word. The essential idea which the author obviously means to emphasize and which the student should try to grasp is that the attainment of the true *Yogic* ideal is the culmination of a long and severe process of character-building and discipline for the unfoldment of our powers and faculties from within, and not the result of chance, stunts, and favours bestowed by anyone or the following of any cheap methods of self-culture in a haphazard manner. This warning is necessary in view of the hidden desire in a very large number of aspirants to enjoy the fruits of *Yogic* practice without undergoing the necessary training and discipline. Instead of taking to the true path of *Yoga* and trying to develop in themselves the necessary qualifications, they are always after easy methods and new teachers who they hope will be able to bestow on them *Siddhis*, etc. as favours.

The four qualifications given by Patañjali are faith, indomitable energy or will, memory and the keen intelligence essential for *Samādhi*. Faith is the firm conviction regarding the presence of the Truth we seek within us and the efficacy of *Yogic* technique in enabling us to reach the goal. It is not ordinary belief which can be shaken by contrary arguments or repeated failures but that state of inner certainty which is present where a purified mind is irradiated by the light of *Buddhi* or spiritual intuition. Without this kind of faith it is impossible for anyone to persevere through many lives which are needed by the ordinary aspirant to accomplish the object of *Yogic* discipline.

The word *Vīrya* in *Saṃskṛta* cannot be translated by any one word in English. It combines in itself the connotations of energy, determination, courage, all aspects of an indomitable will which ultimately overcomes all obstacles and forces its way to the desired goal. Without this trait of character it is not possible for anyone to make the almost superhuman effort which is required in going through the *Yogic* discipline to the end.

The word *Smṛti* is not used here in its ordinary psychological sense of memory but in a special sense. It is the experience of the large majority of aspirants on the path that the lessons of experience are forgotten again and again and the same experiences have therefore to be repeated time after time thus involving tremendous waste of time and effort. The *Yogi* has to acquire the capacity to note the lessons of experience and to retain them in his consciousness for future guidance. Take, for example, a man who is suffering from indigestion. He knows that a particular kind of food which he likes does not agree with him, but when the particular food comes before him he forgets all about the repeated sufferings which he has undergone, yields to the temptation, takes the food and goes through the suffering again. This is a crude example but it illustrates a state of mind which is generally present and which must be changed before progress in *Yoga* is possible. We have been going through all kinds of miseries life after life, the misery of old age, the misery of being torn away from those we love dearly, the misery of unfulfilled desires, and yet we are involving ourselves in these miseries again and again by our desires. Why? Because the lessons of these miseries fail to make a permanent impression on our mind. So the aspirant for Liberation must have the capacity to learn from all experiences quickly and finally, not needing to go through the same experiences over and over again owing to the failure to remember the lessons of these experiences. If we could but retain such lessons in our memory permanently our evolution would be extraordinarily rapid. The capacity to retain such lessons in our consciousness gives a finality to every stage which we cross in our onward journey and prevents our sliding back again and again.

Samādhi-prajñā means the peculiar state of the mind or consciousness which is essential for the practice of *Samādhi*. In this state the mind is turned inwards habitually, bent on the pursuit of the Reality hidden within it, absorbed in the deeper problems of life and oblivious of the external world even though taking part in its activities. *Samādhi-prajñā* cannot obviously mean the state of consciousness *during Samādhi* because it precedes the state of *Samādhi* and *Samādhi* is the objective of *Yoga*.

If *Samādhi* has been attained by following the regular *Yogic* technique (*Upāya-pratyaya*) then it is real *Samādhi* in which the *Yogi* is vividly aware of the realities of the superphysical planes and can bring down with him the knowledge of the higher planes when he returns to the physical body. He is in full control of his vehicles all the time and can pass from one plane to another without suffering any intervening loss of consciousness. On the other hand if the *Samādhi* is the result of mere birth (*Bhava-pratyaya*) then it is not the real *Samādhi* as pointed out previously. This spurious kind of *Samādhi* may, at best, give fitful glimpses of the higher planes which are not reliable and under the control of the will, and even these may disappear as erratically as they have appeared.

२१. तीव्रसंवेगानामासन्नः ।

Tīvra-saṃvegānām āsannaḥ.

तीव्रसंवेगानाम् of those whose wish is intensely strong आसन्नः 'sitting near', near at hand.

21. It (*Samādhi*) is nearest to those whose desire (for *Samādhi*) is intensely strong.

This *Sūtra* and the next define the chief factors upon which depends the rate of progress of the *Yogi* towards his goal. The first factor is the degree of earnestness. The more ardently he desires to reach the object of his search the swifter is his progress. Progress in any line of endeavour is to a great extent determined by earnestness. A great intensity of desire polarizes all the mental faculties and powers and thus helps very greatly the realization of one's aims. But progress in *Yoga* depends upon the earnestness of the aspirant in a far greater degree and for this reason. In the case of objectives which are connected with the external world progress involves changes in the outer world, conditions for which may or may not be as favourable as desired. But in the case of the objective of *Yoga* the changes involved are all within the consciousness of the *Yogi* himself, and the obstacles are more or less of a subjective nature and confined within his own vehicles. There is, therefore, less dependence upon external circumstances and the internal conditions referred to above are more amenable to his control. A man of ambition if he wants to rise to a position of power and influence has to deal with the minds and attitudes of millions of men but the *Yogi* has to deal only with one mind—his own. And it is far easier to deal with one's own mind than that of others *provided one is in earnest.* Nothing really stands between the *Yogi* and his objective except his own desires and weaknesses which can be eliminated easily and quickly provided one earnestly wants to do so. This is so because they are mostly of a subjective nature and merely require understanding and change of attitude.

> Ye suffer from yourselves. None else compels,
> None other holds you that ye live and die
> And whirl upon the wheel and hug and kiss
> Its spokes of agony, —*The Light of Asia*

It has been said by a great sage that it is easier to know your *Ātmā* than to pluck a flower, for in the latter case you have to put forth your hand while in the former you have only to look within.

The student need hardly be reminded that in the essential practice of *Yoga* we are dealing with the recession of consciousness within itself and not with any material change. The process is more of the nature of ' letting go ' than of ' building up ' something which naturally takes time. *Īśvara-praṇidhāna*, for example, which is an independent and self-sufficient means of bringing about *Samādhi* can be developed with extraordinary rapidity when a spiritually mature soul surrenders itself whole-heartedly to *Īśvara.* It is really a process of ' letting go ' our hold on the attractions and pursuits of the worldly life and in such a process progress can be extremely rapid. In fact the whole process can be accomplished instantaneously. Besides being rapid the process is really very easy provided we are in dead earnest. While ' holding ' requires force and effort ' letting go ' does not require any force or effort and can be brought about by merely a change of attitude.

The real trouble with most aspirants is that the degree of earnestness is very feeble and there is not sufficient pressure of will to break down all the hindrances and difficulties which stand in their way. Weaknesses and desires which would simply fade away in an atmosphere of earnestness and realistic approach to the problems of life continue to keep them in bondage, year after year, life after life, because a sufficiently earnest desire for reaching the objective is absent. That is why intensity of desire is a *sine qua non* of rapid progress on the path of *Yoga* and there is no limit to the extent to which the time taken for reaching the goal can be reduced. In fact, Self-realization can be instantaneous if the intensity and earnestness of desire is correspondingly great but it is a big ' if '. Usually, the intensity of desire increases gradually with one's progress and it is only when the aspirant is almost nearing his goal that it attains the required tempo.

It is, however, necessary to mention that this desire to find one's Self is not desire in the ordinary sense and we use the same words in this way for lack of better terms to express our ideas. It has more the quality of indomitable will, that intense concentration of purpose before which all obstacles and difficulties gradually melt away. It is because this *Mumukṣutva* is sometimes reflected in the emotional field of our consciousness and there produces an intense longing for the realization of our aim that there is some justification for calling it a desire.

२२. मृदुमध्याधिमात्रत्वात् ततोऽपि विशेषः ।

Mṛdu-madhyādhimātratvāt tato 'pi viśeṣaḥ.

मृदु- (on account of being) mild; soft मध्य- medium; moderate -आधिमात्रत्वात् (and) intense or powerful ततः from it; after that अपि also; even विशेषः gradation; differentiation; distinction.

22. A further differentiation (arises) by reason of the mild, medium and intense (nature of means employed).

The other factor which determines the rate of the *Yogi's* progress is the nature of the means he adopts in the pursuit of his aim. *Aṣṭānga Yoga* of Patañjali points out only the broad principles of the general method which has to be followed in liberating human consciousness from the limitations of *Avidyā* and gaining Self-realization. It is true that in this system a well-defined technique has been laid down for achieving this end but the different parts of this technique are not rigid in their nature but sufficiently elastic to allow the aspirant to adapt them to his personal needs, temperament and convenience. A system which is meant to subserve the spiritual needs of different types of individuals living in different ages and with different potentialities and capacities could never prove very useful and could not withstand the ravages of time if it demanded adherence to a rigid and uniform course of discipline. The value of Patañjali's system of *Yoga* lies in its elasticity and the capacity to subserve the needs of different types of individuals who share the one common purpose of unravelling the Great Mystery which is hidden within them and are prepared to make the necessary effort and sacrifices to achieve it. It has thus all the advantages of following a definite technique and none of the disadvantages of being confined within a rigid system.

Although Patañjali's system allows great latitude as regards the means which may be adopted in achieving a particular purpose, still, being a scientific system, it is based on following a well-defined technique in tackling the different problems of *Sādhana.* And where technique is involved the progress in achieving any particular purpose must depend upon the nature of the means employed. If we want to be transported to a spot at a distance, however keen we may be to reach it, our progress will depend upon whether we use a bullock-cart, an automobile or an aeroplane. There are processes which do not involve any well-defined technique in the usual sense of the term. In such cases the question of means does not enter the problem at all. For example, if a person is in a fit of temper and wants to become calm he can come back to his normal condition by an adjustment of his attitude which can be so rapid as to appear almost instantaneous. There are certain systems of *Yoga* which do not involve an elaborate technique. Such a path which is based on self-surrender is indicated in the next *Sūtra.* In treading such a path there is really no technique and the progress depends upon intensifying *ad infinitum* one primary fundamental attitude or psychological process either through its own inherent power or by the help of certain subsidiary aids like *Japa.*

Coming back to the question of the rate of progress in cases where some kind of technique is involved let us see how Patañjali has classified these 'means'. He has put them in three classes—mild, moderate and intense—thus following the classical method of classification adopted in Hindu philosophical thought. Wherever it is necessary to classify a number of things belonging to the same category and not differing from one another by sharply defined differences, it is the usual practice to classify these things broadly under three sub-heads as given above. Thus in II-34 also where *Vitarkas* have to be classified the same triple classification has been adopted. This may outwardly appear to be a rather odd system of classification but on closer thought it will be seen that though not strictly scientific it has much to recommend it. It is simple, elastic and takes into account the relative nature of the means employed. What may be considered as 'intense' by a *Yogi* at one stage of evolution may appear 'moderate' to another who is more highly advanced and actuated by greater intensity of desire.

२३. ईश्वरप्रणिधानाद्वा ।

Īśvara-praṇidhānād vā.

ईश्वर God प्रणिधानात् by 'placing oneself' in (God); by devotional dedication to, by self-surrender or resignation to (God) वा or.

23. Or by self-surrender to God.

The attainment of *Samādhi* is possible by following another path in which the aspirant does not bring about the deliberate suppression of the *Citta-Vṛttis* by the force of his will. On this path he simply surrenders himself to the will of *Īśvara* and merges all his desires with the Divine Will. What is *Īśvara-Praṇidhāna* and how it can lead to *Samādhi* is explained at length in dealing with II-32, II-45. We need not, therefore, go into this question here. But let us try to understand the next few *Sūtras* which are meant to give some idea with regard to *Īśvara* to whom the aspirant has to surrender himself in this method of attaining *Samādhi*.

These *Sūtras* bearing upon *Īśvara* have given rise to a controversy among scholars because *Sāṃkhya* is supposed to be an atheistic doctrine and *Yoga* is supposed to be based on *Sāṃkhya*. The relation between *Sāṃkhya* and *Yoga* has not really been definitely settled though the philosophy of *Yoga* is bound up so closely with that of *Sāṃkhya* that the *Yoga* system is sometimes referred to as *Seśvara Sāṃkhya*. The practical student of *Yoga* need not worry himself over these academic questions of philosophy. *Yoga* is a practical science and every practical science has generally a theoretical basis which may or may not in reality correspond exactly with the facts which form the real basis of the science. Since the system of *Yoga* outlined by Patañjali is essentially a scientific system it was inevitable that he should adopt that particular system of philosophy for its theoretical basis which is most scientific in its outlook and comprehensive in its treatment. The choice of *Sāṃkhya* for this purpose was therefore quite natural. But this does not mean necessarily that *Yoga* is based on *Sāṃkhya* or follows that system in toto. The very fact that it differs from *Sāṃkhya* on the most fundamental question of *Īśvara* and has suggested an independent method of attaining *Samādhi* through *Īśvara-Praṇidhāna* shows that this apparent similarity of the two systems should not be taken too seriously. The fact that *Sāṃkhya* while dealing with theoretical questions at great length is almost silent with regard to the practical methods of obtaining release from the bondage of *Avidyā* is also of great significance. It shows that the system was meant to be nothing more than a purely theoretical philosophy offering a scientific and most plausible theory of life and the Universe in terms of the intellect. The real truths of existence were to be discovered directly by each person for himself by following a practical system such as the one outlined in the *Yoga-Sūtras*.

२४. क्लेशकर्मविपाकाशयैरपरामृष्टः पुरुषविशेष ईश्वरः ।

Kleśa-karma-vipākāśayair aparāmṛṣṭaḥ
puruṣa-viśeṣa Īśvaraḥ.

क्लेश (by) afflictions; misery; cause of misery कर्म actions; activities विपाक maturation or fruition आशयैः (and) seed-germs or impressions of desires wherein desires sleep अपरामृष्टः untouched पुरुष- Spirit; an individual unit or centre of Divine Consciousness विशेषः special; particular ईश्वरः Ruler or Presiding Deity of a *Brahmāṇḍa* or Solar system.

24. *Īśvara* is a particular *Puruṣa* who is untouched by the afflictions of life, actions and the results and impressions produced by these actions.

In this *Sūtra* Patañjali has given us two ideas with regard to *Īśvara*. The first is that He is a *Puruṣa*, an individual unit of Divine Consciousness like the other *Puruṣas*. The second is that He is not bound by *Kleśa*, *Karma*, etc. like the other *Puruṣas* who are still involved in the cycle of evolution. As is pointed out later (IV-30) the *Puruṣa* becomes free from *Kleśa* and *Karma* on attaining *Kaivalya* and the vehicle through which *Karma* works (*Karmāśaya*) is destroyed in his case. In what respects then does *Īśvara* differ from the other *Mukta Puruṣas* who have attained *Kaivalya* and become Liberated? The explanation sometimes given that He is a special kind of *Puruṣa* who has not gone through the evolutionary process and who was *ever* free and untouched by the afflictions *at any time* is not very convincing and against the facts as they are known to Occult Science.

The explanation of the discrepancy pointed out above lies in the fact that after the attainment of *Kaivalya* the evolutionary or unfolding process does not come to an end but new vistas of achievement and work open out before the Liberated *Puruṣa.* We can hardly comprehend the nature of this process or the work which it involves but that further stages do exist beyond *Kaivalya* is taken for granted in Occult Science. The further unfoldment of consciousness which takes place in the evolutionary progress beyond *Kaivalya* passes through many stages and culminates ultimately in that tremendously high and glorious stage in which the *Puruṣa* becomes the presiding Deity of a Solar system. During the previous stages He has occupied progressively higher and higher offices in the Hierarchies which govern and guide the various activities in the Solar system. The offices of the *Adhikāri Puruṣas* of different grades like *Buddhas*, *Manus* etc. form, as it were, a ladder the lower end of which rests on the rock of *Kaivalya* and its other end is lost in the unimaginable glory and splendour of Divine Consciousness. The office of *Īśvara* is one of the highest if not the highest rung of this ladder. He is the Supreme Ruler of a Solar system or *Brahmāṇḍa.* It is in His Consciousness that the Solar system lives, moves and has its being. The different planes of the Solar system are His bodies and the powers working the machinery of the Solar system are His powers. In short, He is the Reality whom we generally refer to as God.

How many further stages of unfoldment of consciousness exist between this stage and the undifferentiated Ultimate Reality which is referred to as *Parabrahman* in *Vedānta* we do not know. That such stages exist stands to reason and follows from the facts that the suns do not occupy fixed positions but probably revolve round other stars, that Solar systems are parts of bigger units called galaxies and these in their turn are parts of still bigger units called universes. Whatever the relation which subsists between Solar systems, galaxies, universes and the Cosmos as a whole and their respective Presiding Deities (and astronomy is bringing more and more light to bear on this fascinating question) the conception of the Cosmos being studded with innumerable Solar systems, and each Solar system being presided over by an *Īśvara* is in itself a tremendously grand idea whose truth is based not on mere poetic fancy but definite knowledge of Adepts of Occultism. And to think that the Presiding Deity of each of these Solar systems is a *Puruṣa Viśeṣa* who has passed through the evolutionary cycle like everyone of us and attained to that inconceivably high level imparts a new significance to the idea of human evolution and places it on an entirely new basis. This is a fascinating line of thought which could be pursued in different directions but it is not possible to do so at this point. There is, however, one point which had better be cleared up before we proceed to consider the next *Sūtra*.

What is the relation existing between the *Īśvara* of a Solar system and the innumerable *Puruṣas* who are either undergoing pre-*Kaivalya* evolution or are still associated with the Solar system after attaining Liberation? According to the *Sāṃkhya*, each *Puruṣa* is a separate and independent unit of consciousness and remains so eternally. So the *Puruṣas* who are part of the evolutionary scheme in a Solar system must be quite separate and independent of the *Puruṣa Viśeṣa* who is its presiding Lord according to this philosophy. But according to Occult Science the different *Puruṣas* though separate and independent units of consciousness are yet in some mysterious manner one and share a common Life and Consciousness. The consciousness of the *Īśvara* provides a field in which the consciousness of the other *Puruṣas* in the Solar system can function and unfold. They are nourished by His life and evolve from stage to stage until they themselves become fit to become *Īśvaras* of other newly created Solar systems. So while they are in His Solar system they exist in Him and are one with Him in the most intimate manner and yet they maintain throughout their independent centre and individual uniqueness. This co-existence of Oneness and Separateness upto the last is one of those paradoxes of the inner life which the mere intellect can never understand and which only realization of our true nature can resolve.

But we need not go further into this question. Enough has been said to show that the idea of *Īśvara* has not been artificially grafted on the basic *Sāṃkhyan* philosophy for the sake of convenience but is an integral part of that larger philosophy of the East which is based on the direct experience of an unbroken line of adepts and mystics and of which *Sāṃkhya* shows merely one facet. It should be remembered that the *Yoga-Sūtras* is a book of technical nature giving the technique of *Yoga* and the essential doctrines of this basic philosophy must be understood if that technique is to be mastered properly. It does not mean that what is not given in the *Yoga-Sūtras* does not conform with the *Yogic* philosophy upon which the book is based. The ideas in *Yoga-Sūtras* should be studied against the background of the total Eastern philosophy and there is no justification for isolating them and studying them as if they were based on *Sāṃkhya* or a separate and independent philosophy.

२५. तत्र निरतिशयं सर्वज्ञबीजम्।

Tatra niratiśayaṃ Sarvajña-bījam.

तत्र in Him निरतिशयं the highest; unsurpassed सर्वज्ञ- (of) the Omniscient बीजं the seed; the principle.

25. In Him is the highest limit of Omniscience.

This *Sūtra* gives us another idea with regard to *Īśvara* the Presiding Deity of a Solar system. The meaning of the *Sūtra* is easy to understand but its real significance is generally missed. In order to understand this significance it is necessary to bear in mind that each Solar system is considered to be a separate and, to a great extent, independent manifestation of the One Reality corresponding with its isolation and separation by tremendous distances from other Solar systems in space. We may imagine the innumerable Solar systems scattered throughout the Cosmos as so many centres in the Consciousness of the One Reality in manifestation which is called *Saguṇa Brahman* in Hindu philosophy. Round each such centre manifests the life of the Logos or *Īśvara* of that Solar system much in the same way as the life of a *Puruṣa* manifests round the centre of his consciousness through a set of vehicles. Each Solar system may thus be considered as a sort of reincarnation of its *Īśvara* bringing into each new manifestation on a macrocosmic scale the *Saṃskāras* of the previous Solar systems which have preceded it.

Since each Solar system is the manifestation of the consciousness of its *Īśvara* and each *Īśvara* represents a definite stage in the infinite unfoldment of consciousness in the world of the Relative, it follows that His knowledge though almost unlimited in relation to the other *Puruṣas* in the Solar system must be considered to be limited in relation to the Ultimate Reality of which He is a partial manifestation. We should not forget that manifestation always implies limitation and even an *Īśvara* is in the realm of *Māyā* however thin may be the veil of Illusion which separate His consciousness from that of the *Nirguṇa Brahman* who alone can be considered unlimited in the real sense of the term. So the Omniscience of an *Īśvara* is a relative thing and has a limit and it is this limit which is referred to in this *Sūtra*.

Now all the *Puruṣas* in a particular Solar system or *Brahmāṇḍa* are undergoing a process of evolution and the 'seed' of Omniscience in each *Puruṣa* is unfolding gradually. This unfoldment takes place slowly in the course of ordinary evolution. When *Yoga* is practised and consciousness begins to function on the subtler superphysical planes the unfoldment is accelerated to a remarkable degree and the boundaries of knowledge are suddenly enlarged at each successive stage in *Samādhi*. When *Kaivalya* is attained after *Dharma-Megha-Samādhi* a tremendous expansion of consciousness takes place as pointed out in IV-31. Even after the attainment of *Kaivalya*, as has been pointed out already, the unfoldment of consciousness does not come to an end and such unfoldment must be accompanied by a corresponding expansion of knowledge. Is there any limit to this expansion of knowledge in the case of the *Puruṣas* who are undergoing evolution in a Solar system and whose consciousness is a part of the consciousness of the *Īśvara* of the system? There must be and that limit will naturally be the relative Omniscience of the *Īśvara*, or the knowledge which is contained in His consciousness. No *Puruṣa* can cross that limit as long as he is a part of the Solar system and his consciousness is based, as it were, on the consciousness of the *Īśvara*. His knowledge may go on expanding and may appear infinite but it cannot expand beyond the infinite knowledge of the *Īśvara* of the system just as a fountain cannot rise higher than the reservoir which supplies water to it.

२६. स पूर्वेषामपि गुरुः कालेनानवच्छेदात् ।

Sa pūrveṣām api guruḥ kālenāna-
vacchedāt.

सः He पूर्वेषाम् of the Ancients; of those who came before or first अपि even गुरुः teacher कालेन by time आनवच्छेदात् on acount of not being limited or conditioned.

26. Being unconditioned by time He is Teacher even of the Ancients.

We have seen in the previous *Sūtra* that the knowledge which the *Īśvara* of a *Brahmāṇḍa* carries in His consciousness sets a limit which no one can cross. Not only in knowledge but also in other respects such as power He must be the highest expression in the Solar system and all lesser Entities such as *Manus*, *Buddhas* and *Devatās*, however high their status, must derive their power from Him. That is why He is called *Īśvara*, the Supreme Lord or Ruler. A Solar system, though insignificant as compared with the Cosmos, is still a gigantic phenomenon in time and space. Many planets are born in it, live their life and then disappear, providing during a certain period of their existence a field for the evolution of the innumerable *Jīvātmās* who are part of the Solar System. During all this stupendous period extending over billions of years who guides the different humanities and races which appear and then disappear on the habitable planets? Who inspires and gives knowledge to those who become the Teachers and Leaders of mankind from time to time? Only *Īśvara* can fill this role because He alone survives and continues through all these stupendous changes.

The word *Guruḥ* means both the Teacher as well as the Master, but here, since we are dealing with a treatise on *Yoga*, the emphasis is obviously on the former meaning. This means that He is the Supreme Teacher who not only gives knowledge to the highest teachers but is also the real Teacher, behind all the teachers who are trying to spread the light of knowledge and Divine Wisdom in the world. Scientists and other seekers after knowledge may vainly think that they are wresting the secrets of

Nature and enlarging the boundaries of human knowledge by their own ingenuity and indomitable will but this attitude is utterly wrong, born of egoism and illusion which generally characterize purely intellectual pursuits. It is the pressure of Divine knowledge and will behind the evolutionary progress of humanity which is naturally enlarging the boundaries of human knowledge, and individuals merely become the instruments of the Supreme *Guru* in Whom all knowledge resides. Anyone who has watched with an open mind and a reverent heart the phenomenal progress of Science in modern times and the remarkable manner in which discoveries have been made, one after another, can see the guiding and unseen hand and intelligence behind these discoveries. It is a great pity that this spirit of reverence is lacking in modern Science and puny man, the creature of a day, has taken all the credit for the rapid and phenomenal expansion of knowledge which has taken place during recent times. It is this lack of reverence, the product of blatant materialism which is at the bottom of the wrong direction which Science is gradually taking, making knowledge more and more the instrument of destruction and unhappiness rather than that of ordered progress and true happiness. If this tendency is allowed to grow unchecked the mighty edifice of Science is bound to crash one day in a cataclysm which will destroy the fruits of knowledge garnered through centuries. Where there is no humility and reverence in the pursuit of knowledge it bodes ill for those who are engaged in its pursuit.

Howsoever it may be in the field of Science, in the field of Divine Wisdom *Īśvara* is not only considered to be the fount of all knowledge and wisdom but the real and the only Teacher existing in the world. All great Spiritual Teachers have been considered to be the embodiments of the Great *Guru* and have taught in His name and through His power. The 'Light on the Path' is the light of His knowledge, the 'Voice of the Silence' is His voice. This is a truth which all aspirants treading the path of *Yoga* must burn into their hearts.

२७. तस्य वाचकः प्रणवः ।

Tasya vācakaḥ praṇavaḥ.

तस्य His (of Īśvara) वाचकः designator, indicator; प्रणवः 'Om' pronounced A-U-M as a humming sound.

27. His designator is 'Om'.

Having given in the previous three *Sūtras* some necessary information about *Īśvara* the author points out in the next three *Sūtras* a definite method of establishing direct contact with Him. Before dealing with these three *Sūtras* it is necessary to give very briefly some idea with regard to the theory of *Mantra-Yoga*, for without at least a general idea of this branch of *Yoga* it is not possible to understand adequately the significance of these *Sūtras*.

Mantra-Yoga is that branch of *Yoga* which seeks to bring about changes in matter and consciousness by the agency of 'Sound' the word Sound being used not in its modern scientific sense but in a special sense as we shall see just now. According to the doctrine upon which *Mantra-Yoga* is based the primary manifestation of the Ultimate Reality takes place through the agency of a peculiar and subtle vibration which is called *Śabda* and which means Sound or Word. The world is not only created but maintained by this *Śabda* which differentiates into innumerable forms of vibration which underlie the phenomenal world.

It is necessary first to understand how all the phenomena of Nature can be ultimately based on vibration or peculiar expressions of Energy. First, let us take the material side of these phenomena. Physical matter has been found by Science to consist of atoms and molecules which in their turn are the result of different combinations of still smaller particles like electrons etc. Science has not been able as yet to get a clear picture with regard to the ultimate constitution of physical matter but it has been shown definitely and conclusively that matter and energy are inter-convertible. The Theory of Relativity has shown that mass and energy are not two different entities but are one and the same, the relation between the two being given by the well-known equation of Einstein.

$$E=C^2\ (m'-m)$$

Not only is matter an expression of Energy but the perception of material phenomena depends upon vibrations of various kinds.

Vibrations of different kinds striking the organs of sensation produce the five kinds of sensations and the familiar world of light, sound etc. is thus based on vibration. Modern psychology has not been able to investigate or understand the nature of mental phenomena but the study of these phenomena by Occult methods has shown definitely that their perception is dependent on vibrations in mediums subtler than the physical. There are some phenomena known to modern psychologists such as thought-transference which lend support to this view.

It will be seen, therefore, that there is nothing inherently absurd in the doctrine that the foundation of the whole manifested world existing on many planes and consisting of innumerable phenomena is a tremendously complex and vast aggregate of vibrations of various kinds and degrees. These vibrations or expressions of energy not only constitute the material of the manifested world (using the word material in its widest sense) but by their actions and intereactions produce all the phenomena of the different planes. This conclusion, though startling, is nothing as compared with the still more myserious doctrine of Occult Science according to which all these infinitely complex vibrations of innumerable variety are the expressions of a Single Vibration and this Single Vibration is produced by the Will of the Mighty Being who is the Presiding Deity of the particular manifested world whether this world be a Solar system, Universe or the Cosmos. This tremendous, primary, and integrated vibration from which are derived all the vibrations in manifestation is called *Śabda-Brahman*, i.e. the Ultimate Reality in its aspect of ' Sound ', the word ' Sound ' being used in the most comprehensive and rather mysterious sense as pointed out before. This doctrine put in simple and general terms means that the Ultimate Reality carrying within Itself the *Saṃskāras* of previous manifestations differentiates on manifestation into two primary and complementary expressions—one a composite Integrated Vibration called *Śabda-Brahman* and the other an underlying integrated Consciousness called *Brahma-Caitanya* (i.e. the Reality in its aspect of Consciousness). These two expressions are complementary and mutually dependent since they are the dual expressions of the One Reality and appear or disappear simultaneously.

From this primary relationship of vibration and consciousness existing on the highest level of manifestation flows the relation of these two on all the planes of manifestation down to the physical. So that we find that wherever there is manifestation of consciousness there is vibration associated with it whether we are able to trace it or not. Not only are vibration and consciousness so intimately and indissolubly connected but there is a specific relationship existing between each kind of vibration and the particular aspect of consciousness which it can give expression to, so that each kind of vibration is matched, as it were, by a corresponding state of consciousness. This relation may be understood to a certain extent by considering its expression at the lowest level, namely, sensuous perception. Each particular vibration of light with a definite wavelength produces its corresponding colour perception in consciousness. Each particular vibration of sound produces perception of the corresponding note in consciousness. Although Science has not yet been able to investigate the hidden mechanism of other kinds of sensations it will probably be found when such investigations have been made successfully that each sensation of taste, smell and touch is matched by a corresponding vibration of some kind. What is true on the lowest level is true on all levels of manifestation and therefore there is nothing inherently unreasonable in supposing that consciousness can be influenced or reached by means of vibration or to put it in other words, particular states of consciousness can be brought about by initiating particular kinds of vibrations. Not only can consciousness be affected by vibration, but consciousness by initiating particular vibrations can also influence matter and bring about changes in matter.

The broad and general principles pointed out above form the basis of *Mantra-Śāstra*, the science of using *Mantras* for bringing about certain tangible results, and also of *Mantra-Yoga*, the science of unification or unfoldment of consciousness by the help of *Mantras*. The essential idea underlying both is that by producing a particular kind of vibration through a vehicle it is possible to draw down a particular kind of force through the vehicle or to produce a particular state of consciousness in the vehicle. Such vibrations can be produced by means of *Mantras* each of which represents a particular combination of sounds for bringing about certain specific results.

Since a *Mantra* is a composite thing, a particular combination of sounds arranged in a particular way, it is interesting to enquire what are the basic sounds which are utilized in these combinations. Without going into the details of this question it may be simply stated that the letters of the *Saṃskṛta* alphabet are the elements from which all *Mantras* of *Saṃskṛta* orgin are derived. Each letter is supposed to be the vehicle of a basic eternal power (that is why it is called *Akṣara*) and when introduced into a *Mantra* contributes its specific influence to the total effect which is the objective of the *Mantra*, much in the same way as the different chemical elements contribute their specific properties to the compounds which are derived from them. There are 52 letters of the *Saṃskṛta* alphabet and therefore there are 52 basic elemental powers which are available for producing all kinds of effects through the agency of *Mantras* in their different permutations and combinations. It does not mean, of course, that the *Saṃskṛta* alphabet has some favoured place in the scheme of Nature and the sounds produced by its letters alone can be utilized in constructing *Mantras*. All that is meant is that the effects of sounds produced by letters in the *Saṃskṛta* alphabet have been investigated and evaluated and can thus be used in the construction of *Mantras*. With this brief introduction let us now consider the important *Sūtra* under discussion.

In I-26 it was pointed out that *Īśvara* is the true Teacher of all and the source of the Inner Light by the help of which the *Yogi* treads the path of Liberation. How is that Inner Light to be revealed, to be uncovered so that he may have an unerring and ever-present guide within himself? This Light appears when the mind becomes sufficiently purified by the practice of *Yoga* as is indicated in II-28. But there are certain initial difficulties which must be overcome before the practice of *Yoga* can begin in right earnest. These difficulties are related to the general condition of the mind which in the case of the large majority of aspirants is not at all favourable for the practice of *Yoga*. It is subject to constant and sometimes violent distractions which make it impossible for the aspirant to adopt a life of discipline and to dive within the recesses of his consciousness. How are these distractions to be overcome and the mind steadied sufficiently so that it may become possible for the aspirant to be firmly established on the path of *Yoga*? The next and the subsequent *Sūtras* deal with this important problem.

The first and most effective means which Patañjali prescribed for overcoming this distracted condition of the mind is the *Japa* of *Praṇava* and meditation on its meaning. He calls *Praṇava* as the *Vācaka* of *Īśvara*. What is a *Vācaka*? The literal meaning of *Vācaka* is name or designator but in *Mantra-Yoga* it has a specialized meaning and is used for a name which is essentially of the nature of a *Mantra* and has the power when used in a prescribed manner of revealing the consciousness and releasing the power of a *Devatā* or Divine Being. Being a sound combination which is used to designate a particular Entity it is like a name. But an ordinary name is chosen arbitrarily to indicate somebody and it has no natural or mystic relationship with the person. A *Vācaka*, on the other hand, is a name which has a mystic relationship with the *Vācya* (the Entity designated) and has inherent in it the power of revealing the consciousness and releasing the power of the individual for whom it stands. Such a *Vācaka* is *Om*. It is considered to be the most mystical, sacred and powerful *Mantra* by the Hindus because it is the *Vācaka* of *Īśvara*, the Greatest Power and the Supreme Consciousness as far as our Solar system is concerned.

It may seem preposterous to the ordinary man not familiar with the inner side of life that a mere syllable of three letters can carry hidden within it the potential power which is attributed to it by all *Yogis*, and references to which are found scattered throughout the sacred scriptures of the Hindus. But facts are facts and they are not at all affected by the ignorance and prejudices of people who disbelieve in them. Who could have believed fifty years ago that a mere neutron moving among a number of uranium atoms could produce an explosion powerful enough to blow up a whole city? Anyone who understands the theory of *Mantra-Yoga* and the relation of vibration with consciousness should be able to see that there is nothing inherently impossible in the idea of a mystic syllable possessing such a power. Besides, we should remember that the facts of the inner life with which *Yoga* deals are based upon experience no less than the facts of Science, though it may not be possible or desirable to demonstrate them.

२८. तज्जपस्तदर्थभावनम् ।

Tajjapas tad-artha-bhāvanam.

तत्-जपः its constant repetition तत्-अर्थ (of) its meaning भावनम् dwelling upon in mind; realizing; meditation.

28. Its constant repetition and meditation on its meaning.

How can the power of a *Mantra* like the *Praṇava* be developed? For, it has to be remembered that this power is potential, not active. It is the power of a seed which needs to be developed gradually by providing certain essential conditions, not the power of an electric motor which is available on merely pressing a button. This is a fact frequently lost sight of by many people. They think that by merely repeating a *Mantra* a few times they can obtain the desired result. They cannot. A *Mantra* can no more give in this way the result for which it is devised than a seed of a mango tree can satisfy a man who is hungry. The seed must be sown, watered and the tender plant tended for years before it can bear fruit and satisfy the hungry. In the same way the potential power which resides in a *Mantra* must be developed slowly by the application of the right methods before it can become available for the spiritual advancement of the *Sādhaka*. The process generally takes years of the most strenuous and one-pointed discipline and practice and even then the *Sādhaka* may not be quite successful if he has not provided the right conditions. The higher the object of the *Mantra* the more difficult and prolonged the process of unfolding the power which is latent in it.

The two principal means of developing the power which is latent in *Praṇava* which are equally applicable to other similar *Mantras* are given in the *Sūtra* we are considering. The first means is *Japa*. This is a well-known technique of *Mantra-Yoga* in which the *Mantra* is repeated again and again (first audibly, then silently and lastly mentally) in a prescribed manner until the desired results begin to appear. The repetition of the *Mantra* is necessary and sometimes the *Sādhakas* are required to repeat it such an enormous number of times that it becomes a test of their patience and endurance. But though generally this number is great the number by itself is not the most important factor. The other conditions—mental and emotional—are equally important. *Japa* begins in a mechanical repetition but it should pass by stages into a form of meditation and unfoldment of the deeper layers of consciousness.

The efficacy of *Japa* is based upon the fact that every *Jīvātmā* is a microcosm thus having within himself the potentialities of developing all states of consciousness and all powers which are present in the active form in the macrocosm. All the forces which can help this Divine spark within each human heart to become a roaring fire are to be applied. And the unfoldment of consciousness takes place as a result of the combined action of all these forces rather than the mere repetition of the *Mantra*. Still, the *Mantra* must be there to integrate and polarize these forces as the tiny seed must be there to utilize the soil, water, air and sunshine in the development of the tree. It is not possible to deal here with the *modus operandi* of *Japa* and the manner in which it arouses the potentialities of the microcosmic *Jīvātmā*. It may be merely pointed out that its potency depends upon its capacity to arouse subtle vibrations within the vehicles which it affects. A *Mantra* is a sound combination and thus represents a physical vibration which is perceptible to the physical ear. But this physical vibration is its outermost expression and hidden behind the physical vibration and connected with it are subtler vibrations much in the same way as the dense physical body of man is his outermost expression and is connected with his subtler vehicles. These different aspects of *Vāk* or 'speech' are called *Vaikharī*, *Madhyamā*, *Paśyanti* and *Parā*. *Vaikharī* is the audible sound which can lead through the intermediate stages to the subtlest form of *Parā Vāk*. It is really through the agency of these subtler forms of 'sound' that the unfoldment of consciousness takes place and the hidden potentialities become active powers. This release of powers takes a definite course according to the specific nature of the *Mantra* just as a seed grows into a tree, but into a particular kind of tree according to the nature of the seed.

The other means of utilizing the power which is latent in *Praṇava* is *Bhāvanā*. This word literally means 'dwelling upon in mind'. Let us try to understand its significance in the present context. The object of the dual practice prescribed in this *Sūtra* is to contact the Divine Consciousness of *Īśvara*. The *Japa* has the effect of attuning the vehicles. But something more is necessary in order to bring down the Divine influence and establish contact with the Divine Consciousness. If an electric current is to flow into a mechanism we need not only conductance or capacity to transmit the current but also voltage, pressure to make the current flow. In the same way in order to make it possible for the individual consciousness to draw nearer to the Divine Consciousness we need not only attunement of the vehicles but a drawing force, an attraction which corresponds to voltage in the flow of the electric current. This force which draws together the two—the *Jīvātmā* and the *Paramātmā*—may take different forms. In *Bhakti-Yoga*, for example, it takes the form of intense devotion or love. In *Mantra-Yoga* it takes the form of *Bhāvanā* or intense meditation on the significance of the *Mantra* and the object which is sought to be gained. This *Bhāvanā* is not merely an intellectual process like the one we employ in finding the solution of a mathematical problem. It is a joint action of all our faculties in the pursuit of a common goal. So that not only the spirit of intellectual enquiry is there but also the deep yearning of the lover who wants to find the Beloved and the will of the *Haṭha-Yogi* who wants to break through all the barriers which separate him from the object of his search. This kind of *Bhāvanā* polarizes all our powers and faculties and produces the necessary concentration of purpose. Thus gradually the distractions which take the mind of the aspirant away from the object of his search are removed and he is able to turn his attention inwards.

२९. ततः प्रत्यक्चेतनाधिगमोऽप्यन्तरायाभावश्च ।

Tataḥ pratyak-cetanādhigamo
'py antarāyā-bhāvaś ca.

ततः from it (this practice) प्रत्यक् (of) in-turned; in the opposite direction चेतना consciousness अधिगमः attainment अपि also अन्तराय (of) hindrances; obstacles अभावः absence; disappearance च and.

29. From it (result) the disappearance of obstacles and turning inward of consciousness.

In this *Sūtra* Patañjali has given the two results which ensue from the practice prescribed in the previous *Sūtra*. First, the awakening of a new kind of consciousness which is called *Pratyak Cetanā*, and second, the gradual disappearance of the 'obstacles'.

Let us first try to understand what is meant by *Pratyak Cetanā*. There are two kinds of consciousness of diametrically opposite nature—*Pratyak* and *Parāṅga* or inward-turned and outward-turned. If we study the mind of the ordinary individual we shall find that it is entirely outward-turned. It is immersed in the outer world and is occupied all the time with the procession of images which pass continuously in the field of consciousness. This outward-turned consciousness is caused by *Vikṣepa*, the projection outward by the lower mind of what is present within it at the centre. As we shall deal with the question of *Vikṣepa* fully in discussing the next *Sūtra* let us leave it here and try to understand what *Pratyak Centanā* is. As has been pointed out above *Pratyak Cetanā* is the inward-turned consciousness or consciousness directed towards its centre. It is thus the exact opposite of the outward-turned or *Parāṅga Cetanā* as illustrated in the following figures.

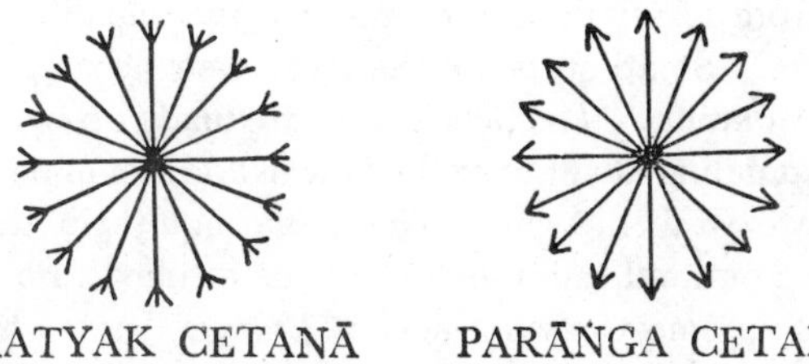

PRATYAK CETANĀ PARĀṄGA CETANĀ

FIG. 2

The whole aim and process of *Yoga* consists in withdrawing the consciousness from without to within, for the ultimate mystery of life is hidden in the very heart or centre of our being and can be found only there and nowhere else. In the case of the *Yogi* the tendency of the lower mind to run outwards and to keep itself busy with the objects of the outer world must therefore be replaced gradually by a tendency to return automatically to its 'centred' condition without effort. It is only under these conditions that it can be 'joined', as it were, with the higher principles. But it may be pointed out that this mere tendency to be pointed towards the centre is not *Pratyak Cetanā* although it is a necessary stage in its attainment. It is the actual contact with the higher principles resulting in the irradiation of the personality by the influence of these higher principles (*Ātmā-Buddhi-Manas*) which is the essence of *Pratyak Cetanā*. The contact is no doubt indirect but it is sufficiently effective and real to enable the personality to derive from it many advantages. The strength of the *Ātmā*, the illumination of *Buddhi* and the knowledge of the higher mind gradually filter down into the personality in an ever-increasing measure and provide the necessary guidance and momentum for treading the path of *Yoga*. The contact becomes direct only in *Samādhi* when consciousness leaves one vehicle after another and becomes centred at deeper and deeper levels.

The other result of *Japa* and meditation on *Praṇava* is the gradual disappearance of the obstacles which lie in the path of the *Yogi*. These obstacles are of various kinds—impurities and disharmonies in the vehicles, weaknesses of character, lack of development etc. But *Praṇava* as we have seen touches the very heart of our being, arouses in the microcosm vibrations which can bring out from it all the latent powers and faculties which lie sleeping there. So all obstacles whatever their nature, yield to its dynamic stimulation. The deficiencies are made up by the growth of the corresponding faculties or the flow of additional power. The impurities are washed away. The disharmonies in the vehicles are smoothed out and the vehicles become attuned to one another and to the Supreme Consciousness of *Īśvara*. And so a complete regeneration of the individuality takes place, a regeneration which makes it fit to tread the path of *Aṣṭāṅga Yoga* or *Īśvara-Praṇidhāna*.

It is obvious that an instrument so effective and powerful in its action cannot be used in a haphazard and careless manner without involving the *Sādhaka* in all kinds of difficulties and dangers. A careful consideration of the necessary conditions and their strict regulation is therefore absolutely necessary. This is not the place to deal with these conditions in detail. It is enough to point out that purity, self-control and a very cautious and gradual use of the power are some of the essential conditions. So the practice can be taken up usefully and safely only after *Yama* and *Niyama* have been mastered to a considerable extent.

The seven *Sūtras* from 1-23 to 1-29 form, in a way, a separate set giving the technique of the path of mysticism on which the aspirant goes direct to his goal without studying and mastering the intermediate planes which separate him from the object of his search. On this path self-surrender is the only weapon and in using this weapon, *Japa* and meditation on *Praṇava* constitute the sole technique. The *Japa* and meditation turn the consciousness of the aspirant right about in the direction of his goal, remove all the obstacles and self-surrender does the rest.

३०. व्याधिस्त्यानसंशयप्रमादालस्याविरतिभ्रान्तिदर्शनालब्धभूमिकत्वानवस्थितत्वानि चित्तविक्षेपास्तेऽन्तरायाः ।

Vyādhi-styāna-saṃśaya-pramādālasyā-
virati-bhrānti-darśanālabdhabhūmi-
katvānavasthitatvāni citta-vikṣepās
te 'ntarāyāḥ.

व्याधि- disease स्त्यान- dullness; languor; drooping state संशय- doubt प्रमाद- carelessness आलस्य- laziness अविरति- hankering after objects भ्रान्तिदर्शन- delusion; erroneous view अलब्धभूमिकत्व- non-achievement of a stage; inability to find a footing अनवस्थितत्वानि (and) unsteadiness; instability चित्त (of) mind विक्षेपाः distractions (causes of distraction) ते they (are) अन्तरायाः obstacles; hindrances.

30. Disease, languor, doubt, carelessness, laziness, worldly-mindedness, delusion, non-achievement of a stage, instability, these (nine) cause the distraction of the mind and they are the obstacles.

It was pointed out in the last *Sūtra* that the turning outward of consciousness is caused by *Vikṣepa*. In this *Sūtra* Patañjali gives a number of conditions which cause the mind to be distracted and which consequently make the successful practice of *Yoga* impossible. This distracted condition of the mind in which it is constantly flung about in all directions, away from the centre, is called *Vikṣepa*. Since this condition of the mind is the opposite of that needed for the practice of *Yoga* we have to understand clearly the nature of *Vikṣepa* and the means to avoid it. To enable us to do this let us first cast a glance at the mind of the average man of the world. There are two general characteristics which we are likely to find in the large majority of people. The first is the lack of purpose. They drift through life being carried along on its currents in a helpless manner. There is no directive force within them which can modify their circumstances and give a certain direction to their life. Even when they decide to pursue any particular objective they are easily thrown off the track by any obstacles that may come in their path. In short, they have not developed concentration of purpose which enables a man to pursue an aim relentlessly until he has achieved it. Of course, there are some exceptional people who have developed a strong will and have the capacity to pursue a fixed aim till success is gained. Such people generally rise to the top in their respective spheres of work and become captains of industry, great inventors, scientists and political leaders.

Now, though the *Yogi* has no ambitions and the pursuit of any worldly aims does not form part of his life, still, he does need concentration of purpose like any ambitious man working in the outer world. The pursuit of *Yogic* ideals requires in fact more concentration of purpose than that of any worldly aim can, because in the first place, the difficulties are greater and in the second place, the sphere of work is inside and the objective is to a great extent unknown and intangible. The *Yogi* has generally to work against great odds, the results of his efforts take a long time to appear and even when they do appear do not bring with them the kind of satisfactions for which the lower nature of man generally craves. So, only an extraordinary concentration of purpose can enable him to keep to his course in the face of difficulties and obstacles. If this is not present he is likely to suffer from frustration and the disintegration of his mental forces to which such frustration generally leads. Under these circumstances distractions of all kinds such as those mentioned in the present *Sūtra* are likely to arise and cause the mind to be thrown constantly off the track.

The second general characteristic of the ordinary mind is that it is constantly and completely turned outwards. It is used to taking interest only in the objects of the outer world and this habit has become so strong that any effort to reverse the direction of consciousness and to make the mind withdraw from the periphery to the centre is accompanied by a mental struggle. Even in the case of people who are generally called introverts the tendency is merely to keep oneself occupied with one's mental images in disregard of what is happening in the outer world. This is rather an abnormal condition of the mind and is quite different from that condition in which the mind is directed to its centre and is thus attuned to the higher principles.

This centrifugal tedency of the mind does not matter in the case of the ordinary man because his interest and field of work is in the external world and the question of drawing the mind within does not arise. But the *Yogi* has to draw the mind within and the centrifugal tendency must therefore be replaced by a centripetal tendency so strong that it requires definite force of will to keep the mind directed outwards. These two tendencies which make the mind inward-turned or outward-turned correspond to *Pratyak* and *Parāṅga Cetanā* and may be illustrated by the same diagrams which were used in representing the two forms of consciousness in dealing with the last *Sūtra*.

This condition of the mind in which it is turned outwards and is subject to distractions is also called *Vikṣepa*. It is the normal condition in the case of the ordinary man and is taken as a matter of course by him because he grows up with it and it does not interfere with the kind of work he is required to do. The word *Vikṣepa* is used generally only in this ordinary sense and it is very probable that it has been used by Patañjali in this sense in the present context. But there is a mystery underlying this natural tendency of the mind to remain outward-turned which throws some light on the nature of *Vikṣepa*. It is worthwhile referring to it briefly here.

If we are to understand this mystery let us first consider the formation of a virtual image by a mirror. We all know that if an object is placed in front of a plain mirror an exact image of it is seen in the mirror and the image appears to be on the other side of the mirror at the same distance as the object is in front of it. The formation of such an image can be illustrated by the following diagram.

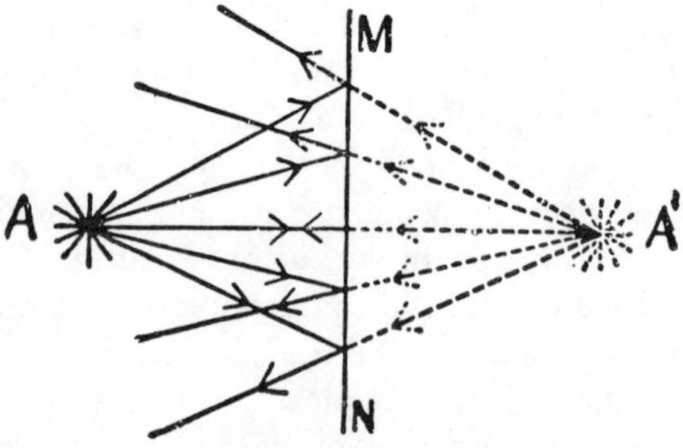

FIG. 3

A is the object and A′ is its image formed by the mirror MN. It will be seen that all the rays coming from the object and striking the mirror are reflected in such a manner that if the reflected rays are produced backwards they would meet at the point A′ where the image of the object is seen. It is because the reflected rays all *seem* to come from the point A′ that the virtual image of the object is seen at that point. It is easy to see that this virtual image is a pure illusion produced by the peculiar reflection of light rays. But the important point to note in this phenomenon is that an object can be seen at a place where there exists nothing at all corresponding to it.

In a similar manner the familiar world of forms, colours, sounds etc. which we see outside us and in which we live our life is formed by a mysterious process of mental projection. The vibrations which are conveyed through the sense-organs to our brain produce through the instrumentality of the mind an image in our consciousness but the mind projects this image outwards and it is this projection which produces the impression of a real world outside us. As a matter of fact, this impression of the familiar solid and tangible world outside us is a pure illusion. The world image we see is a virtual image in the sense that the objects we see outside us are not there at all. Their appearance there is based on the external world of atoms and molecules and their vibrations which stimulate the sense-organs as well as on the inner world of Reality which is the ultimate basis of the mental image. The mind brings about the interaction of spirit and matter and in addition projects the result of this interaction outside as a virtual image as shown in the following diagram:

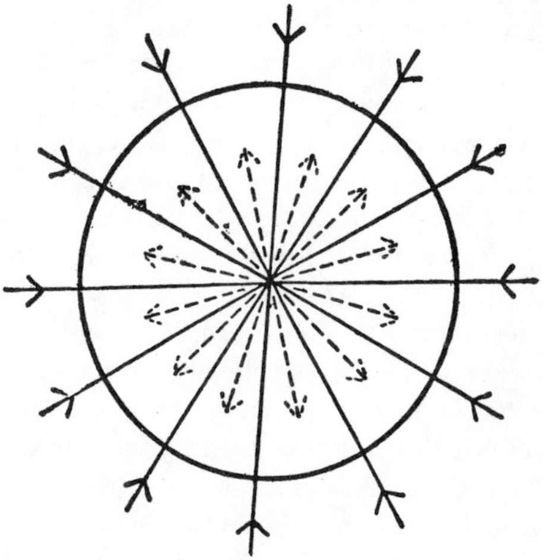

FIG. 4

It is this projection outwards by the lower mind of what is really within which constitutes the fundamental nature of *Vikṣepa* and which lies at the basis of this outward-turned condition of the mind.

The fact that the world image which we see outside us is an illusion does not necessarily mean the denial of the physical world. The physical world is the stimulator of the world image but the image is the mind's own creation (in the light of Reality). This is not in contravention of modern scientific ideas. Take, for example, the question of colour. All that Science knows is that light vibrations of a certain frequency give the impression of a certain colour. It knows only the objective side of the phenomenon but as to why a certain frequency of vibration gives the impression of a particular colour it cannot say. The physical world of Science is merely a world of whirling atoms and molecules and the play of various kinds of energies. The mental world which springs forth in our consciousness through the instrumentality of the physical world is something quite apart from, though dependent upon, the physical world. There is a gulf between the two which Science has not been able to bridge and will not be able to bridge until it takes into account the world of Reality which expresses itself through the phenomena of consciousness.

Patañjali has enumerated nine conditions of the mind or body which cause *Vikṣepa* and thus serve as obstacles in the path of the *Yogi*. Let us briefly consider these before we proceed further.

(1) Disease: This is obviously a hindrance in the path of the *Yogi* because it draws the mind again and again to the physical body and makes it difficult to keep it directed inwards. Perfect health is a necessity for treading the path of *Yoga* and that is, no doubt, one of the reasons why the author has included *Āsana* and *Prāṇāyāma*, two practices of *Haṭha-Yoga*, in his system.

(2) Languor: Some people have an apparently healthy physical body but lack nerve power so that they always feel below par and disinclined to take up any work requiring prolonged exertion. This chronic fatigue is in many cases psychological in origin and due to the absence of any definite and dynamic purpose in life. In other cases it is due to some defect in the *Prāṇamaya Kośa* which results in an inadequate supply of vital force to the physical body. Whatever its cause it acts as an obstacle because it undermines all efforts to practise *Sādhanā*.

(3) Doubt: An unshakeable faith in the efficacy of *Yoga* and its methods is a *sine qua non* for its successful practice. Such faith

is needed in achieving success in any line of endeavour but more so in this line because of the peculiar conditions under which the *Yogi* has to work. In the Divine adventure which he has undertaken the objective is unknown and there are no clearly defined standards by which he can judge and measure his progress. Doubts of various kinds are therefore liable to arise in his mind. Is there really any Reality to be realized or is he merely pursuing a mirage? Are the methods he is using really effective? Are those methods the right methods for him? Has he the capacity to go through all the obstacles and reach the goal? These and other doubts of a similar nature are liable to assail his mind from time to time especially when he is passing through the periods of depression which come inevitably in the path of every aspirant. It is at these times that he needs *Śraddhā*—unshakeable faith in his objective, in himself and in the methods which he has adopted. It may not be possible to avoid these periods of depression and doubt especially in the early stages but it is his behaviour and reaction to them which show whether he has true faith or not. If he can ignore them even though he feels them, he comes out of the shade into the sunshine again and resumes his journey with renewed enthusiasm. If he allows these doubts and moods to interfere with his *Sādhanā* and relaxes his efforts, they acquire an increasing hold on his mind until he is completely side-tracked and abandons the path altogether.

(4) CARELESSNESS: This is another obstacle which besets the path of many aspirants for the *Yogic* life. It has the effect of relaxing the mind and thus undermines its concentration. Some people are careless by nature and when they come into the field of *Yoga* they bring their carelessness with them. Carelessness is a weakness which prevents a man from achieving eminence in any line of endeavour and condemns him to a mediocre life. But in the field of *Yoga* it is not only an obstacle but a great danger and the careless *Yogi* is like a child who is allowed to play with dynamite. He is bound to do himself serious injury sooner or later. No one should think of treading this path who has not conquered the habit of carelessness and learnt to pay careful attention not only to important things of life but also to those which are considered unimportant.

(5) Laziness: This is another habit which results in a distracted condition of the mind. Although it results in the same kind of ineffectiveness in life as in the case of languor it is yet different. It is a bad mental habit acquired by continued yielding to the love of comfort and ease and tendency to avoid exertion. If we may say so, languor is a purely physical defect while laziness is generally a purely psychological condition. A restoration to health automatically cures the former but a prolonged discipline based on the execution of hard and difficult tasks is the only means of curing the latter.

(6) Worldly-mindedness: The worldly man is so immersed in the interests pertaining to his outer life that he does not get time even to think about the real problems of life. And there are many people who pass through life without having ever given any serious thought to these problems. When a person takes to the path of *Yoga* as a result of the dawning of *Viveka* and of his becoming alive to the illusions of life the momentum of the past is still behind him and it is not so easy to shut out the interests of the worldly life suddenly and completely. These hankerings after the objects of the world still continue to trouble him and cause serious distraction in his mind. Of course, all depends upon the reality of the *Viveka*. If we *really* see the illusions which are inherent in the pursuit of worldly objects like wealth, honour, name etc. then we lose all attraction for them and naturally give up their pursuit. But if the *Viveka* is not real—is of the pseudo-variety—the result of mere 'thinking', then there is constant struggle between the desires which drag the mind outside and the will of the *Yogi* who tries to make the mind dive within. Thus, worldly-mindedness can be a serious cause of *Vikṣepa*.

(7) Delusion: This means taking a thing for what it is not. It is due generally to lack of intelligence and discrimination. A *Sādhaka* may, for example, begin to see lights and hear sounds of various kinds during his early practices. These things are very spurious and do not mean much and yet there are many *Sādhakas* who get excited about these trivial experiences and begin to think they have made great progress. Some think that they have reached high states of consciousness or are even foolish enough to

think that they have seen God. This incapacity to assess our supernormal experiences at their proper worth is basically due to immaturity of soul and those who cannot distinguish between the essential and non-essential things in spiritual unfoldment find their progress blocked at a very early stage. They tend to get entangled in these spurious experiences of a psychic nature and are soon side-tracked. It is easy to see that the unhealthy excitement which accompanies such undesirable conditions of the mind will cause great distraction and prevent it from diving inwards.

(8) NON-ACHIEVEMENT OF A STATE: The essential technique of *Yoga* consists, in the earlier stages, in establishing the mind firmly in the stages of *Dhāraṇā*, *Dhyāna* and *Samādhi*, and after *Samādhi* has been attained, in pushing steadily, step by step, into the deeper levels of consciousness. In all these stages change from one state to another is involved and this is brought about by persistent effort of the will. Sometimes this passage is easy and comes after a reasonable amount of effort. At other times the *Yogi* seems to make no progress and a dead wall appears to be facing him. This failure to obtain a footing in the next stage can cause distraction and disturb the perfect equanimity of the mind unless the *Yogi* has developed inexhaustible patience and capacity for self-surrender.

(9) INSTABILITY: Another kind of difficulty arises when the *Yogi* can get a foothold in the next stage but cannot retain it for long. The mind reverts to its previous stage and a considerable amount of effort has to be put forth in order to regain the foothold. Of course, in all such mental processes reversions of this nature are to a certain extent unavoidable. But it is one thing to lose one's foothold in the next stage because only practice makes perfect and another thing to lose it because of the inherent fickleness of the mind. It is only when the instability is due to the inherent unsteadiness of the mind that *Vikṣepa* can be said to be present and special treatment is called for.

It should be noted that the nine obstacles enumerated in this *Sūtra* are of a particular type—those which cause *Vikṣepa* and thus hinder the *Yogi* in the practice of *Dhāraṇā*, *Dhyāna* and *Samādhi*. There can be other kinds of obstacles also. Every serious defect of character can become an obstacle. *Karma* can place obstacles in the path of the aspirant which make the practice of *Yoga* for the time being impossible. Attachments to objects, persons or ideas frequently stand in the way of many aspirants taking to the life of *Yoga*. These different kinds of obstacles are dealt with in their proper places. Defects of character, for example, in the treatment of *Yama-Niyama*.

The reason why Patañjali has dealt here with this class of obstacles in particular lies, of course, in the fact that this is the *Samādhi Pāda* and he is dealing with all the essential factors involved in understanding this important subject. He gives in this *Sūtra* some idea with regard to the nature of obstacles which cause *Vikṣepa* before dealing in eight subsequent *Sūtras* (I-32-39) with the various methods which may be adopted for overcoming this tendency.

३१. दुःखदौर्मनस्याङ्गमेजयत्वश्वासप्रश्वासा विक्षेपसहभुवः ।

Duḥkha-daurmanasyāṅgamejayatva - śvāsa - praśvāsā vikṣepa-sahabhuvaḥ.

दुःख- pain दौर्मनस्य- despair, depression etc., caused by mental sickness अङ्गमेजयत्व- shaking of the body; lack of control over the body; nervousness श्वासप्रश्वासाः (and) inspiration and expiration; hard breathing विक्षेप distraction सहभुवः accompanying (symptoms).

31. (Mental) pain, despair, nervousness and hard breathing are the symptoms of a distracted condition of mind.

After enumerating in the last *Sūtra* those conditions which cause *Vikṣepa* the author gives in this *Sūtra* a number of symptoms by which the presence of *Vikṣepa* can be recognized. The first of these is pain. The presence of pain either physical or mental always shows some serious defect or disharmony in the vehicle. Physical pain is a sign of positive disease while mental pain shows definitely that the mind is not in a natural healthy state. It is either in a state of inner conflict, torn between opposite desires or under the domination of *Kleśas*. Pain is an indication provided by Nature to bring to the notice of the person concerned that all is not well with him. But while most people would run to a doctor if there is any physical pain very few people think of having their mind examined or examining it themselves even when they are suffering excruciating mental pain. But that is what is needed really.

When pain is combined with a consciousness of impotence or incapacity to remove it effectively it leads to despair, despair then leads to nervousness which is merely an outer physical symptom of despair. Nervousness when it reaches a certain degree of intensity disturbs the breathing because it disorganizes the flow of *Prāṇic* currents. So these four symptoms really represent the four stages which follow one another when the mind is in that undesirable condition which causes *Vikṣepa*.

Since they are mere symptoms the proper way to deal with them is to treat the mind for the fundamental disease which afflicts it. And this will involve a long and tedious course of discipline of our whole nature because all parts of our nature are inter-related. The whole problem of human suffering and misery has been dealt with in Section II by Patañjali in a masterly manner in his theory of *Kleśas*. It will be clear to anyone who has understood this theory that there can be no cheap but effective solution of the problem of human suffering except through the conquest of the Great Illusion. As long as this is not achieved and the mind remains subject to the illusions of the lower life, suffering and misery must remain and the outer symptoms which reflect the disordered condition of the mind must continue to appear in greater or lesser degree.

But as has been pointed out already, Patañjali is not dealing here with the fundamental problem of human suffering and misery but with those particular conditions of the mind which produce *Vikṣepa* and interfere with the practice of *Dhāraṇa*, *Dhyāna* and *Samādhi*. This problem is of a more limited nature and has to be tackled by adopting means of a more limited and specific nature. These are dealt with in the following eight *Sūtras*.

३२. तत्प्रतिषेधार्थमेकतत्त्वाभ्यासः ।

Tat-pratiṣedhārtham eka-tattvābhyāsaḥ.

तत् that (there) प्रतिषेधार्थम् for removal; for checking एक (of) one तत्त्व principle; truth अभ्यासः practice; intense application.

32. For removing these obstacles there (should be) constant practice of one truth or principle.

Some commentators have introduced quite unnecessary mystification in the interpretation of this *Sūtra*, some going to the absurd length of suggesting that the exercises recommended in the six subsequent *Sūtras* for removing *Vikṣepa* and developing concentration of purpose are methods of practising *Samādhi*! In one sense, since Reality touches life at every point, theoretically, there can be no limit to the depth into which we can penetrate in pursuing any one truth and this can lead to *Samādhi.* But the context in which this *Sūtra* occurs and the nature of the illustrative methods which are given in the subsequent *Sūtras* leave no room for doubt with regard to its meaning. The object of these exercises is not the attainment of *Samādhi*, for that is sought to be achieved by a different clearly defined series of steps outlined in *Āṣṭāṅga Yoga.* The object is obviously the reversal of the tendency of the mind to run constantly after a multitude of objects in the outer world and to develop the capacity to pursue constantly one objective inside within the realm of consciousness.

It has been pointed out previously that the average man lacks not only concentration of purpose but also the capacity to keep the mind directed within. Both these are *sine qua non* for the practice of *Yoga* and hence the necessity of developing these capacities in a high degree for the aspirant. The removal of the obstacles follows naturally when concentration of purpose has been developed to a sufficient degree. When a dynamic purpose enters the life of a person who has been leading a purposeless life, his mental and other forces become gradually polarized and all difficulties like those mentioned in I-30 tend to disappear. But, of course, the aspirant for *Yogic* life has not only to acquire the capacity to pursue an objective with energy and perseverance but in addition his objective must be within. The exercises which Patañjali has recommended are such that both these capacities are developed simultaneously.

३३. मैत्रीकरुणामुदितोपेक्षाणां सुखदुःखपुण्यापुण्यविषयाणां भावनातश्चित्तप्रसादनम् ।

Maitrī-karuṇā-muditopekṣāṇāṃ sukha-duḥkha-puṇyāpuṇya-viṣayāṇaṃ bhāvanātaś citta-prasādanam.

मैत्री friendliness करुणा compassion मुदिता (and) gladness उपेक्षाणां indifference सुख joy; happiness दुःख sorrow; misery पुण्य virtue अपुण्य (and) vice विषयाणां (having for their) objects भावनातः by cultivating attitudes (towards); by dwelling in mind (upon) चित्त (of) mind प्रसादनम् clarification; purification.

33. The mind becomes clarified by cultivating attitudes of friendliness, compassion, gladness and indifference respectively towards happiness, misery, virtue and vice.

In giving a number of alternative exercises for overcoming *Vikṣepa*, the author begins with two *Sūtras* the relevancy of which, in relation to the subject being considered, is not sometimes quite clear to students. In the *Sūtra* we are considering Patañjali defines the correct attitude of the would-be *Yogi* in the various kinds of situations that may arise in his relationship with those amongst whom he lives. One of the greatest sources of disturbance to the mind is our uncontrolled reactions to our human environment, to what people do around us and to the pleasant or unpleasant conditions in which we get involved. The ordinary man has no well-defined principle for the regulation of these reactions. He reacts to these things in a haphazard manner according to his whims and moods with the result that he is being constantly disturbed by all kinds of violent emotions. Some people, finding these emotional reactions unpleasant, decide not to react at all and gradually become cold, hard-hearted and indifferent to those around them. Both these attitudes are undesirable and cannot lead to acquiring a calm, gentle and compassionate nature in accordance with the requirements of the higher life. Spiritual life can go neither with violent reactions nor with cold indifference which some misguided stoics recommend to their followers. It requires a balanced nature in which our reactions are correctly regulated by the highest motives and are in harmony with the Great Law. The point to note here is that the development of a hard and callous nature, which is indifferent to the happiness and suffering of others, is no real solution of the problem of mental equilibrium and the freedom from disturbances which is thus acquired is more apparent than real because it is artificial and against the law of Love. Besides, there is the danger of the *Yogi* who allows himself to become callous drifting into the Left-hand path and creating for himself and others untold suffering.

Patañjali has not only pointed out the necessity for the *Yogi* of controlling and regulating his reactions to his environment but has also laid down the general principle on which this regulation is to be based. This principle is, of course, derived from the laws of psychology and practical experience in dealing with the problem of adjusting ourselves to our environment. It ensures for the *Yogi* both the equilibrium of mind and freedom from entanglements which he needs for the steady pursuit of his object.

The principle on the basis of which the *Yogi* has to regulate his attitudes and reactions is quite clear from the *Sūtra* but there is one point on which doubt may arise in the mind of the student. Patañjali prescribes indifference towards vice. To some it may appear that this is not in accordance with the highest ideals of spiritual life and an attitude of active help and compassion towards the wicked would be better than that of mere indifference. This objection seems quite reasonable and incidents may be quoted from the lives of great spiritual teachers and saints in support of this argument. But we have to remember that this *Sūtra* is not meant to prescribe a code of conduct for people in general or for those who have become enlightened and are thus in a position to serve as spiritual teachers. It is a code of conduct recommended for the practical student of *Yoga* who is an aspirant for enlightenment. He is engaged in the pursuit of an objective of an extraordinarily difficult nature and he cannot afford to divert his energies for the purpose of reforming others. According to the Eastern tradition and conception of spirituality, active work for the spiritual regeneration of others comes after a person has gained at least a certain degree of enlightenment himself. If we go out to reform others while we ourselves are bound by all kinds of illusions and limitations, we are not likely to gain much success in our endeavour and may seriously jeopardize our own progress. The aspirant for *Yoga* cannot frown upon the wicked because that would tend to arouse hatred and have undesirable repercussions on his own mind. He cannot show sympathy towards them because that would be encouraging vice. So the only course left open to him is to adopt an attitude of indifference.

The result of following the rule given in this *Sūtra* is to bring about clarification of the mind and to remove one of the causes of mental disturbance for the beginner. All those distortions and complexes which the average man develops in his conflicting relations with others must be combed out and the psyche made healthy and harmonious. Otherwise, *Vikṣepa* will continue to trouble him and make the practice of *Yoga* impossible.

Besides a clarified mind, another essential requisite for the practice of *Yoga* is a strong and restful nervous system. How this can be ensured is indicated in the next *Sūtra*.

३४. प्रच्छर्दनविधारणाभ्यां वा प्राणस्य ।

Pracchardana-vidhāraṇābhyāṃ vā
prāṇasya.

प्रच्छर्दन (by) ejection; expiration -विधारणाभ्यां (and) retention; holding वा or प्राणस्य of breath.

34. Or by the expiration and retention of breath.

The subject of *Prāṇāyāma* has been dealt with in II-49-53. In the *Sūtra* given above Patañjali has referred only to some preliminary practices which have only a limited objective, namely the purification of the *Nādīs*. These *Nādīs* are channels along which the currents of *Prāṇa* or vitality flow in the *Prāṇamaya Kośa*. If these channels are not quite clear and the currents of *Prāṇa* do not flow in them smoothly various kinds of nervous disturbances are produced. These manifest chiefly in a general feeling of physical and mental restlessness which causes *Vikṣepa*. This condition can be removed by practising one of the well-known breathing exercises for the purification of the *Nādīs* (*Nādī Śuddhi*). Since *Kumbhaka* does not play any part in these exercises and no strain of any kind is involved they are quite harmless though highly beneficial for the nervous system. If they are practised correctly for long periods of time and the *Yogic* regime of life is followed at the same time, the physical body becomes light and full of vitality and the mind calm and restful.

These exercises should, however, not be taken as variants of deep-breathing which has no other effect except that of increasing the intake of oxygen in the body and thus promoting health. They come somewhere between deep-breathing and *Prāṇāyāma* proper which aims at gaining complete control of the *Prāṇic* currents in the body. This point will become clear when we are dealing with the subject of *Prāṇāyāma* in Section II.

It should be noted that Patañjali does not consider these preliminary exercises for the purification of *Nādīs* as *Prāṇāyāma*. He defines *Prāṇāyāma* in II-49 and according to that definition *Kumbhaka*, the cessation of inspiration and expiration, is an essential part of *Prāṇāyāma*.

३५. विषयवती वा प्रवृत्तिरुत्पन्ना मनसः स्थितिनिबन्धनी ।

Viṣayavatī vā pravṛttir utpannā manasaḥ sthiti-nibandhanī.

विषयवती sensuous वा or प्रवृत्तिः functioning; occupation; pursuit उत्पन्ना arisen; born मनसः of the mind स्थिति steadiness निबन्धनी binder (of) ; helpful in establishing.

35. Coming into activity of (higher) senses also becomes helpful in establishing steadiness of the mind.

The next means which Patañjali gives for making the mind steady is its absorption in some superphysical sensuous cognition. Such cognition may be brought about in a variety of ways, for example, by concentrating the mind on certain vital centres in the body. A typical example of this method is *Laya-Yoga* in which the mind is concentrated on *Nāda* or superphysical sounds which can be heard at certain points within the body. In fact, this method of bringing the mind to rest is considered so effective that a separate branch of *Yoga* based on this principle has grown up.

How far this unification of the mind with *Nāda*, which forms the basis of *Laya-Yoga*, can take the *Sādhaka* in his search for Reality, it is difficult to say. Since this method forms the basis of a separate and independent branch of *Yoga*, it is possible some *Yogis* were able to make considerable advance in their search by this method. But it is very probable that *Laya-Yoga* merges with *Rāja-Yoga* at one stage or another like many other minor systems of *Yoga* and is useful only in the preliminary work of making the mind steady and tranquil and giving the *Sādhaka* direct experience of some superphysical phenomena. Anyhow, the usefulness of this method in overcoming *Vikṣepa* and preparing the mind for the advanced stages of *Yogic* practice is beyond question.

३६. विशोका वा ज्योतिष्मती ।

Viśokā vā jyotiṣmatī.

विशोका sorrowless; serene वा or; also ज्योतिष्मती luminous.

36. Also (through) serene or luminous (states experienced within).

In *Laya-Yoga* the mind is made steady by absorbing it in *Anāhata Śabda*. The same object can be gained by bringing it in contact with other superphysical sensations or states of consciousness. Man's constitution, including both the physical and superphysical bodies, is very complex and there are a large number of methods available for establishing partial contact between the lower and the higher vehicles. Some of these methods depend upon purely artificial aids, others on the *Japa* of a *Mantra* and still others on meditation of a particular type. Which of these methods will be adopted by a *Sādhaka* will depend upon the *Saṃskāras* which he brings from previous lives and the capacity and temperament of the teacher who initiates him in these preliminary practices. As a result of such practice the *Sādhaka* may begin to see an unusual light within him or feel an utter sense of peace and tranquillity. These experiences while of no great significance in themselves can hold the mind by their attractive power and gradually bring about the required condition of steadiness.

The *Sādhaka* should, however, keep in his mind the purpose of these practices. In the first place, he should not attach to them undue importance and significance and begin to imagine that he is making great progress on the path of *Yoga*. He is learning merely the ABC of *Yogic* science. In the second place, he should not allow these experiences to become a mere source of emotional and mental satisfactions. Many people begin to use such practices as a dope and an escape from the stress and strain of ordinary life. If such wrong attitudes are adopted these practices frequently become a hindrance instead of a help in the path of the *Sādhaka*.

३७. वीतरागविषयं वा चित्तम् ।

Vīta-rāga-viṣayaṃ vā cittam.

वीतराग a human being who has transcended human passions or attachment -विषयम् (having for its) object वा or; also चित्तम् the mind.

37. Also the mind fixed on those who are free from attachment (acquires steadiness).

Vītarāgas are those souls who have conquered human passions and risen above *Rāga-Dveṣa*. Meditation on the life and character of such a soul will naturally help the *Sādhaka* to acquire freedom from *Rāga-Dveṣa* himself and thus develop serenity and steadiness of mind. It is a well-known law of life that we tend to reproduce in our life the ideas which constantly occupy our mind. The effect is heightened very greatly if we deliberately select some virtue and meditate upon it constantly. The rationale of this law used in character-building has been discussed in dealing with III-24 and it is unnecessary to elaborate the point here. But we should note that Patañjali recommends meditation not on an abstract virtue but on the virtue as embodied in a human personality. There is a definite reason for this. In the first place, a beginner who is still trying to acquire steadiness of mind is not likely to derive much benefit from meditation on an abstract virtue. The association of a beloved human or divine personality with a virtue increases enormously the attractive power of that virtue and hence its influence on our life. Secondly, earnest meditation on such a personality puts us in rapport with that personality and brings about a flow of power and influence which accelerates our progress. The object of meditation may be one's Master, or a great Spiritual Teacher or one of the Divine Incarnations.

३८. स्वप्ननिद्राज्ञानालम्बनं वा ।

Svapna-nidrā-jñānālambanaṃ vā.

स्वप्न dream state निद्रा state of dreamless sleep ज्ञान (and) knowledge -आलम्बनम् (having for its) support; that on which a thing rests or depends वा also.

38. Also (the mind) depending upon the knowledge derived from dreams or dreamless sleep (will acquire steadiness).

This *Sūtra* giving another method of overcoming *Vikṣepa* seems to have been completely misunderstood and many commentators have tried to explain it away with a lot of rigmarole. The clue to the meaning of the *Sūtra* lies in the significance of the two words *Svapna* and *Nidrā*. If we interpret the *Sūtra* as " meditating on the knowledge obtained in dreams or dreamless sleep " it seems to be meaningless. What useful purpose will be served by meditation on the chaotic images which pass through the brain in the dream state nobody has cared to enquire. And even if we concede the point in relation to the dream state in which there are some images, though chaotic, what shall we say about the dreamless state in which the mind appears to be utterly blank? How is the *Sādhaka* troubled with *Vikṣepa* to utilize this blank condition of the mind for developing one-pointedness?

The fact is that *Svapna* and *Nidrā* do not refer to the condition of the brain during sleep but to the subtler vehicles into which consciousness passes during the period of sleep. When we go to sleep the *Jīvātmā* leaves the physical body and begins to function in the next subtler vehicle. Very partial contact is maintained with the physical body to enable it to carry on its normal physiological activities, but the conscious mind is really functioning in the subtler vehicle. Many people called psychics have a natural capacity for passing out of the physical body into the next subtler world and bringing back into the physical brain more or less vague knowledge of their experiences in that world. The common man, though he is in the same subtler world during sleep cannot generally bring back any memory of his experiences because his brain is not in that peculiar condition required for this purpose. If any mental images are transmitted they become distorted and mixed up with the images which are produced by the automatic activity of the brain and the ordinary chaotic and meaningless dream is the result. Sometimes, the *Jīvātmā* is able to impress some idea or experience on the brain and a significant dream results but this is very rare. All such mental activity is included in the *Svapna* state.

There is a deeper state of consciousness underlying the *Svapna* state corresponding to a still more subtler world into which a person may slip during sleep. This corresponds to the higher sub-planes of the astral world or in rare cases to the lower sub-planes of the mental world. When this happens the physical brain is completely cut off from the activities of the mind and naturally becomes a blank. This state is called technically *Nidrā*. It will be seen that though in this state the brain is blank the mind is working at a higher level and dealing with phenomena of a subtler nature.

Now, it is possible by special training and practice to bring down into the physical brain a memory of experiences undergone in these subtler worlds corresponding to the *Svapna* and *Nidrā* states. Under these conditions the brain is able to transmit the mental images without any distortion and the knowledge obtained under these circumstances is reliable. When this can be done a great deal of useful information can be gathered and work done on these subtler planes during the period of sleep. The waking life gradually merges with the life in so-called sleep and there is no abrupt break which usually takes place on leaving the body or coming back to it after sleep. It is this definite and useful knowledge about these superphysical planes which can be acquired during sleep that is referred to in this *Sūtra* and not the chaotic dreams or the condition of void which are experienced by the ordinary man. The gathering and bringing down of this knowledge into the waking state becomes a matter of absorbing interest and provides one method of overcoming the condition of *Vikṣepa*. In this case also the mind becomes more and more one-pointed and engrossed in an objective which is 'inside'.

It should be remembered, however, that this kind of mental activity has nothing to do with *Samādhi*. It is allied to psychism and differs from it in the fact that it is the result of definite training and therefore the knowledge which is acquired is more useful and reliable.

३९. यथाभिमतध्यानाद्वा ।

Yathābhimata-dhyānād vā.

यथा as अभिमत desired; agreeable ध्यानात् by meditation वा or.

39. Or by meditation as desired.

After giving a number of methods for overcoming the condition of *Vikṣepa* Patañjali concludes this subject by saying that the *Sādhaka* may adopt any method of meditation according to his predilection. This should bring home to the student that the practices recommended by the author are merely means to a definite end which should always be kept in mind. Any other method which serves to make the mind steady and one-pointed can be adopted.

Another idea which is implicit in the *Sūtra* is that the method chosen for this purpose should be in accordance with one's temperament. In that way the mind is helped to acquire the habit of one-pointedness by the natural attraction for the object of pursuit. Thus a *Sādhaka* with clairvoyant tendencies will find the method given in I-38 not only attractive but helpful. Another with an emotional temperament will feel a natural predilection for the method given in I-37. Such predilections are the result of training and experiences in previous lives and generally point to the 'ray' of the individual or the fundamental type to which he belongs.

A little experimentation may be permissible in the selection of the method but trying one method after another should not be allowed to become a habit, for this will aggravate the very malady which is sought to be cured.

४०. परमाणुपरममहत्त्वान्तोऽस्य वशीकारः ।

Paramāṇu-parama-mahattvānto 'sya
vaśīkāraḥ.

परम- ultimate; smallest अणु atom परम- (and) ultimate; greatest महत्व largeness; infinity अन्तः ending (in); extending (up to) अस्य his (of the yogi) वशीकारः mastery.

40. His mastery extends from the finest atom to the greatest infinity.

In this *Sūtra* Patañjali has summed up the powers which can be acquired by the practice of *Yoga*. He says, in fact, that there is no limit to the powers of the *Yogi*. This may appear to the modern man a tall claim and he may dismiss it as another illustration of the hyperboles found scattered in Eastern books like the *Purāṇas*. That *Yoga* confers some powers on its votaries he will be prepared to concede, to deny this would be to fly in the face of facts within the experience of a large number of intelligent people. But to claim for the *Yogi* omnipotence—which is what the statement in this *Sūtra* really amounts to—will appear an absurd exaggeration of facts.

Taken by itself the statement made in this *Sūtra* does appear too sweeping. But we must remember that Patañjali has devoted almost one whole Section to the subject of *Siddhis* or powers acquired through *Yoga*. The present *Sūtra* is therefore expected to be read in the light of all that is said later about *Siddhis* in Section III. The generalization contained in it is therefore not an unqualified statement and if studied along with Section III and the general remarks made in dealing with III-16 will appear quite rational and intelligible

४१. क्षीणवृत्तेरभिजातस्येव मणेर्ग्रहीतृग्रहणग्राह्येषु तत्स्थतदञ्जनता समापत्तिः ।

Kṣīṇa-vṛtter abhijātasyeva maṇer grahītṛ-grahaṇa-grāhyeṣu tatstha-tadañjanatā samāpattiḥ.

क्षीणवृत्तेः of him in whose case the modifications of the mind have been almost annihilated अभिजातस्य of transparent; well-polished इव like मणेः of the jewel or crystal ग्रहीतृ (in) cognizer; subject ग्रहण cognition; the relation between the subject and object ग्राह्येषु (and) cognized objects तत्स्थ on which it rests तदञ्जनता the taking of the form or colour of that समापत्तिः consummation; outcome; fusion.

41. In the case of one whose *Citta-Vṛttis* have been almost annihilated, fusion or entire absorption in one another of the cognizer, cognition and cognized is

brought about as in the case of a transparent jewel (resting on a coloured surface).

This is one of the most important and interesting *Sūtras* in the book for many reasons. Firstly, it throws light on the nature of *Samādhi* as perhaps no other *Sūtra* does; secondly, it enables us to get some insight into the nature of consciousness and mental perception, and lastly, it provides a clue to the *modus operandi* of the many powers which can be wielded by the *Yogi*.

If we are to understand the underlying significance of the *Sūtra* we should first recall the philosophical conception upon which it is based. According to this conception the manifested Universe is an emanation of an Ultimate Reality and its different planes, visible and invisible, may be considered to be formed by a sort of progressive condensation or involution of consciousness. At each stage of the progressive condensation a subjective-objective relationship is established between the more condensed and less condensed aspects of consciousness, the less condensed assuming the subjective and the more condensed the objective role. The Ultimate Reality at the basis of the manifested Universe is the only purely subjective principle while all other partial expressions of that Reality in the realm of manifestation have a double subjective-objective role, being subjective towards those expressions which are more involved and objective towards those less involved. Not only is there at each point the possibility of this meeting of subjective and objective but wherever and whenever such meeting takes place a definite relation is established between the two. So the manifested Universe is really not a duality but a triplicity and that is how every manifestation of Reality at any level or in any sphere has three aspects. These three aspects corresponding to the subjective and objective sides of manifestation and the relation which must exist between them are referred to in the present *Sūtra* as *Grahītṛ*, *Grahaṇa* and *Grāhya* and may be translated into English by sets of words such as knower, knowing, known or cognizer, cognition, cognized or perceiver, perception, perceived.

This fundamental fact underlying manifestation, that the One has become the Three, is the basis of the mysterious identity which exists between these three apparently different components of the triplicity. It is because the One Reality has become the Three that it is possible to bring about a fusion of the Three into One, and it is this kind of fusion which is the essential technique and secret of *Samādhi.* This fusion can take place at four different levels of consciousness corresponding to *Vitarka, Vicāra, Ānanda* and *Asmitā* stages of *Saṃprajñāta Samādhi* but the principle underlying the fusion of the Three into One is the same at all the levels and the result also is the same, namely the attainment by the knower of perfect and complete knowledge of the known.

Before we take up the question of bringing about this fusion at different levels let us first consider the very apt simile used by Patañjali to bring home to the student the essential nature of *Samādhi.*

If we place a small piece of ordinary stone on a sheet of coloured paper the stone is not at all affected by the coloured light coming from the paper. It stands out against the paper as it was owing to its imperviousness to this light If we place a colourless crystal on the same piece of paper we immediately see a difference in its behaviour towards the light coming from the paper. It absorbs some of the light and thus appears at least partially assimilated with the paper. The degree of absorption will depend upon the transparency of the crystal and the freedom from defects in its substance. The more perfect the crystal the more completely will it transmit the light and become assimilated with the coloured paper. A crystal of perfectly transparent glass with no internal defects or colour will become so completely assimilated with the paper as almost to disappear in the light coming from it. It will be there but in an invisible form and emitting only the light of the paper upon which it is placed. We should note that it is the freedom of the crystal from any defects, characteristics, marks or qualities of its own which enables it to become completely assimilated with the paper on which it is placed. Even a trace of colour in an otherwise perfect crystal will prevent its perfect assimilation.

The behaviour of a mind in relation to an object of contemplation is remarkably similar to the behaviour of the crystal in relation to the coloured paper. Any activity, impression, or bias which the mind has apart from the object of contemplation will stand in the way of its becoming fused with it completely. It is only when the mind has, as it were, annihilated itself completely and destroyed its independent identity that it can become assimilated with the object of contemplation and shine with the pure truth enshrined in that object.

Let us consider for a while the various factors which prevent this process of assimilation. First of all come the various tendencies, some almost instinctive in character, which impart strong biases to the mind and make it flow naturally and powerfully along certain predetermined lines. Such tendencies are, for example, those of accumulating possessions, indulging in all kinds of enjoyments, attractions and repulsions. Such tendencies which are derived from desires of various kinds tend to throw up in the mind mental images and temptations in accordance with their own nature. All such tendencies are sought to be eliminated from the mind of the aspirant by the practice of *Yama*, *Niyama* and *Vairāgya*. Then come the sensuous impressions derived from the contact of the sense-organs with the external world. Along the avenues of the sense-organs flows a continuous current of impressions into the mind, modifying it continually into a never ending series of images. These impressions are cut off when *Samādhi* is to be practised by means of *Āsana*, *Prāṇāyāma* and *Pratyāhāra*. The *Yogi* has now to deal only with the inherent activity of the mind itself, the activity which it can carry on with the help of the images stored in its memory and its power to arrange and re-arrange those images in innumerable patterns. This kind of activity is sought to be controlled and canalized in *Dhāraṇā* and *Dhyāna* and the mind made to direct its activity solely in one channel. There is nothing left now in the mind, there is nothing which can arise in the mind except the ' seed ' of *Saṃyama* or the object of contemplation. But the mind is still separate from the object and as long as it retains its subjective role it cannot become one with the object. This awareness of the mind of itself which stands in its way of becoming fused with the object of contemplation and ' shining ' solely with the truth hidden within the object is eliminated in *Samādhi*. How this self-awareness is dissolved to bring about the complete fusion of the knower, known and knowing is the subject of the subsequent *Sūtras*.

In considering the simile of the perfectly transparent crystal which is placed on coloured paper we should note that though the crystal is free from its own defects and can thus become assimilated with the coloured paper, still, the coloured light from the paper colours it. So, it is still not quite free from defect. An external influence still modifies it though this is of a very subtle nature. It is only when it is placed on a piece of white paper which is giving out white light that the crystal will shine with white light which includes all colours in harmonious blending and is the symbol of the Whole Truth or Reality.

Similarly, in *Sabīja Samādhi* although all the other defects of the mind have been eliminated one defect is still there. This defect is its permeation with the partial truth of the 'seed' of contemplation. Compared with the Whole Truth which includes and integrates all partial truths, the partial truth of the 'seed' acts as a hindrance and prevents the mind from shining with the Whole Truth. So, as long as the partial truth of any 'seed', gross or subtle, occupies the mind the Whole Truth of the One Reality cannot shine through it. For the realization of the Whole Truth which can be found only in the consciousness of *Puruṣa*, according to *Yogic* terminology, it is necessary to remove even the impression of any partial truth realized in *Sabīja Samādhi*. This is accomplished by the practice of *Nirbīja Samādhi* or '*Samādhi* without seed'. The transparent and perfect crystal of the mind can then shine with the pure white Light of Truth. It will be seen, therefore, that in *Sabīja Samādhi* the *Vṛttis* of the mind are replaced by pure but partial knowledge of a particular aspect of Reality but in *Nirbīja Samādhi* this pure but partial knowledge is replaced by the Reality or consciousness of *Puruṣa* itself. The mind has merged in the One Reality and exists unperceived only to radiate its unimaginable effulgence.

What has been said above with regard to the conditions which must be fulfilled before the fusion of the knower with the known can be brought about in *Samādhi* should make it clear that the *Yogic* technique has to be adopted as a whole and not piecemeal. If, for example, the ordinary desires have not been eliminated and merely curbed, it is impossible to practise *Samādhi*. These desires will continue to exert unconscious pressure and throw up all kinds of images in the mind and it will not be possible to maintain under these conditions the uninterrupted and tranquil state of the mind in which alone *Samādhi* can be practised. This state cannot be brought about by the mere exertion of will-power as some people suppose, for the exertion of will-power on a mind agitated by even sub-conscious desires is bound to produce mental strain, and a mind under strain which may be inappreciable, is quite unfit for the practice of *Samādhi*. The tranquillity which is a pre-requisite for *Samādhi* is a condition of extraordinary and habitual stability, and real stability cannot exist where there is strain. It is necessary to emphasize these facts again and again because aspirants who are not familiar with the realities of *Yogic* life plunge directly into the practice of meditation without any preparation whatsoever and then begin to fret and wonder why they do not make any progress. The practice of higher *Yoga* requires a thorough and all-round preparation extending over long periods of time. This does not mean, of course, that the aspirant should not make a beginning with only a few simple practices and gradually extend the area of his endeavour until he has mastered the preparatory lessons.

There is one word in this *Sūtra* whose significance should be noted. This is *Kṣīṇa*. This word means 'attenuated' or 'weakened'. It does not mean 'annihilated' or completely 'dead'. In performing *Saṃyama* in *Sabīja Samādhi* there is always a 'seed' present in the mind. So the mind cannot be said to be without *Vṛtti* or modification. It is only when *Nirbīja Samādhi* is practised that the mind becomes without *Vṛtti*. It is true that in the ultimate phase of each of the *Vitarka*, *Vicāra*, *Ānanda* and *Asmitā* stages of *Saṃprajñāta Samādhi* the partial truth which shines forth through the mind can hardly be called a *Vṛtti* in the ordinary sense. Still, we cannot say that the mind is present in an unmodified condition for the light of the partial truth as explained above still colours the mind. The change from the ordinary condition of the mind in which all kinds of transformation are continually taking place to the condition in which only one object continues to occupy the mind is called *Samādhi Pariṇāma* in III-11 and the final state reached in the transformation can best be described as one in which the *Vṛttis* of the mind have become *Kṣīṇa*. But it should be obvious that this does not mean complete annihilation or disappearance of the *Vṛttis* as suggested by some commentators.

४२. तत्र शब्दार्थज्ञानविकल्पैः संकीर्णा सवितर्का ।

Tatra śabdārtha-jñāna-vikalpaiḥ saṃkīrṇā savitarkā.

तत्र there; in it शब्द (with) word अर्थ real meaning; true knowledge of the object which the *Yogi* wants ज्ञान ordinary knowledge based on sense perceptions and reasoning विकल्पैः (and) alternation between different alternatives owing to doubt or uncertainty संकीर्णा mixed up; confused; unresolved; involved सवितर्का a state of *Samādhi* characterized by *Vitarka* (see I-17 and II-19).

42. *Savitarka Samādhi* is that in which knowledge based only on words, real knowledge and ordinary knowledge based on sense perception or reasoning are present in a mixed state and the mind alternates between them.

In dealing with the first three *Sūtras* of Section III the three purely mental processes of *Dhāraṇā*, *Dhyāna* and *Samādhi* have been explained in detail. In I-41 the essential nature of *Samādhi* has been discussed. But it is necessary to note that the word *Samādhi* is not used for any specific or definite state of the mind. It stands for a very wide range of super-conscious states of the mind which lead to and end in *Kaivalya*. The state of *Samādhi* must be attained before entry into the higher realms of consciousness is possible. It ushers the *Yogi* into those realms but the investigation of those realms and the mastery of the forces and powers which work on those realms has still to be accomplished by the *Yogi*. It will be seen therefore that the mental state defined in III-3 is merely a preliminary condition which qualifies the *Yogi* to enter upon this task of investigation and control just as a Master's degree of a university qualifies a student to enter upon a course of independent scientific research. In the ten *Sūtras* beginning with I-42 some further light is thrown upon the technique of *Samādhi* which has to do with the investigation and mastery of these realms on the one hand and the realization of Reality which lies beyond those realms on the other. *Samādhi* with the former objective is called *Sabīja Samādhi* and that with the latter objective *Nirbīja Samādhi.*

When the *Yogi* has mastered the technique of *Samādhi* as given in I-3 and can perform *Saṃyama* on anything which can become an object of *Saṃyama,* and of which the inner reality has to be discovered, the question arises: How does he make further progress? How does he utilize the power which he has so far acquired for the investigation and mastery of the higher realms of existence which he can now contact through his subtler vehicles?

The technique of these further stages of progress is hinted at in I-42-51. It is not given in detail because no one who has not gone through the *Yogic* discipline and reached the advanced stage where he can perform *Saṃyama* can really understand these things even theoretically. The *Sūtras* mentioned above should therefore be understood not to embody the technique of the higher stages of *Samādhi* but merely as pointing to these stages which exist and their relative position in the line of progress. They are suggestive, not explanatory. They are like the sketch map of a country which a traveller may intend to explore. Such a sketch map merely gives the relative position of the different parts of the country and the direction in which the traveller should proceed in order to reach his goal. But something more is needed for exploring a country than a mere sketch map.

Before we proceed to consider the above mentioned *Sūtras* let us first try to understand the distinction between *Sabīja* and *Nirbīja Samādhis.* In connection with I-17 on *Saṃprajñāta Samādhi* it was pointed out that this kind of *Samādhi* has four stages. These stages represent, as has been explained already, the four distinct and distinguishable levels at which consciousness functions through the four subtler vehicles and corresponding to the four stages of *Guṇas* mentioned in II-9. It is also pointed out in connection with III-5 that the higher consciousness functioning at those levels in a state of *Samādhi* is quite different from the ordinary mental consciousness with which we are familiar and is called *Prajñā*.

That is why *Samādhi* of this class is called *Saṃprajñāta.* All these four stages of *Saṃprajñāta Samādhi* are comprised in *Sabīja Samādhi* as pointed out in I-46.

Why is *Samādhi* pertaining to these four stages called *Sabīja Samādhi*? The clue to this question lies in the meaning of the word *Bīja* or seed. What is the essential form of a seed? It is a conglomeration of different kinds of matter arranged in different layers, the outermost layer forming the protective and least essential part and the innermost layer or core forming the real or essential part of the whole set. So that, in order to get at the essential part or real substance of the seed we have to tear open the different layers one after another until we reach the core.

The general constitution of a seed described above will show at once the appropriateness of calling any *Samādhi* of the *Saṃprajñāta* type *Sabīja Samādhi. Saṃyama* in *Saṃprajñāta Samādhi* is always performed on some 'object' which is called a 'seed' because it has different layers of meaning, etc. covering an essential core which is the reality of the object. We can come into touch with the different layers of the object or 'seed' by splitting it open, as it were, mentally through the technique of *Samādhi.* Each successive stage of *Samādhi* reveals to our consciousness a different and deeper layer of the reality of the object and by continuing the process of *Saṃyama* through the successive stages we ultimately arrive at the innermost reality of the object. Each stage of *Samādhi* lays bare only one layer of the total reality hidden within the object and the process of penetration may have to be pushed in some cases through all the four stages before the ultimate reality hidden within the object is revealed.

But though there are four stages in *Sabīja Samādhi* and it may be necessary to pass through all these four stages before the object on which *Saṃyama* is performed is revealed in its totality, this does not mean that every object on which *Saṃyama* can be performed is sufficiently complex to require going through all the four stages. Different objects differ in their complexity or subtlety, some being more complex and having more subtle counterparts than others as is explained in dealing with III-6. Patañjali has not discussed systematically and in detail the different types of 'seeds' on which *Saṃyama* can be performed and the method of "splitting them open" in *Samādhi* but a study of the *Sūtras* given in the latter portion of Section III will give the student a fairly good idea of the large variety of objects which are taken up for *Saṃyama* in *Yogic* practice. A careful study of these *Sūtras* will not only give the student some idea with regard to the different purposes of *Sabīja* and *Nirbīja Samādhi* but also throw some light on the technique of *Samādhi*. It will help him to get a clearer insight into the meaning of the two rather enigmatic *Sūtras* I-42-43 in which alone Patañjali has given some definite information with regard to the mental processes involved in *Samādhi*.

Before we proceed to discuss these two *Sūtras* let us first consider a few conclusions which may be drawn from a general study of the objects (*Viṣayā*) upon which *Saṃyama* is performed and the results which accrue from this practice. These conclusions may be stated very briefly as follows:

(1) If two things are related as cause and effect then by performing *Saṃyama* on the effect it is possible to have knowledge of the underlying cause or vice versa as for example in III-16.

(2) If certain phenomena leave an impression on any medium it is possible to come into touch with the phenomena by reviving the impressions through *Saṃyama* as for example in III-18.

(3) If a particular principle in nature finds expression in a particular phenomenon then by performing *Saṃyama* on the phenomenon, it is possible to know directly the underlying principle, as for example in III-28 or III-29.

(4) If a particular object is the expression of an archetype then by performing *Saṃyama* on the object it is possible to have direct knowledge of the archetype as for example in III-30.

(5) If a particular centre in the body is an organ of a higher vehicle, faculty etc. then by performing *Saṃyama* on the centre direct contact is established with the vehicle, faculty etc. as for example in III-33 or III-35.

(6) If a thing exists in several degrees of subtlety, one derived from the other in a series, then by performing *Saṃyama* on the outermost or least subtle form it is possible to gain knowledge of all the forms, step by step, as for example in III-45.

A careful consideration of the facts mentioned above will show that *Saṃyama* is really a means of passing from the outer expression to the reality within whatever may be the nature of the relationship between the outer expression and the inner reality. Since the reality underlying all objects is contained in the Divine Mind and the object of *Saṃyama* in *Sabīja Samādhi* is to know this reality it follows that what the *Yogi* does in *Saṃyama* is to sink into his own consciousness until he reaches the level of Divine Mind in which the reality of the object is to be found. The 'seed' on which *Saṃyama* is performed merely determines the line along which consciousness has to sink. This may be illustrated by the following diagram:

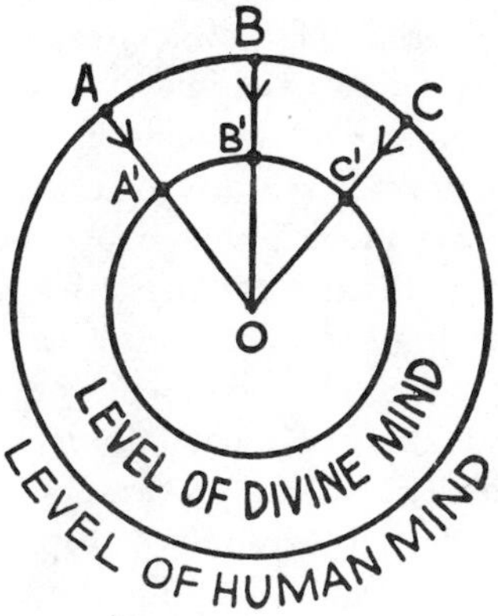

FIG. 5

A, B, C are different objects which can serve as 'seeds' of *Sabīja Samādhi.* A′, B′, C′ are respectively the realities of these objects which can be found in the Divine Mind through *Saṃyama.* O is the Centre of Divine Consciousness. It will be seen that in every case the essential process is the same, namely proceeding from the periphery along a radius to the centre until the intervening circle is reached. But different objects which are represented by different points on the outer circle make it necessary to proceed along different radii to the centre. In proceeding in this manner consciousness automatically touches the reality of the particular object when it reaches the level of the Divine Mind. So the 'seed' merely determines the direction along which consciousness has to sink in order to reach the corresponding reality in the Divine

Mind. It does not make any difference as far as the essential process of *Saṃyama* is concerned but merely guides the consciousness to the reality which is the object of the search.

In *Nirbīja Samādhi* the aim of the *Yogi* is the Centre of Divine Consciousness represented by O in the diagram. In reaching the point O he must proceed along a radius and must cross the intervening states of consciousness. That is why *Nirbīja Samādhi* can come only after *Sabīja Samādhi* when all the stages of *Saṃprajñāta Samādhi* have been crossed.

Having cleared the ground to a certain extent let us now proceed to consider I-42 which throws some light on the technique of splitting open the ' seed ' of ' *Sabīja* ' *Samādhi*. This *Sūtra* deals with the mental processes involved in the very first stage of *Samādhi* and may best be understood in relation to a concrete object having a name and form. We are so used to taking all things which come within the range of our experience for granted that we never pay any attention to the mysteries which are obviously hidden within the simplest of objects. Every physical object which we can perceive through our sense organs is really a conglomerate of several kinds of mental impressions which can be sorted out to a certain extent by a process of mental analysis on the basis of our knowledge of sensuous perception and other facts discovered by Science. Let us take for the sake of illustration a simple concrete object like a rose. Our knowledge regarding a rose is a mixture in which facts like those given below enter:

(1) It has a name which has been chosen arbitrarily and has no natural relationship with the object.

(2) It has a form, colour, odour etc. which we can perceive through our sense-organs. These will vary from rose to rose but there is an irreducible minimum of qualities which are common to all roses and which make a rose, a rose.

(3) It is a particular combination of certain atoms and molecules (or electrons at a deeper level) distributed in a certain manner in space. The mental image which is formed in our mind on the basis of this scientific knowledge is quite different from the mental image derived from the sense-organs.

(4) It is a particular specimen of an archetype, all roses which come into being conforming to this archetypal rose.

A consideration of some of the facts given above will show to the student how mixed up our ideas are regarding even common objects with which we come in contact every day. Our true knowledge with regard to the real object is mixed up or confused with all kinds of mental images and it is not possible for us to separate the pure knowledge from these mental images by ordinary processes of mental analysis or reasoning. The only way in which this can be done is by performing *Saṃyama* on the object and fusing the mind with it as explained in I-41. The pure, real, internal knowledge regarding the object is isolated from the mixed external knowledge and the *Yogi* can then know the real object by making the mind one with it.

It is obvious that there must be two stages in this process of ' knowing by fusing '. In the first stage the heterogeneous knowledge regarding the object must be separated into its different constituents. In this stage all the constituents of the knowledge, internal and external, are present but from an undifferentiated and confused state they are resolved more and more into a state of clearly-defined and differentiated constituents. In the second stage the mind is fused with the pure knowledge which has been isolated in the first stage. In this process of selective fusion, naturally, all the other constituents which depend upon memory drop out automatically and the mind shines only with the pure knowledge of the object, nothing else. I-42 deals with the first stage and I-43 with the second stage.

Let us now consider the significance of the words used in I-42 to indicate this resolution and differentiation of this composite knowledge with regard to the object into its clearly defined constituents. The word *Tatra* refers to the state of *Samādhi* described in the previous *Sūtra* and is obviously used to point out that this process of resolution is carried out in a state of *Samādhi* and cannot be accomplished by an ordinary process of mental analysis. It is only when the mind has been completely isolated from external influences and has reached the concentrated state of *Dhyāna* that it can successfully tackle this problem of resolution. *Śabda-Artha-Jñāna* define the three categories of knowledge which are inextricably mixed up in the mind of the ordinary man and can be resolved only in *Savitarka-Samādhi*. *Śabda* refers to knowledge which is based only on words and is not connected in any way with the object which is being considered. Much of our thinking is of this superficial nature, based merely on words and not touching the object at all. *Artha* refers to the true knowledge about the object or its real meaning which the *Yogi* wants. And *Jñāna* refers to the ordinary knowledge based on the perception of the sense-organs and the reasoning of the mind. The condition of not being able to distinguish clearly between these three kinds of knowledge with the result that the mind hovers between them is sought to be conveyed by the word *Vikalpaiḥ*. This is inevitable as long as the three kinds of knowledge have not separated out, as it were, in three separate layers but are present in a state of mixture or *con-fusion* which is indicated by the word *Saṃkīrṇā*. It will perhaps help the student to understand this progressive resolution of the three kinds of knowledge if we illustrate the process diagrammatically as follows:

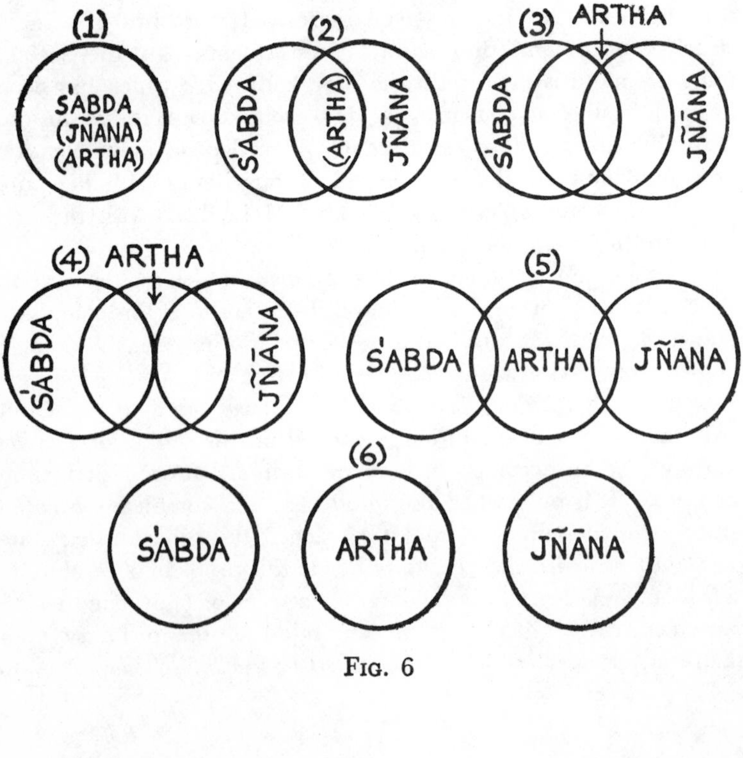

FIG. 6

It will be seen that while in the first step knowledge based on Śabda only covers the other two, the progressive resolution results in the last step in the complete separation of the three. Students of Science will also find the analogy of an emulsion helpful in understanding this progressive resolution and separation into two separate and distinct constituents. If two immiscible liquids are shaken together vigorously it is possible to prepare an emulsion in which both appear to be present in a homogeneous condition though they really remain separate. But if the emulsion is allowed to stand for some time the two liquids will gradually separate out into two separate layers. This analogy is especially apt because it is the absence of agitation which leads to the separation of the two layers just as in *Savitarka Samādhi* it is really the extreme tranquillization of the mind which brings about the separation of the different kinds of knowledge.

When the different mental components have separated and are seen in their correct relationship then there can be no confusion or going from one to the other. It is because they are mistaken for one another and the proper province of each is not defined that there is confusion and consequent *Vitarka* (see also in this connection III-17). When the mental picture clears up and each component is seen in true perspective *Vitarka* must come to an end.

४३. स्मृतिपरिशुद्धौ स्वरूपशून्येवार्थमात्रनिर्भासा निर्वितर्का ।

Smṛti-pariśuddhau svarūpa-śūnyevārtha-mātra-nirbhāsā nirvitarkā.

स्मृति (of) memory परिशुद्धौ on clarification स्वरूप own form; essential nature; self-awareness शून्य devoid (of) इव as if अर्थ- object; real meaning; true knowledge of the object मात्र- only निर्भासा presenting; shining (with); appearing (as) निर्वितर्का a state of *Samādhi* characterized by absence of *Vitarka*.

43. On the clarification of memory, when the mind loses its essential nature (subjectivity), as it were,

and the real knowledge of the object alone shines (through the mind) *Nirvitarka Samādhi* is attained.

The *Savitarka* stage of *Samādhi* which has been dealt with in the previous *Sūtra* prepares the ground for the *Nirvitarka* stage. The confused state of the mind in which different kinds of knowledge were mixed up has been gradually replaced by a clarified state in which the three kinds of knowledge are seen separate and clearly distinguishable. This clarification is called *Smṛti-pariśuddhi* in the present *Sūtra*. Why is this resolution of knowledge present in the mind of the *Yogi* called 'clearing up of memory'? To understand the reason for the use of the word *Smṛti* in this connection the student should recall I-6 in which the *Vṛttis* or modifications of the mind are classified under five heads and *Smṛti* or memory is one of these. If he has understood the basis of this classification he will see at once that the modification of the mind in *Savitarka Samādhi* comes under *Smṛti* or memory. As the *Yogi's* mind is cut off completely from the external world, the modification cannot come under 'right knowledge' or 'wrong knowledge'. As he is not asleep but fully conscious it cannot come under 'sleep'. As he is performing *Saṃyama* not on any imaginary thing but on a definite thing of which the *reality* it to be known, the modification cannot come under 'imagination'. The modification is really of the nature of memory because it is a reproduction in the mind of a thing which has been experienced before. That is why Patañjali calls the process of clearing up as 'clarification of memory'.

When the memory has become clarified the mind is ready for the next step, viz. reducing the self-awareness to the utmost limit. This mental process which is called *Svarūpa-Śūnya* has been explained in dealing with III-3 and it is not necessary to go into this question here, but two facts may be pointed out in this connection. The first point we should note is that the dissolution of the mental self-awareness can come only after the resolution of the composite and complex knowledge with regard to the object into its three clearly defined constituents. This is clear from the word *Pari-śuddhau* which means 'on the clearing up of'. The second point to which attention may be drawn is the significance of the word *Iva* after *Śūnya*. The word *Iva* means 'as if' and it is used to signify that though the mind seems to disappear it is still there. The very fact that the 'object' is 'shining' in it points to the presence of the mind. It is only its subjective nature which has disappeared in the object, as it were, thus bringing about a fusion of the subjective and objective which is necessary for attaining the *Samādhi* state. It is this fusion which brings about the disappearance of the other two constituents *Śabda* and *Jñāna* leaving the pure knowledge or *Svarūpa* of the object alone to fill the mind. The object is then seen in its naked reality. The use of the word *Nirbhāsā* which means 'shining' for describing the filling of the mind with the *Svarūpa* or real knowledge of the 'object' follows naturally from the simile used in I-41 for illustrating the fusion of subjective and objective. The mind though itself imperceptible like the transparent jewel yet shines with the light of true knowledge of the object. The use of the word *Nirvitarka* for a state of *Samādhi* in which there is no *Vitarka* also requires some explanation. One can understand the use of the word *Savitarka* in the previous *Sūtra* because the state of *Samādhi* is accompanied by *Vitarka*. But why use the word *Nirvitarka* for a state in which there is no *Vitarka*? Simply to indicate the nature of the state which has gone before. When one says that his mind is unburdened, it means not only that there is no burden on it now but also that it was burdened before. The use of the word *Nirvitarka* in this *Sūtra* means, therefore, that the state indicated is arrived at after passing through the *Savitarka* state and is merely the consummation or culmination of the previous state. The consciousness is still functioning at the same level and in the same vehicle though it has reached the utmost limit as far as knowledge with regard to that object on that plane is concerned. Any further change in this state can only be a repetition of itself as explained in connection with III-12. It is only by the practice of *Nirodha* that consciousness can pass on into the next vehicle and a new series of changes at a higher level can begin.

An interesting question that may arise in the mind of the student is: Who brings about the fusion of subjective and objective and also the further transformations which take place in the further stages of *Samādhi*? Upto the point where *Vitarka* is present the transformations may be supposed to take place through the agency of the subjective mind which is still active. But who provides the guiding and propelling force after the subjective mind has merged in the object? Obviously, the *Puruṣa* who is present all the time in the background and who is the lord of the mind as pointed out in IV-18. The mind itself is inert and it is the constant presence of the *Puruṣa* in the background which endows it not only with the capacity to perceive but also the will to change. The mind is always an instrument. The real *Draṣṭā* and the *Kartā* is the *Puruṣa* always. So when the lower mind merges with the object in *Nirvitarka Samādhi* it is the *Puruṣa* working *in his higher principles* who really is in charge and is ultimately responsible for the continuous and delicate transformations which take place in the further stages of *Samādhi*. In fact, throughout the continuous unfoldment which takes place in *Yoga* upto the point of attaining *Kaivalya*, it is the *Puruṣa* who has to be considered as guiding the evolution. It is true that this view is not in conformity with the conceptions of *Sāṃkhya* philosophy in which the *Puruṣa* is considered to be a mere *Draṣṭā*, spectator, but *Yogic* technique, as pointed out elsewhere, is not based solely on *Sāṃkhya* and without assuming a guiding role for the *Puruṣa* this technique would be unintelligible. This is not the place, however, to enter into this philosophical question.

४४. एतयैव सविचारा निर्विचारा च सूक्ष्मविषया व्याख्याता ।

Etayaiva savicārā nirvicārā ca sūkṣma-viṣayā vyākhyātā.

एतया by this एव even; alone; itself सविचारा *Samādhi* involving *Vicāra* or reflection (see I-17 and II-19) निर्विचारा *Sāmādhi* not involving *Vicāra* च and सूक्ष्मविषया *Samādhi* involving (still more) subtle 'objects' व्याख्याता described or explained.

44. By this (what has been said in the two previous (*Sūtras*) *Samādhis* of *Savicāra*, *Nirvicāra* and subtler stages (I-17) have also been explained.

The difficulty of comprehending *Samādhi* even in the lowest *Savitarka-Nirvitarka* stage, in spite of the fact that we are living in a world of names and forms and are familiar to some extent with the working of the concrete mind, should make it easy to understand why Patañjali has not dealt with the higher stages of *Samādhi* in detail and has disposed of the whole subject in two *Sūtras*. I-44 merely points out that the mental processes in *Savicāra-Nirvicāra* and other higher stages of *Samādhi* are analogous to those of *Savitarka-Nirvitarka Samādhi*, i.e. the *Samādhi* in relation to *Sūkṣma-Viṣayās* or subtle objects, begins with *Saṃyama* on the outermost aspect of the object which is the most complex and ending with the isolation of the object in its real state which is the simplest. It may be mentioned here that the progressive involution of consciousness in matter is generally accompanied by the increasing complexity of the functions and the reverse process of release of consciousness from the limitations of matter means simplification of functions. An example will serve to throw some light on this general principle. The process of perceiving an external world requires the agency of sense-organs on the physical plane, there being a separate sense-organ for contacting each *Bhūta*. But on the higher spiritual planes perception takes place through a single faculty which is called *Pratibhā* and which performs the functions of all the five sense-organs in an integrated manner.

A clear grasp of this fundamental principle will help the student in understanding the role of *Samādhi* in this process of unveiling the subtler and more profound aspects of objects in the manifested Universe. *Samādhi* does nothing more than reverse this involution of consciousness and this evolution or unfoldment of consciousness automatically reveals the subtler aspects of these objects. What the *Yogi* really does is to sink deeper and deeper into his own consciousness. This brings into action the more comprehensive faculties of the increasingly subtler planes which alone can reveal the subtler aspects of objects. What the intellect may strain to the utmost to understand without much success becomes self-evident in the light of these higher faculties. That is why Patañjali has not tried to deal with matters which are really beyond the comprehension of the brain-bound intellect.

४५. सूक्ष्मविषयत्वं चालिङ्गपर्यवसानम् ।

Sūkṣma-viṣayatvaṃ cāliṅga-pary-
avasānam.

सूक्ष्मविषयत्वं the state of *Samādhi* concerned with subtle objects च and अलिङ्ग- the last stage of the *Guṇas* (II-19), -पर्यवसानम् extending (up to).

45. The province of *Samādhi* concerned with subtle objects extends up to the *Alinga* stage of the *Guṇas*.

If different objects are subtle to different degrees how can these degrees of subtlety be classified? The different degrees of subtlety can be classified in the most comprehensible manner by assigning them to the planes on which they exist. But for reasons which have been pointed out in dealing with I-17 Patañjali has adopted a functional and not a structural basis for classifying phenomena and so the degrees of subtlety have been classified according to the stages of the *Guṇas* given in II-19. As the subject has been dealt with thoroughly in that context it is not necessary to discuss it here. It may, however, be pointed out that according to *Sāṃkhya* all objects are the result of different combinations of *Guṇas* and so the classification of objects in four categories according to the four stages of the *Guṇas* is perfectly logical. The last stage of the *Guṇas* is called *Alinga* and so naturally the limit of subtlety corresponds with the *Alinga* stage.

४६. ता एव सबीजः समाधिः ।

Tā eva sabījaḥ samādhiḥ.

ताः those एव only सबीजः with 'seed'; having an object; objective समाधिः *Samādhi*.

46. They (stages corresponding to subtle objects) constitute only *Samādhi* with 'seed'.

All objects within the realm of *Prakṛti* upon which *Saṃyama* may be performed to discover their relative reality have been summed up in I-45. *Samādhi* which deals with any of these objects is called *Sabīja Samādhi* for reasons explained in connection with I-42. An object on which *Saṃyama* is performed is technically called a ' seed ' whether it is gross or subtle. So *Sabīja Samādhi* may also be called objective *Samādhi* as opposed to *Nirbīja Samādhi* or subjective *Samādhi* in which there is no ' object ' or ' seed ' of meditation. The Seeker Himself is the object of His search. The Seer who has gained the capacity to see truly all objects within the realm of *Prakṛti* now wants to see Himself as He really is.

What distinguishes *Sabīja Samādhi* from *Nirbīja Samādhi* is therefore the presence of an object associated with *Prakṛti* whose relative reality has to be realized. In *Nirbīja Samādhi*, *Puruṣa* who is beyond the realm of *Prakṛti* is the ' objectless ' objective. He is the Seeker as well as the object of the search. In *Sabīja Samādhi* also he is really seeking Himself but a veil, howsoever thin, still obscures his vision. In *Nirbīja Samādhi* He attempts to tear off the last veil in order to obtain a completely unobstructed vision of Himself. This is what is meant by Self-Realization.

४७. निर्विचारवैशारद्येऽध्यात्मप्रसादः ।

Nirvicāra-vaiśāradye 'dhyātma-prasādaḥ.

निर्विचार *Samādhi* (of) the *Nirvicāra* stage वैशारद्ये on the refinement; on attaining the utmost purity अध्यात्म spiritual प्रसादः lucidity, clarity.

47. On attaining the utmost purity of the *Nirvicāra* stage (of *Samādhi*) there is the dawning of the spiritual light.

I-47 is meant to draw a distinction between the lower and higher stages of *Samādhi* and to emphasize that spirituality is not necessarily associated with all the stages. We have seen already that *Sabīja Samādhi* begins on the plane of the lower mind and its province extends upto the *Ātmic* plane. At which point in these successive stages of *Samādhi* does the light of spirituality begin to dawn in consciousness? To be able to answer this question we should recall that the intellect is the separative and constrictive principle in man which distorts his vision and is responsible for the common illusions of the lower life. As long as consciousness is functioning within the realms of the intellect alone it must remain bound by those illusions. *Samādhi* in the realm of the intellect, while it reveals the lower aspect of the reality which is hidden behind the objects on which *Saṃyama* is performed, does not necessarily bring with it perception of the higher truths of a spiritual nature, does not for instance give a vision of the fundamental unity of life. It is conceivable, for example, that a scientist may discover many of the truths underlying the physical world by means of *Samādhi* and yet remain absolutely unaware of the deeper spiritual truths which are associated with spirituality. Some of the lower *Siddhis* such as those dealt with in III-28-32 can be obtained in this manner. In fact the black magicians who are called Brothers of the Shadow, are all *Yogis* who are proficient in the technique of lower *Yoga* and undoubtedly possess many of the lower *Siddhis*. But their work is confined within the realm of the intellect and they remain ignorant of the higher truths of existence. Their selfish outlook and evil ways debar them from entering into the deeper and spiritual realms of consciousness and thus acquiring true wisdom and spiritual illumination.

This *Sūtra* points out that spiritual illumination begins to flood the mind when the *Yogi* has reached the last stage of *Nirvicāra Samādhi* and is in the borderland which separates the intellect from the next higher spiritual principle, *Buddhi* or Intuition. In this stage the light of *Buddhi* which is the source of wisdom and spirituality begins to shed its radiance on the intellect. Illuminated in this manner the intellect ceases to be a slave of the lower self and becomes a willing instrument of the Higher Self working through *Ātmā-Buddhi-Manas*. For, the distortions and illusions associated with the intellect are not really inherent in this principle. They are due to the absence of spiritual illumination. An intellect illuminated by the light of *Buddhi* and under the control of the *Ātmā* is a magnificent and powerful instrument which even the Adepts use constantly in Their work.

४८. ऋतम्भरा तत्र प्रज्ञा ।

Ṛtambharā tatra prajñā.

ऋतम्भरा Truth-bearing; Right-bearing तत्र there प्रज्ञा higher state of consciousness (experienced in *Samādhi*).

48. There, the consciousness is Truth-and-Right-bearing.

In the previous *Sūtra* the stage at which the purely intellectual consciousness is converted into spiritual consciousness in *Samādhi* was pointed out. The present *Sūtra* gives an important attribute of the new type of consciousness which emerges as a result of this change. This is called *Ṛtambharā*. This word is derived from two *Saṃskṛta* roots *Ṛtam* which means 'the Right' and *Bhara* which means 'to bear' or 'to hold'. *Ṛtambharā* therefore literally means Right-bearing. *Ṛtam* and *Satyam* (the True) are two words of very profound significance in the scripture of the Hindus and being correlatives are generally used together. Although they are sometimes used synonymously there is a subtle distinction in their meaning which many people find it difficult to grasp. To understand this we should recall the well-known doctrine of Eastern philosophy according to which the Universe, both seen and unseen, is a manifestation of a Divine Reality or Spirit which abides within it and is the ultimate cause and source of all that takes place in it in terms of time and space. That Reality is referred to as *Sat* and Its existence in the Universe manifests in two fundamental ways. In the first place, It constitutes the truth or the very essence of all things. This is called *Satyam*. In the second place, It determines the ordered course of things both in their material and moral aspect. This is called *Ṛtam*. *Satyam* is thus the relative truth underlying manifestation constituting the realities of all things. *Ṛtam* is the cosmic order including all laws—natural, moral or spiritual—in their totality which are eternal and inviolable in their nature. *Satyam* and *Ṛtam* will therefore be seen to be two aspects of *Sat* in manifestation, one static the other dynamic. They are inseparable and together constitute the very foundation of the manifested Universe. *Ṛtambharā Prajñā* is thus that kind of consciousness which gives an unerring perception of the Right and the True underlying manifestation. Whatever is perceived in the light of this *Prajñā* must be Right and True.

In dealing with the previous *Sūtra* the distorting influence of the intellect was referred to and we saw how the intellect, without the illumination of *Buddhi* is incapable of perceiving the deeper truths of life. Let us consider briefly how this obscuration which is brought about by the intellect works. In our search for knowledge we want the truth as a whole but the intellect allows us to see only a part of the truth at a time. So the knowledge derived through the intellect is never perfect, can by its very nature be never perfect. The manner in which our inellect brings about this fragmentation of truth and prevents us from seeing things as they are is realized only when we transcend the intellect in *Samādhi* and penetrate into the deeper realms of consciousness lying beyond the intellect. Not only is nothing seen as a whole by the intellect, but nothing is seen in its correct perspective in its relation to other things and other truths which exist at the same time. This results in exaggerating the importance of partial truths, misusing knowledge concerning natural forces, adopting wrong means to gain right ends and so many other evils of which the modern civilization based on intellect provides so many and such glaring instances. This lack of wholeness and lack of perspective must characterize all knowledge and action based on intellect divorced from wisdom.

The knowledge obtained in *Samādhi* when the light of *Buddhi* illuminates the mind is not only free from error and doubt but also related to the underlying Cosmic Law which governs manifestation. It is based not only on Truth but also on Right. That is why the *Prajñā* or consciousness functioning in these higher stages of *Samādhi* is called *Ṛtambharā*. The knowledge which the *Yogi* gets is not only perfectly true but he is incapable of misusing that knowledge, as knowledge obtained through the intellect alone can be misused. Life and action based on such knowledge must be righteous, and in accordance with the Great Law which governs the whole Universe.

४९. श्रुतानुमानप्रज्ञाभ्यामन्यविषया विशेषार्थत्वात् ।

Śrutānumāna-prajñābhyām anya-viṣayā viśeṣārthatvāt.

श्रुत heard; (based on) revelation or testimony अनुमान (based on) inference -प्रज्ञाभ्याम् from (these) two (levels of) higher consciousness अन्यविषया having another object or content विशेषार्थत्वात् because of having a particular object.

49. The knowledge based on inference or testimony is different from direct knowledge obtained in the higher states of consciousness (I-48) because it is confined to a particular object (or aspect).

In the previous *Sūtra* one prominent characteristic of the new consciousness which dawns on the refinement of *Nirvicāra Samādhi* was pointed out. This *Sūtra* clarifies still further the distinction between intellectual and intuitive knowledge. As was pointed out in I-7, there are three sources of right knowledge—direct cognition, inference and testimony. All these three are available in the realm of the intellect. Direct cognition, however, plays a very limited part in this realm because it is confined to the unreliable reports received through the sense-organs. These reports by themselves do not give us right knowledge and have to be constantly checked and corrected by the other two methods mentioned above. We see the Sun rising in the East every morning, moving across the sky and sinking in the West but by inference we know that this is a mere illusion and the Sun appears to move on account of the rotation of the earth on its axis. In the same way the familiar world of forms, colours etc. which we cognize with our sense-organs has no real existence. It is all a play of electrons, atoms, molecules and various kinds of energies which Science has discovered. We hardly realize what an important part inference and testimony play in our life until we try to analyse our ordinary knowledge and the means of obtaining it. These two instruments of obtaining and correcting knowledge are peculiarly intellectual and are not necessary in the higher realms of the mind which transcend the intellect. A person who is obliged to discover objects in a room which is utterly dark is obliged to feel them carefully but he does not need to adopt this crude method of discovery and investigation if he is able to get a light. He can see them directly. Knowledge on the spiritual planes beyond the intellect is based neither on inference nor on testimony but only on direct cognition. But this direct cognition, unlike the direct cognition through the sense-organs, is not subject to error and does not require correction by means of inference and testimony.

What does the phrase *Viśeṣārthatvāt* mean? Literally, it means ' because of having a particular object '. It has been pointed out already that the intellect is capable of grasping only one thing at a time, either one object or one aspect of an object. It is this fragmentation of knowledge, this inability to see things in the background of the whole which is the greatest limitation of intellectual perception, and intuitive perception is free from this limitation. In the higher realms of consciousness each object is seen not in isolation but as part of a whole in which all truths, laws and principles have their due place. The intellect is like a telescope which can be directed only on a particular star and can see it in isolation from other stars. Intuitive consciousness is like the eye which can see the whole heavens simultaneously and in true perspective. The analogy is no doubt crude but it may help the student to grasp the difference between the two types of consciousness.

The need for taking the help of inference and testimony arises because of the insufficiency of knowledge and this insufficiency is due to the absence of the whole in the background. It is true that intuitive knowledge may not be perfect and may lack the precision and detail of intellectual knowledge but as far as it goes it is free from the possibility of error and distortion. A dim light in a big room may not give a clear picture of its contents but it enables things to be seen in their proper proportion and perspective. As the light becomes stronger all things are seen more clearly but in the same proportion and perspective. On the other hand, a man who is groping in the dark, feeling one object after another, may get an entirely wrong idea with regard to any object and will have to revise his uncertain conclusions constantly and sometimes drastically.

५०. तज्जः संस्कारोऽन्यसंस्कारप्रतिबन्धी ।

Taj-jaḥ saṃskāro 'nya-saṃskāra-prati-bandhī.

तज्जः (तत्+जः) born of it संस्कारः impression अन्य (of) other संस्कार impressions प्रतीबन्धी preventer; that which stands in the way of.

50. The impression produced by it (*Sabīja Samādhi*) stands in the way of other impressions.

In *Sabīja Samādhi* the *Citta* is always moulded upon a particular pattern, this pattern being determined by the 'seed' which is the object of *Saṃyama*. The control of the will over the mind is so complete that it is impossible for any external distraction to produce the slightest alternation in the impression created by the object. The nature of the object will be different according to the stage of *Samādhi* but an object must always be there and this prevents other ideas from taking possession of the mind. Even in ordinary life we find that if the mind is busy in thinking deeply along a particular line it is more difficult for any distracting idea to get into it, the deeper the concentration the greater the difficulty of any such idea gaining entrance into the mind. But the moment the mind ceases to function under the control of the will and is in a relaxed condition all kinds of ideas which were kept in abeyance in the sub-conscious mind begin to appear in the conscious mind. Something similar, though at a much deeper level, would take place if the impression created by the 'seed' in *Saṃprajñāta Samādhi* is removed before the capacity to keep the mind equally alert and concentrated in the condition of void is acquired. The sudden entry of all kinds of ideas in an uncontrolled manner on account of the vacuum which would be produced may lead to all kinds of serious complications.

It will be seen therefore that *Saṃprajñāta Samādhi* is not only a means of acquiring knowledge and power in the different realms of *Prakṛti* but also for gaining the final objective of Self-realization. For, it is only after sufficient practice of *Saṃprajñāta Samādhi* that the corresponding *Asaṃprajñāta Samādhi* can be practised and it is only after sufficient practice of *Sabīja Samādhi* in the four stages that *Nirbīja Samādhi* can be practised. This should serve to remove the misconception common among a certain class of over-enthusiastic aspirants that it is possible to dive directly into the realms of Reality without going through long and tedious mental discipline and acquiring the capacity to perform *Sāṃyama* on any object. This will also explain why spiritual teachers generally prescribe *Saguṇa Upāsanā* and discourage aspirants from taking to *Nirguṇa Upāsanā* in the early stages. The problem of spiritual life and Self-realization would be all too easy if aspirants had only to sit down and make their minds empty in the ordinary way!

५१. तस्यापि निरोधे सर्वनिरोधान्निर्बीजः समाधिः ।

Tasyāpi nirodhe sarva-nirodhān nirbījaḥ samādhiḥ.

तस्य of that अपि also निरोधे on suppression; inhibition सर्व (of) all निरोधात् by suppression निर्बीजः 'Seedless'; subjective समाधिः *Samādhi*.

51. On suppression of even that owing to suppression of all (modifications of the mind) 'Seedless' *Samādhi* (is attained).

When the capacity to perform *Saṃyama* has been acquired and the *Yogi* can pass easily into the last stage of *Sabīja Samādhi* corresponding to the *Asmitā* stage of *Saṃprajñāta Samādhi* (I-17) and the *Aliṅga* stage of the *Guṇas* (II-19) he is ready for taking the last step, namely, transcending the realm of *Prakṛti* altogether and attaining Self-realization. In the *Asmitā* stage consciousness is functioning in the subtlest form of *Citta* and enlightenment has reached the highest degree, but since consciousness is still in the realm of *Prakṛti* it must be limited to some extent. The veils of illusion have been removed one after another but there is still present one last, almost imperceptible veil which prevents complete Self-realization and the object of *Nirbīja Samādhi* is to remove this. In the earlier stages of *Saṃprajñāta Samādhi* the dropping of the 'seed' leads to the emergence of consciousness into the next subtler plane but after the *Asmitā* stage has been reached and the consciousness is centred on the *Ātmic* plane the dropping of the 'seed' will lead the emergence of consciousness into the plane of *Puruṣa* himself. The Light which was upto this stage illuminating other objects now illuminates Itself, for it has withdrawn beyond the realm of these objects. The Seer is now established in his own Self (I-3).

It is impossible to imagine this state in which the light of consciousness illuminates itself instead of illuminating other objects outside itself but the student, at least, should not make the mistake of imagining it as a state in which the *Yogi* finds himself immersed in a sea of nebulous bliss and knowledge. Each successive stage of unfoldment of consciousness increases tremendously its vividness and clarity and brings about an added influx of knowledge and power. It is absurd to suppose therefore that in the last stage which marks the climax of this unfoldment consciousness lapses suddenly into a vague and nebulous state. It is only the limitations of the vehicles through which we try to visualise this state which prevent us from comprehending it even to a limited extent. When the vibrations of sound become too rapid they appear as silence. When the vibrations of light become too fine they appear as darkness. In the same way the extremely subtle nature of this transcendent consciousness of Reality appears as a void to the mind.

The explanation given above should enable the student to understand clearly the relation between *Nirbīja Samādhi* and *Asaṃprajñāta Samādhi*. It will be seen that *Nirbīja Samādhi* is nothing but the last stage of *Asaṃprajñāta Samādhi.* It differs from the previous *Asaṃprajñāta Samādhis* in that there is no deeper level of *Citta* into which consciousness can withdraw. Any further withdrawal now must be into the consciousness of the *Puruṣa* himself. The consciousness of the *Yogi* is, as it were, poised on the brink of the manifested Universe and has to plunge from the last foothold in the realm of *Prakṛti* into the Ocean of Reality. The *Yogi* is like a swimmer standing on a high cliff abutting on the sea. He jumps down from one ledge to another and then comes to the lowest level from which he has to plunge directly into the sea. The last jump is different from all the preceding jumps in that he passes into an entirely different kind of medium.

Nirbīja Samādhi is so called not only because there is no ' seed ' in the field of consciousness but also because in this kind of *Samādhi* no new *Saṃskāra* is created. One characteristic of a ' seed ', namely its complex and multi-layer nature, has already been referred to in I-42 and provides the reason for calling the object of *Saṃyama* in *Samādhi* a ' seed '. But another characteristic of a seed is that it reproduces itself when sown in the ground. This potentiality to reproduce themselves under favourable conditions is also present in the ' seeds ' of *Saṃprajñāta Samādhi.* In *Nirbīja Samādhi,* there being no ' seed ' no *Saṃskāras* can be produced. Not only no fresh *Saṃskāras* can be produced but the old *Saṃskāras* of *Sabīja Samādhi* are gradually dissipated by *Para-Vairāgya* and partial contact with the *Puruṣa* (IV-29). The consciousness thus gradually becomes free to function unburdened by the kind of *Saṃskāras* which tend to draw it back into the realm of *Prakṛti.* *Nirbīja Samādhi* is therefore not only a means of passing out of the realm of *Prakṛti* but also of exhausting the subtle *Saṃskāras* which still remain and which must be destroyed completely before *Kaivalya* can be attained.

SECTION II

SĀDHANA PĀDA

SĀDHANA PĀDA

१. तपःस्वाध्यायेश्वरप्रणिधानानि क्रियायोगः ।

Tapaḥ-svādhyāyeśvara-praṇidhānāni kriyā-yogaḥ.

तपः asceticism; austerity स्वाध्याय self-study; study which leads to the knowledge of the Self through *Japa* ईश्वरप्रणिधानानि (and) self-surrender, or resignation to God क्रियायोगः preliminary (practical) *Yoga.*

1. Austerity, self-study and resignation to *Īśvara* constitute preliminary *Yoga.*

The last three of the five elements of *Niyama* enumerated in II-32 have been placed in the above *Sūtra* under the title of *Kriyā-Yoga.* This is rather an unusual procedure and we should try to grasp the significance of this repetition in a book which attempts to condense knowledge to the utmost limit. Obviously, the reason why *Tapas*, *Svādhyāya* and *Īśvara-praṇidhāna* are mentioned in two different contexts lies in the fact that they serve two different purposes. And since the development of the subject of self-culture in Section II of the *Yoga-Sūtras* is progressive in character it follows that the purpose of these three elements in II-1 is of a more preliminary nature than that in II-32. Their purpose in II-32 is the same as that of the other elements of *Niyama* and has been discussed at the proper place. What is the purpose in the context of II-1? Let us see.

Anyone who is familiar with the goal of *Yogic* life and the kind of effort it involves for its attainment will realize that it is neither possible nor advisable for anybody who is absorbed in the life of the world and completely under the influence of *Kleśas* to plunge all at once into the regular practice of *Yoga*. If he is sufficiently interested in the *Yogic* philosophy and wants to enter the path which leads to its goal he should first accustom himself to discipline, should acquire the necessary knowledge of the *Dharma-Śāstras* and especially of the *Yoga-Śāstras* and should reduce the intensity of his egoism and all the other *Kleśas* which are derived from it. The difference between the outlook and the life of the ordinary worldly man and the life which the *Yogi* is required to live is so great that a sudden change from the one to the other is not possible and if attempted may produce a violent reaction in the mind of the aspirant, throwing him back with still greater force into the life of the world. A preparatory period of self-training in which he gradually assimilates the *Yogic* philosophy and its technique and accustoms himself to self-discipline makes the transition from the one life to the other easier and safer. It also incidentally enables the mere student to find out whether he is sufficiently keen to adopt the *Yogic* life and make a serious attempt to realize the *Yogic* ideal. There are too many cases of enthusiastic aspirants who for no apparent reason cool off, or finding the *Yogic* discipline too irksome, give it up. They are not yet ready for the *Yogic* life.

Even where there is present the required earnestness and the determination to tread the path of *Yoga* it is necessary to establish a permanent mood and habit of pursuing its ideal. Mere wishing or willing is not enough. All the mental powers and desires of the *Sādhaka* should be polarized and aligned with the *Yogic* ideal. Many aspirants have very confused and sometimes totally wrong ideas with regard to the object and technique of *Yoga*. Many of them have very exaggerated notions with regard to their earnestness and capacity to tread the path of *Yoga*. Their ideas become clarified and their capacity and earnestness are tested severely in trying to practise *Kriyā-Yoga*. They either emerge from the preliminary self-discipline with a clearly defined aim and a determination and capacity to pursue it to the end with vigour and single-minded devotion, or they gradually realize that they are not yet ready for the practice of *Yoga* and decide to tune their aspiration to the lower key of mere intellectual study.

This preparatory self-discipline is triple in its nature corresponding to the triple nature of a human being. *Tapas* is related to his will, *Svādhyāya* to the intellect and *Īśvara-praṇidhāna* to the emotions. This discipline, therefore, tests and develops all the three aspects of his nature and produces an all-round and balanced growth of the individuality which is so essential for the attainment of any high ideal. This point will become clear when we consider the significance of these three elements of *Kriyā-Yoga* in dealing with II-32.

There exists some confusion with regard to the meaning of the *Saṃskṛta* word *Kriyā*, some commentators preferring to translate it as 'preliminary', others as 'practical'. As a matter of fact *Kriyā-Yoga* is both practical and preliminary. It is preliminary because it has to be taken up in the initial stages of the practice of *Yoga* and it is practical because it puts to a practical test the aspirations and earnestness of the *Sādhaka* and develops in him the capacity to begin the practice of *Yoga* as distinguished from its mere theoretical study however deep this might be.

२. समाधिभावनार्थः क्लेशतनूकरणार्थश्च ।

Samādhi-bhāvanārthaḥ kleśa-tanūkaraṇārthaś ca.

समाधि trance भावनार्थः for bringing about क्लेश afflictions तनूकरणार्थः for reducing; for making attenuated च and.

2. (*Kriyā-Yoga*) is practised for attenuating *Kleśas* and bringing about *Samādhi*.

Although the practice of the three elements of *Kriyā-Yoga* is supposed to subserve the preparatory training of the aspirant it should not therefore be assumed that they are of secondary importance and have only a limited use in the life of the *Sādhaka*. How effective this training is and to what exalted stage of development it is capable of leading the aspirant will be seen from the second *Sūtra* which we are considering and which gives the results of practising *Kriyā-Yoga*. *Kriyā-Yoga* not only attenuates the *Kleśas* and thus lays the foundation of the *Yogic* life but it also leads the aspirant to *Samādhi*, the essential and final technique of *Yoga*. It is, therefore, also capable of building to a great extent the superstructure of the *Yogic* life. The importance of *Kriyā-Yoga* and the high stage of development to which it can lead the *Sādhaka* will be clear when we have considered the ultimate results of practising *Tapas*, *Svādhyāya* and *Īśvara-praṇidhāna* in II-43-45.

The ultimate stage of *Samādhi* is, of course, reached through the practice of *Īśvara-praṇidhāna* as indicated in I-23 and II-45. Although the two results of practising *Kriyā-Yoga* enumerated in II-2 are related to the initial and ultimate stages of *Yogic* practice they are really very closely connected and in a sense complementary. The more the *Kleśas* are attenuated the greater becomes the capacity of the *Sādhaka* to practise *Samādhi* and the nearer he draws to his goal of *Kaivalya*. When the *Kleśas* have been reduced to the vanishing point he is in habitual *Samādhi* (*Sahaja-Samādhi*), at the threshold of *Kaivalya*.

We shall take up the discussion of these three elements of *Kriyā-Yoga* as part of *Niyama* in II-32.

३. अविद्यास्मितारागद्वेषाभिनिवेशाः क्लेशाः ।

Avidyāsmitā-rāga-dveṣābhiniveśāḥ kleśāḥ.

अविद्या ignorance; lack of awareness; illusion अस्मिता 'I-am-ness' egoism; राग attraction; liking द्वेष repulsion; dislike -अभिनिवेशाः (and) clinging (to life); fear of death क्लेशाः pains; afflictions; miseries; causes of pain.

3. The lack of awareness of Reality, the sense of egoism or 'I-am-ness', attractions and repulsions towards objects and the strong desire for life are the great afflictions or causes of all miseries in life.

The philosophy of *Kleśas* is really the foundation of the system of *Yoga* outlined by Patañjali. It is necessary to understand this philosophy thoroughly because it provides a satisfactory answer to the initial and pertinent question, 'Why should we practise *Yoga*?' The philosophy of *Kleśas* is not peculiar to this system of *Yoga*. In its essential ideas it forms the substratum of all schools of *Yoga* in India though perhaps it has not been expounded as clearly and systematically as in the *Sāṃkhya* and *Yoga Darśanas*.

Many Western scholars have not fully understood the real significance of the philosophy of *Kleśas* and tend to regard it merely as an expression of the pessimism which they think characterizes Hindu philosophical thought. At best they take it in the light of an ingenious philosophical conception which provides the necessary foundation for certain systems of philosophy. That it is related to the hard facts of existence and is based upon a close and scientific analysis of the phenomena of human life, they would be hardly prepared to accept.

Purely academic philosophy has always been speculative and the essential task of the expounder of a new philosophical system is considered to be to provide a plausible explanation of the fundamental facts of life and existence. Some of these explanations which form the basis of certain philosophical systems are extraordinarily ingenious expositions and illustrations of reasoned thought, but they are purely speculative and are based on the superficial phenomena of life observed through the senses. Philosophy is considered to be a branch of learning concerned with evolving theories about life and the Universe. Whether these theories are correct and help in solving the real problems of life is not the concern of the philosopher. He has only to see that the theory which he puts forward is intellectually sound and provides an explanation of the observed facts of life with the maximum of plausibility. Its value lies in its rationality and ingeniousness and possibly intellectual brilliance, not in its capacity to provide a means of overcoming the miseries and sufferings incidental to human life. No wonder, academic philosophy is considered barren and futile by the common man and treated with indifference, if not with veiled contempt.

Now, in the East, though many ingenious and purely speculative philosophies have been expounded from time to time, philosophy has been considered, on the whole, as a means of expounding the real and deeper problems of human life and providing clear-cut and effective means for their solution. There is not much demand for purely speculative systems of philosophy and such as exist are treated with a kind of amused tolerance as intellectual curiosities —nothing more. The great problem of human life is too urgent, too serious, too profound, too awful to leave any room for the consideration of mere intellectual theories, however brilliant these might be. If your house is on fire you want a means of escape and are not in a mood to sit down and read a brilliant thesis on architecture at that time. Those who can remain satisfied with purely speculative philosophies have not really understood the great and urgent problem of human life and its deeper significance. If they see this problem as it really is then they can be interested only in such philosophies as offer effective means for its solution.

Although the perception of the inner significance of the real problem of human life is dependent upon an inner change in consciousness and awakening of our spiritual faculties and cannot be brought about by an intellectual process of reasoning imposed from without, still, let us consider man in time and space and see whether his circumstances justify the extraordinary complacency which we find not only among the common people but also among the so-called philosophers.

Let us first consider man in space. In giving us a true picture of man in the physical Universe of which he is a part nothing has helped us so much as the discoveries of modern Science. Even before man could use a telescope the vision of the sky at night filled him with awe and wonder at the immensity of the Universe of which he was an insignificant part. But the researches of astronomers have shown that the physical Universe is almost unbelievably larger than what it appears to the naked eye. The 6,000 stars that are within the range of our unaided vision form, according to Science, a group which is only one among at least a billion other groups which stretch out to infinity in every direction. Astronomers have made a rough calculation of the number of stars that are within the range of the high-powered telescopes available these days and think there may be as many as 100 billion stars in our galaxy alone, some smaller than our sun and others very much bigger. This galaxy which is only one of 100,000 already definitely known to astronomers is so vast that light with a speed of 186,000 miles per second takes about 100,000 years to travel from one side to the other. In this vast 'known' Universe even our Solar system with its maximum orbital (of planets) diameter of 7 billion miles occupies an insignificant place by comparison. Narrowing down our vision to the Solar system we again find that the earth occupies only an insignificant place in the huge distances that are involved. It has a diameter of 8,000 miles compared with 865,000 miles of the sun and moves slowly in its orbit round the sun at an approximate distance of 93 million miles. Coming down still further to our earth we find man occupying an insignificant position as far as his physical body is considered. A microbe moving over the surface of a big school globe is physically a formidable object in comparison with man moving over the surface of the earth.

This is the awful picture that Science gives of man in the physical Universe, but so great is the illusion of *Māyā* and the complacence which it engenders that we not only do not wonder about human life and tremble at our destiny but go through life engrossed in our petty pursuits, and sometimes even obsessed with a sense of self-importance. Even the scientists who scan this vast Universe every night with their telescopes remain unaware of the profound significance of what they see.

The picture which Science presents of our physical world in its infinitesimal aspect is no less disconcerting. That physical matter constituting our bodies consisted of atoms and molecules has been known for quite a long time. But the recent researches of Science in this field have led to some startling discoveries. The hard and indestructible atoms which constituted the bed-rock of modern scientific materialism have been found to be nothing more than different permutations and combinations of two fundamental types of positive and negative charged particles—protons and electrons. The protons form the core of the atom with electrons in varying numbers revolving round it in different orbits with tremendous speed, an atom being thus a Solar system in miniature. And what is still more startling, it has been found that these electrons may be nothing but charges of electricity with no material basis because mass and energy become indistinguishable at the high speed at which electrons move in their orbits. In fact, the conversion of matter into energy which has now become an accomplished fact shows that matter may be nothing more than an expression of locked-up energy. This conclusion which really means that matter disappears into energy has been arrived at, by an irony of fate, by the efforts of materialistic science which was responsible for giving a tremendous materialistic bias to our thinking and living. This hard fact means—and let the reader ponder carefully over this problem—that the well-known and so-called real world which we cognize with our sense-organs, a world of forms, colour, sound, etc., is based upon a phantom world containing nothing more than protons and electrons. These facts have become matters of common knowledge but how many of us, even scientists who work on these problems, seem to grasp the significance of these facts. How many are led to ask the question which should so naturally arise in the light of these facts 'What is man?' Is there any further proof needed that the mere intellect is blind and is incapable of seeing even the obvious truths of life, much less the Truth of truths?

Leaving the world of space let us glance for a while at the world of time. Here again we are faced with tremendous immensities of a different nature. An infinite succession of changes seems to extend on both sides into the past and the future. Of this endless expanse of time a period of a few thousand years just behind us is all that is reliably known to us while we have only a vague and hazy conception of what lies in the lap of the uncertain future. For aught we know the sun may explode the very next moment and destroy all life in the Solar system before we know what has happened. We are almost certain that millions and millions of years lie behind us but what has happened in those years we cannot know except by inference from what we observe in the visible Universe of stars around us. The past is like a huge tidal wave advancing and devouring everything in its path. Magnificent civilizations on our earth of which only traces are left and even planets and solar systems have disappeared in this tidal wave never to appear again and a similar relentless fate awaits everything from a grain of dust to a Solar system. Time, the instrument of the Great Illusion devours everything. And yet, look at puny man, whose achievements and glories are also to disappear in this void, how he struts about on the world stage clothed with brief authority or glory in the few moments which have been allotted to him. Surely, this awful panorama of ceaseless change which is unfolding before his eyes should make him pause and at least wonder what is all this about. But does it?

The above picture of man in time and space is not at all over-drawn. A man has only to isolate himself for a while from his engrossing environment and ponder over these facts of life to realize the illusory nature of his life and to feel the so-called zest of life melt away. But few of us have the eyes to look at this awful vision, and if by any chance our eyes open accidently for a while, we find the prospect too terrifying and shut them again, and completely oblivious and unaware of the real nature of life continue to live with our joys and sorrows until the flame of life is snuffed out by the hand of Death.

Now, the above picture of man in space and time has been given not with a view to provide entertainment for the intellectually curious, or even food for thought for the thoughtful, but to prepare the ground for the consideration of the philosophy of *Kleśas* which forms the foundation of the *Yogic* philosophy. For the philosophy of *Yoga* is based on the hard realities of life, harder than the realities of Nature given to us by Science. Those who are not aware of these realities, or are aware only superficially in their intellectual aspects can hardly appreciate the goal or the technique of *Yoga*. They may find *Yoga* a very interesting subject for study, even fascinating in some of its aspects, but they cannot have the determination to go through the tremendous labour and ordeals which are required to rend asunder the veils of illusion created by Time and Space, and to contact the Reality which is hidden behind these veils.

With this brief introduction let us now turn to consider the philosophy of *Kleśas* as it is outlined in the *Yoga-Sūtras*. Let us first take the *Saṃskṛta* word *Kleśa*. It means pain, affliction or misery but gradually it came to acquire the meaning of what causes pain, affliction or misery. The philosophy of *Kleśas* is thus an analysis of the underlying and fundamental cause of human misery and suffering and the way in which this cause can be removed effectively. This analysis is not based upon a consideration of the superficial facts of life as observed through the senses. The *Ṛṣis* who expounded this philosophy were great Adepts who combined in themselves the qualifications of a religious teacher, scientist and philosopher. With this triple qualification and synthetic vision they attacked the great problem of life, determined to find a solution of the riddle which Time and Space have created for the illusion-bound man. They observed the phenomena of life not only with the help of their senses and the mind, but in the full conviction that the solution lay beyond even the intellect they dived deeper and deeper into their own consciousness, tearing aside veil after veil, until they discovered the ultimate cause of the Great Illusion and the misery and suffering which are its inevitable results. They discovered, incidentally, in their search other subtler worlds of entrancing beauty hidden beneath the visible physical world. They discovered new faculties and powers within themselves—faculties and powers which could be utilized for studying these subtler worlds and pursuing their enquiry into still deeper layers of their own consciousness. But they did not allow themselves to be entangled by these subtler worlds and did not rest content until they had penetrated deep enough within their consciousness to find an effective and permanent solution of the great problem of life. They discovered in this way not only the ultimate cause of human misery and suffering but also the only effective means of destroying these afflictions permanently.

It is very necessary for the student to realize the experimental nature of this philosophy of *Kleśas* and the greater philosophy of *Yoga* of which it is an integral part. These are not the results of speculation or reasoned thought as many systems of philosophy are. The philosophy of *Yoga* claims to be derived from the results of scientific experiments, guided by the spirit of philosophic enquiry, inspired by religious devotion. We cannot, obviously, verify this essentially scientific system by the ordinary methods of Science and say to the sceptic: 'Come I will prove it before your eyes.' We cannot judge it by the ordinary academic standards of philosophers who apply purely intellectual criteria for judging these things. The only way in which it can be verified is to follow the path which was taken by the original discoverers and which is outlined in this system of *Yoga*. The sceptic might feel that it is unfair to ask him to assume the validity of what he wants to get proved, but this, from the very nature of things, cannot be helped. Those who have seen the fundamental problem of life in its true aspects will consider the gamble worth taking, for that provides the only way out of the Great Illusion. For others it does not matter whether they do or do not believe in the teachings of *Yoga*. They are not yet ready for the Divine Adventure.

Before discussing in detail the philosophy of *Kleśas* as outlined in Section II of the *Yoga-Sūtras* it will be desirable to give an analysis of the whole subject in the form of a table. This will show at a glance the different aspects of the subject and their relation to one another. It will be seen from the summary given in this table—a fact which is difficult to grasp otherwise—that the whole subject has been dealt with in a systematic and masterly manner. The student who wants to get a clear insight into the philosophy of *Kleśas* will do well, therefore, to go through the following summary carefully and ponder over it before taking up the detailed study of the subject.

PHILOSOPHY OF KLEŚAS—SYNOPSIS

	Question dealt with	*Subject*	*Numbers of* Sūtras *in which the subject is dealt with in Section II*
1.	What are *Kleśas*?	Enumeration and definitions.	3, 4, 5, 6, 7, 8, 9.
2.	How are they destroyed?	General methods of destroying them.	10, 11.
3.	Why should *Kleśas* be destroyed?	They involve us in a never-ending cycle of births and deaths and miseries of life.	12, 13, 14, 15.
4.	Can their result—miseries of life—be destroyed?	Yes, those that are still in the future.	16.
5.	What is the fundamental cause of these miseries?	Union and identification of the Knower with the Known.	17.

	Question dealt with	*Subject*	*Numbers of* Sūtras *in which the subject is dealt with in Section II*
6.	What is the nature of the Known?	Interactions of *Bhūtas, Indriyas* and *Guṇas* which result in experience and liberation.	18, 19.
7.	What is the nature of the Knower?	The Knower is pure consciousness.	20, 21, 22.
8.	Why have the Knower and the Known been brought together?	For the evolution of powers of *Prakṛti* and for Self-realization of the *Puruṣa*.	23.
9.	How have the Knower and Known been brought together?	Through a veil of illusion caused by *Avidyā*.	24.
10.	How can the Knower and Known be separated?	By destroying the veil of *Avidyā*.	25.
11.	How can this veil of *Avidyā* be destroyed?	By *Viveka* which leads to increasing awareness of his own nature by the *Puruṣa* in 7 stages.	26, 27.
12.	How can *Viveka* be developed?	By the practice of *Yoga*.	28.

The author opens the subject with an enumeration of the five *Kleśas* in II-3. The English equivalents of the *Saṃskṛta* words do not correctly and fully convey the ideas implied and the English words which come nearest to the *Saṃkṛta* names of the *Kleśas* have been given. The underlying significance of the five *Kleśas* will be explained in dealing with the subsequent *Sūtras*.

४. अविद्या क्षेत्रमुत्तरेषां प्रसुप्ततनुविच्छिन्नोदाराणाम् ।

Avidyā kṣetram uttareṣāṃ prasupta-tanu-
vicchinnodārāṇām.

अविद्या ignorance or lack of awareness of Reality क्षेत्रं field; source उत्तरेषाम् of the following ones प्रसुप्त (of) dormant; sleeping तनु attenuated; thin विच्छिन्न scattered; dispersed; alternating उदाराणाम् (and) expanded; fully operative.

4. *Avidyā* is the source of those that are mentioned after it, whether they be in the dormant, attenuated, alternating or expanded condition.

This *Sūtra* gives two important facts concerning the nature of the *Kleśas*. The first is their mutual relationship. *Avidyā* is the root-cause of the other four *Kleśas* which in their turn produce all the miseries of human life. A closer study of the nature of the other four *Kleśas* will show not only that they can grow only on the soil of *Avidyā* but also that the five *Kleśas* form a connected series of causes and effects. The relation existing between the five *Kleśas* may be likened to the relation of root, trunk, branches, leaves and fruit in a tree. The conclusion that the five *Kleśas* are related to one another in this manner is further strengthened by II-10 but we shall discuss this question in dealing with that *Sūtra*.

The other idea in this *Sūtra* is the classification of the states or conditions in which these *Kleśas* may exist. These four states are defined as (1) dormant, (2) attenuated, (3) alternating, (4) expanded. The dormant condition is that in which the *Kleśa* is present but in a latent form. It cannot find expression for lack of proper conditions for its expression and its kinetic energy has become potential. The attenuated condition is that in which the *Kleśa* is present in a very feeble or tenuous condition. It is not active but can become active in a mild degree on a stimulus being applied. In the fully expanded condition the *Kleśa* is fully operative and its activity is all too apparent like the waves on the surface of the sea in a storm. The alternating condition is that in which two opposite tendencies overpower each other alternately as in the case of two lovers who sometimes become angry and affectionate alternately. The feelings of attraction and repulsion alternate, though fundamentally they are based on attachment.

It is only in the case of the advanced *Yogis* that the *Kleśas* are present in the dormant form. In the case of ordinary people, the *Kleśas* are present in the other three conditions, depending upon external circumstances.

५. अनित्याशुचिदुःखानात्मसु नित्यशुचिसुखात्मख्यातिरविद्या ।

Anityāśuci-duḥkhānātmasu nitya-śuci-sukhātmakhyātir avidyā.

अनित्य (of) non-eternal अशुचि impure दुःख misery; pain; evil अनात्मसु (and) non-*Ātman*; not-Self नित्य eternal शुचि pure सुख happiness; pleasure; good आत्म (and) Self ख्यातिः knowledge; consciousness, (taking) अविद्या ignorance.

5. *Avidyā* is taking the non-eternal, impure, evil and non-*Ātman* to be eternal, pure, good and *Ātman* respectively.

This *Sūtra* defines *Avidyā* the root of the *Kleśas*. It is quite obvious that the word *Avidyā* is not used in its ordinary sense of ignorance or lack of knowledge, but in its highest philosophical sense. In order to grasp this meaning of the word we have to recall the initial process whereby, according to the *Yogic* philosophy, consciousness, the Reality underlying manifestation, becomes involved in matter. Consciousness and matter are separate and utterly different in their essential nature but for reasons which will be discussed in the subsequent *Sūtras* they have to be brought together. How can *Ātmā*, which is eternally free and self-sufficient, be made to assume the limitations which are involved in the association with matter? It is by depriving it of the knowledge or rather the awareness of its eternal and self-sufficient nature. This deprivation of knowledge of its true nature which involves it in the evolutionary cycle is brought about by a transcendent power inherent in the Ultimate Reality which is called *Māyā* or the Great Illusion.

Of course, this simple statement of a transcendent truth can give rise to innumerable philosophical questions such as 'Why should it be necessary for the *Ātmā* which is self-sufficient to be involved in matter?' 'How is it possible for the *Ātmā* which is eternal to become involved in the limitations of Time and Space?' There is no real answer to such ultimate questions although many answers, obviously absurd, have been suggested by different philosophers from time to time. According to those who have come face to face with Reality and know this secret, the only method by which this mystery can be unravelled is to *know* the Truth which underlies manifestation and which by its very nature is incommunicable.

As a result of the illusion in which consciousness gets involved it begins to identify itself with the matter with which it becomes associated. This identification becomes increasingly fuller as consciousness descends further into matter until the turning point is reached and the upward climb in the opposite direction begins. The reverse process of evolution in which consciousness gradually extricates itself, as it were, from matter results in an increasing realization of its Real nature and ends in complete Self-realization in *Kaivalya.* It is this fundamental privation of knowledge of its Real nature, which begins with the evolutionary cycle, is brought about by the power of *Māyā,* and ends with the attainment of Liberation in *Kaivalya,* which is called *Avidyā.* *Avidyā* has nothing to do with the knowledge which we acquire through the intellect and which refers to the things concerning the phenomenal worlds. A man may be a great scholar, a walking encyclopaedia as we say, and yet may be so completely immersed in the illusions created by the mind that he may stand much below a simple-minded *Sādhaka* who is partially aware of the great illusions of the intellect and the life in these phenomenal worlds. The *Avidyā* of the latter is much less than that of the former in spite of the tremendous difference in knowledge pertaining to the intellect. This absence of awareness of our true nature results in the inability to distinguish between the eternal, pure, blissful Self and the non-eternal, impure and painful not-Self.

The word 'eternal' here means as usual the state of consciousness which is above the limitation of time as we know it as a succession of phenomena. 'Pure' refers to the purity of consciousness as it exists unaffected and unmodified by matter which imposes upon it the limitation of the three *Guṇas* and consequent illusions. 'Blissful', of course, refers to the *Ānanda* or bliss of the *Ātmā* which is inherent in it and which is independent of any external source or circumstance. The privation of this *Sukha* or bliss which is inevitable when consciousness is identified with matter is *Duḥkha* or misery. All these three attributes, which have been mentioned in the distinction between the Self and the not-Self, are merely illustrative and not exhaustive because it is impossible to define the nature of the Self and to distinguish it from the not-Self in terms of the limited conceptions of the intellect. The central idea to be grasped is that the *Ātmā* in its purity is fully conscious of its Real nature. Progressive involution in matter deprives it of this Self-knowledge in increasing degree and it is the privation of this knowledge which is called *Avidyā*. As the matter is one pertaining to the realities beyond the scope of the intellect it is not possible to understand it through the medium of the intellect alone.

६. दृग्दर्शनशक्त्योरेकात्मतेवास्मिता ।

Dṛg-darśana-śaktyor ekātmatevāsmitā.

दृक्(शक्ति) (of) power of consciousness; seer; *Puruṣa* दर्शनशक्त्योः (and) power of seeing; cognition; *Buddhi* एकात्मता identity; blending together; इव as if अस्मिता 'I-am-ness'.

6. *Asmītā* is the identity or blending together, as it were, of the power of consciousness (*Puruṣa*) with the power of cognition (*Buddhi*).

Asmitā is defined in this *Sūtra* as the identification of the power of consciousness with the power of cognition, but as the power of cognition always works through a vehicle, in its wider and more intelligible meaning it may be considered as the identification of consciousness with the vehicle through which it is being expressed. This is a very important and interesting idea which we should understand thoroughly if we want to master the technique of liberating consciousness from the limitations under which it works in the ordinary individual. The *Saṃskṛta* word *Asmitā* is derived from *Asmi* which means literally ' I am '. ' I am ' represents the pure awareness of Self-existence and is therefore the expression or *Bhāva*, as it is called, of pure consciousness or the *Puruṣa*. When the pure consciousness gets involved in matter and owing to the power of *Māyā*, knowledge of its Real nature is lost the pure ' I am ' changes into ' I am this ' where ' this ' may be the subtlest vehicle through which it is working, or the grossest vehicle, namely the physical body. The two processes, namely the loss of awareness of its Real nature and the identification with the vehicles are simultaneous. The moment consciousness identifies itself with its vehicles it has fallen from its pure state and it becomes bound by the limitations of *Avidyā*, or we may say that the moment the veil of *Avidyā* falls on consciousness its identification with its vehicles results immediately, though philosophically *Avidyā* must precede *Asmitā*.

The involution of consciousness in matter is a progressive process and for this reason though *Avidyā* and *Asmitā* begin where the thinnest veil of *Māyā* involves pure consciousness in the subtlest vehicle, the degree of *Avidyā* and *Asmitā* goes on increasing as the association of consciousness with matter becomes more and more strengthened. As consciousness descends into one vehicle after another the veil of *Avidyā* becomes, as it were, thicker and the tendency to identify oneself with the vehicle becomes stronger and grosser. On the other hand, when the reverse process takes place and consciousness is released from its limitations in its evolutionary upward climb, the veil of *Avidyā* becomes thinner and the resulting *Asmitā* weaker and subtler. This evolution on the upward arc takes place in seven definite and clearly marked stages as is indicated in II-27. These stages correspond to the transference of consciousness from one vehicle to a subtler vehicle.

Let us now come down from the abstract principles and consider the problem in relation to things with which we are familiar and which we can understand more easily. Let us consider the problem of the expression of consciousness through the physical body. We should remember, in considering this question that the consciousness which is normally expressed through the physical body is not pure unmodified consciousness being involved in a vehicle. It has already passed through several such involutions and it is already heavily loaded, as it were, when it seeks expression through the outermost or grossest vehicle. It is therefore consciousness conditioned by the limitations of all the intervening vehicles which form a kind of bridge between it and the physical body. But as the process of involution and consequent identification is in essence the same at each stage of involution, we can get some idea of the underlying principles even though the expression of consciousness through the physical body is complicated by the factors referred to above.

Coming back to our problem we then see that the association of consciousness, conditioned as mentioned above, with the physical body must lead to this identification with the vehicle and the language which is used by all of us in common intercourse reflects this fully. We always use such expressions as 'I see', 'I hear', 'I go', 'I sit'. In the case of the savage and the child this identification with the body is so complete that there is not the slightest feeling of discrepancy in using such language. But the educated and intelligent man, whose identification with the body is not quite complete and who feels to a certain extent that he is different from the body, is aware at least in a vague manner that it is not he who sees, hears, walks and sits. These activities belong to the physical body and he is merely witnessing them through his mind. Still, from force of habit and disinclination to go deeper into the matter, or from fear of appearing odd in using the correct language he continues to use the common phraseology. So deep-rooted is this identification that even physiologists, psychologists and philosophers, who are supposed to be familiar with the mechanism of sense-perception and intellectually recognize the mere instrumentality of the physical body, are hardly actively aware of this tendency and may identify themselves with the body completely. It is worth noting that mere intellectual knowledge with regard to such patent facts does not by itself enable a person to separate himself from his vehicles. Who has more detailed knowledge with regard to the physical body and its functions than a doctor who has dissected hundreds of bodies and knows that it is a mere mechanism. One would expect that a doctor at least, from whom nothing inside the body is hidden, will be above this tendency to regard himself as the body. But is a doctor in any way better off in this respect than a layman? Not at all. This is not a matter of ordinary seeing and understanding at all.

Asmitā or identification with a vehicle is not a simple but a very complex process and has many aspects. The first aspect we may consider is identification with the powers and faculties associated with the vehicles. For example, when a person says 'I see' what really happens is that the faculty of sight is exercised by the body through the eye and the in-dwelling entity becomes merely aware of the result, i.e. the panorama presented before the eye. Again, when he says, 'I walk' what really happens is that the will working through the mind moves the body on its legs like a portable instrument and the in-dwelling entity identifying himself with the movement of the body says, 'I walk'.

The second aspect is the association of the subtler vehicle in this process of identification where a compound *Asmitā*—if such a phrase can be used—is produced. Thus when a person says he has a headache what is really happening is that there is a slight disorder in the brain. This disorder by its reaction on the next subtler vehicle through which sensations and feelings are felt produces the sensation of pain. The in-dwelling entity identifies himself with this joint product of these two vehicles and this results in 'his' having a headache, although a little thought will show him that it is not he but the vehicle which is having the pain of which he is aware. The same thing working at a somewhat higher level produces such reactions as 'I think', 'I approve'. It is the mind which thinks and approves and the consciousness becomes merely aware of the thought process which is reflected in the physical body. Ambition, pride and similar unpleasant traits of human character are merely highly developed and perverted forms of this tendency to identify ourselves with the workings of the mind.

A third aspect which may be considered in this process of identification is the inclusion of other accessories and objects in the environment. The physical body becomes a centre round which get associated a number of objects which in smaller or greater degree become part of the ' I '. These objects may be animate or inanimate. The other bodies which are born of one's body become ' my children '. The house in which one's body is kept becomes ' my house '. So round the umbra (total shadow) created by *Asmitā* with the body is a penumbra (partial shadow) containing all those objects and persons which ' belong ' to the ' I ' working through the body and they produce the attitude or *Bhāva* of ' my ' and ' mine '.

The above brief and general discussion of *Asmitā* associated with the physical body will give some idea to the student with regard to the nature of this *Kleśa*. Of course, *Asmitā* manifesting through the physical body is the grossest form of the *Kleśa* and as we try to study the working of this tendency in the subtler vehicles we find it more and more elusive and difficult to deal with. Any thoughtful man can separate himself *in thought* from his physical body and see that he is not the bag of flesh, bones and marrow with the help of which he comes in contact with the physical world. But few can separate themselves from their intellect and realize that their opinions and ideas are mere thought patterns produced by their mind just like the thought patterns produced by other minds. The reason why we take interest in and attach so much importance to our opinions lies, of course, in the fact that we identify ourselves with our intellect. Our thoughts, opinions, prejudices and predilections are part of our mental possessions, children of our mind, and that is why we feel and show such undue and tender regard for them.

Of course, there are levels of consciousness even beyond that of the intellect. In all these *Asmitā* is present though it becomes subtler and more refined as we leave one vehicle after another. It is no use dealing with these subtler manifestations of *Asmitā* here because unless one can transcend the intellect and function in these super-intellectual fields one cannot really understand them.

Although the question of destroying the *Kleśas* will be dealt with later in subsequent *Sūtras* there is one fact which may be usefully pointed out here. Many methods have been suggested whereby this tendency to identify ourselves with our vehicles may be gradually attenuated. Many of these methods are quite useful and do help us in a certain measure to disentangle our consciousness from our vehicles. But it has to be borne in mind that complete dissociation from a vehicle takes place only when consciousness is able to leave the vehicle deliberately and consciously and function in the next subtler vehicle (of course, with all the still subtler vehicles present in the background). When the *Jīvātmā* is able to leave a vehicle at will and 'see' it separate from himself then only is the false sense of identification completely destroyed. We may meditate for years trying to separate ourselves in thought from the body but the result of this will not be as great as one experience of leaving it consciously and seeing it actually separate from ourselves. We shall, of course, re-enter that body and assume all its limitations but it can never again exercise on us the same illusory influence as it did before. We have *realized* that we are different from the body. For the advanced *Yogi* who can and does leave his body every now and then and can function independently of it in a routine manner, it is just like a dwelling house. The very idea of identifying himself with the body will appear absurd to him. It will be seen, therefore, that practice of *Yoga* is the most effective means of destroying *Asmitā* completely and permanently. As the *Yogi* leaves one vehicle of consciousness after another in *Samādhi* he destroys progressively the tendency to identify himself with those vehicles and with the destruction of *Asmitā* in this manner the veil of *Avidyā* automatically becomes thinner.

७. सुखानुशयी रागः ।

Sukhānuśayī rāgaḥ.

सुख pleasure; happiness अनुशयी accompanying; resulting (from) रागः attraction; liking.

7. That attraction, which accompanies pleasure, is *Rāga*.

Rāga is defined in this *Sūtra* as the attraction which one feels towards any person or object when any kind of pleasure or happiness is derived from that person or object. It is natural for us to get attracted in this manner because the soul in bondage, having lost the direct source of *Ānanda* within, gropes after *Ānanda* in the external world and anything which provides even a shadow of this in the form of ordinary happiness or pleasure becomes dear to it. If we are attracted to any person or object we shall always find on scrutiny that the attraction is due to some kind of pleasure, physical, emotional or mental. We may be addicted to a particular kind of food because we find it pleasant. We may be attached to a person because we derive from him some kind of pleasure, physical or emotional. We may be devoted to a particular pursuit because it gives us intellectual satisfaction.

८. दुःखानुशयी द्वेषः ।

Duḥkhānuśayī dveṣaḥ.

दुःख pain; अनुशयी accompanying; resulting (from), द्वेषः repulsion.

8. That repulsion which accompanies pain is *Dveṣa*.

Dveṣa is the natural repulsion felt towards any person or object which is a source of pain or unhappiness to us. The essential nature of the Self is blissful and therefore anything which brings pain or unhappiness in the outer world makes the outer vehicles recoil from that thing. What has been said about *Rāga* is applicable to *Dveṣa* in an opposite sense because *Dveṣa* is only *Rāga* in the negative, the two together forming a pair of opposites.

As these two *Kleśas* form the most prominent part of the fivefold tree which provides the innumerable fruits of human misery and suffering it is worthwhile taking note of a few facts concerning them.

(1) The attractions and repulsions which bind us to innumerable persons and things, in the manner indicated above, condition our life to an unbelievable extent. Unconsciously or consciously we think, feel and act according to hundreds of these biases

produced by these invisible bonds and there is hardly any freedom left for the individual to act, feel and think freely. The conditioning of the mind which takes place when we are under the domination of any overpowering attraction or repulsion is recognized, but few people have any idea of the distortion produced in our life by the less prominent attractions and repulsions or the extent to which our life is conditioned by them.

(2) These attractions and repulsions bind us down to the lower levels of consciousness because it is only in these levels that they can have free play. It is a fundamental law of life that we find ourselves sooner or later where our conscious or unconscious desires can be satisfied. Since these attractions and repulsions are really the breeders of desires pertaining to the lower life they naturally keep us tied down to the lower worlds where consciousness is under the greatest limitations.

(3) The repulsions bind us as much as the attractions. Many people are vaguely aware of the binding nature of the attractions but few can understand why repulsions should bind an individual. But repulsions bind as much as the attractions because they also are the expression of a force connecting the two components which are repelled from each other. We are tied to the person we hate perhaps more firmly than to the person we love, because the personal love can be transformed into impersonal love easily and then loses its binding power. But it is not so easy to transmute the force of hatred and the poison generated by it is removed from one's nature with great difficulty. As *Rāga* and *Dveṣa* form a pair of opposites we cannot transcend one without transcending the other. They are like two sides of a coin. In the light of what is said above it will be seen that *Vairāgya* is not only freedom from *Rāga* but also freedom from *Dveṣa*. A free and unconditioned mind does not oscillate from side to side. It remains stationary at the centre.

(4) Attractions and repulsions really belong to the vehicles but owing to the identification of consciousness with its vehicles we feel that we are being attracted or repelled. When we begin to control and eliminate these attractions and repulsions we gradually become aware of this fact and this knowledge then enables us to control and eliminate them more effectively.

(5) That *Rāga* and *Dveṣa* in their gross form are responsible for much of human misery and suffering will become apparent to anyone who can view life dispassionately and can trace causes and effects intelligently. But only those who systematically try to attenuate the *Kleśas* by means of *Kriyā-Yoga* can see the subtler workings of these *Kleśas*, how they permeate the whole fabric of our worldly life and prevent us from having any peace of mind.

९. स्वरसवाही विदुषोऽपि तथा रूढोऽभिनिवेशः ।

Svarasavāhī viduṣo 'pi tathā rūḍho 'bhiniveśah.

स्वरसवाही sustained by its own forces; flowing on automatically विदुषः the learned (or wise) अपि even तथा in that way रूढः riding; dominating अभिनिवेशः great fear of death; strong desire for life; thorough infiltration (of the mind); will-to-live.

9. *Abhiniveśa* is the strong desire for life which dominates even the learned (or the wise).

The last derivative of *Avidyā* is called *Abhiniveśa*. It is generally translated as desire for life or will-to-live. That every human being, in fact every living creature, wants to continue to live is, of course, a fact with which everyone is familiar. We sometimes see people who have nothing to gain from life. Their life is one long drawn-out misery and yet their attachment to life is as great as ever. The reason for this apparent anomaly is, of course, that the other four *Kleśas* which result in desire for life or *Abhiniveśa* are in full operation even in the absence of unfavourable external circumstances.

There are two points in this *Sūtra* which require some explanation. First, that this strong attachment to life which is universal is well established even in the learned. One may expect ordinary people to feel this attachment but a wise man at least who knows all about the realities of life may be expected to sit lightly on life. But as a matter of fact, this is not so. The philosopher who is well versed in all the philosophies of the world and knows intellectually all the deeper problems of life is as much attached to life as the ordinary person who is ignorant about these things. The reason why Patañjali has pointed out this fact definitely lies perhaps in his intention to bring to the notice of the would-be *Yogi* that mere knowledge of the intellect (*Viduṣaḥ* here really means the learned and not the wise) is in itself inadequate for freeing a man from this attachment to life. Unless and until the tree of *Kleśas* is destroyed, root and branch, by a systematic course of *Yogic* discipline the attachment to life in smaller or greater degree will continue in spite of all the philosophies we may know or preach. The would-be *Yogi*, therefore, places no reliance on such theoretical knowledge. He treads the path of *Yoga* which alone can bring freedom from the *Kleśas*.

The second point to be noted in this *Sūtra* is contained in the phrase *Svarasavāhī* which means sustained by its own inherent force or potency. The universality of *Abhiniveśa* shows that there is some constant and universal force inherent in life which automatically finds expression in this ' desire to live '. The desire to live is not the result of some accidental development in the course of evolution. It seems to be an essential feature of that process. What is this all-powerful force which seems to underlie the current of life and which makes every living creature stick to life like a leech all the time? According to the *Yogic* philosophy this force is rooted in the very origin of things and it comes into play the moment consciousness comes in contact with matter and the evolutionary cycle begins. As was pointed out in II-4 *Avidyā* is the root of all the *Kleśas* and *Abhiniveśa* is merely the fruit or the final expression of the chain of causes and effects set in motion with the birth of *Avidyā* and the involution of consciousness in matter.

It was pointed out earlier that the different *Kleśas* are not unconnected with one another. They form a sort of series beginning with *Avidyā* and ending with *Abhiniveśa*. This view is supported by II-10 according to which the method by which the subtle forms of *Kleśas* can be destroyed is by reversing the process by which they are produced. According to this view, then, *Abhiniveśa* is merely the final phase in the development of the *Kleśas* and that is why it is *Svarasavāhī*. Until the initial cause disappears the subsequent effects must continue to appear in an unending flow.

In the connected series of *Kleśas*, *Rāga* and *Dveṣa* appear as the immediate cause of attachment to life. It follows from this that the greater the play of attractions and repulsions in the life of an individual the greater must be his attachment to life. Observation of life shows that this is to a great extent true. It is people who are under the domination of most violent attractions and repulsions who are most attached to life. We also find that in old age these attractions and repulsions temporarily lose their force to some extent and *pari passu* the desire for life also becomes comparatively feebler.

१०. ते प्रतिप्रसवहेयाः सूक्ष्माः ।

Te pratiprasava-heyāḥ sūkṣmāḥ.

ते they प्रतिप्रसव re-absorption; re-mergence; resolution into respective cause or origin हेयाः capable of being reduced or avoided or abolished सूक्ष्माः subtle.

10. These, the subtle ones, can be reduced by resolving them backward into their origin.

In II-10 and II-11 Patañjali gives the general principles of first attenuating the *Kleśas* and finally destroying them. The *Kleśas* can exist in two states, active and potential. In their active state they can be recognized easily by their outer expressions and the definite awareness which they produce in the mind of the *Sādhaka*. In the case of a person who is in a fit of anger it is easy to see that *Dveṣa* is in full operation. The same person when he subjects himself to a rigid self-discipline acquires the capacity to keep himself absolutely calm and without repulsion towards any one and thus reduces this *Kleśa* to a potential condition. *Dveṣa* has ceased to function but its germs are still there and, given very favourable conditions, can be made active again. Their power has become potential but not completely destroyed. The transition from the fully active to the perfectly dormant condition takes place through a number of stages which have been pointed out in II-4. Through the practice of *Kriyā-Yoga* they can be attenuated progressively until they become quite dormant, incapable of being aroused by ordinary stimuli from the external world. But given extraordinary conditions they can be made active again. So we have to deal with two problems in the complete elimination of the *Kleśas*, first to reduce them to the inactive or *Sūkṣma* state and then to destroy even their potential power. The first is referred to generally as reducing the *Kleśas* to the form of 'seeds' which under favourable conditions have still the power to grow into a tree, and the second as 'scorching the seeds' so that while they may retain the outer form of the 'seeds' they have really become incapable of germinating and growing into a tree.

The problem of reducing the *Kleśas* to the condition of 'seeds' is itself divisible under two sub-heads, that of reducing the fully active forms to the attenuated forms (*Tanu*) and then reducing the latter to the extremely inactive condition (*Prasupta*) from which they cannot be aroused easily. Since the first of these two problems is the more important and fundamental in its nature Patañjali has dealt with it first in II-10. The second problem of reducing the active forms of the *Kleśas* to the partially latent condition, being comparatively easier, is dealt with in II-41, though in *Sādhanā* it really precedes the first problem.

In II-10 the method of reducing the *Kleśas* which have been attenuated to the dormant stage has been hinted at. The phraseology used by Patañjali is extremely apt and expressive but many people find it difficult to understand the meaning of this pregnant *Sūtra*. The phrase *Pratiprasava* means involution or re-absorption of effect into cause or reversing the process of *Prasava* or evolution. If a number of things are derived in a series from a primary thing by a process of evolution they can all be reduced to the original thing by a counter-process of involution and such a counter process is called *Pratiprasava*. Let us consider the underlying significance of this phrase in the present context.

We have seen already that the five *Kleśas* mentioned in II-3 are not independent of each other but form a series beginning with *Avidyā* and ending with *Abhiniveśa*. The process of the development of *Avidyā* into its final expression *Abhiniveśa* is a causal process, one stage naturally and inevitably leading to the next one. It is therefore inevitable that if we want to remove the final element of this fivefold series we must reverse the process whereby each effect is absorbed in its immediate cause and the whole series disappears. It is a question of removing all or none. This means that *Abhiniveśa* should be traced back to *Rāga-Dveṣa*, *Rāga-Dveṣa* to *Asmitā*, *Asmitā* to *Avidyā*, and *Avidyā* to Enlightenment. This tracing backward is not merely an intellectual recognition but a realization which nullifies the power of the *Kleśas* to affect the mind of the *Yogi*. This realization can come to a certain extent on the physical plane but is attained in its fullness on the higher planes when the *Yogi* can rise in *Samādhi* to those planes. It will, therefore, be seen from what has been said above that there is no short-cut to the attenuation and final destruction of the *Kleśas*. It involves the whole technique of *Yogic* discipline.

The fact that the subtle forms of *Kleśas* remain in their 'seed' form even after they have been attenuated to the extreme limit is of great significance. It means that the *Sādhaka* is not free from danger until he has crossed the threshold of *Kaivalya* and reached the final goal. As long as these 'seeds' lurk within him there is no knowing when he may become their victim. It is these unscorched 'seeds' of *Kleśas* which account for the sudden and unexpected fall of *Yogis* after they have reached great heights of illumination and power. This shows the necessity of exercising the utmost discrimination right up to the very end of the Path.

When the latent forms of *Kleśas* have been attenuated to the utmost limit and the resulting tendencies have been made extremely feeble—brought almost to the zero level—the question arises, 'How to destroy the potentiality of these tendencies so that there may be no possibility of their revival under any circumstances?' How to scorch the 'seeds' of *Kleśas* so that they cannot germinate again? This is a very important question for the advanced *Yogi* because his work has not been completed until this has been done. The answer to this question follows from the very nature of the *Kleśas* which has been discussed previously. If the *Kleśas* are rooted in *Avidyā* they cannot be destroyed until *Avidyā* is destroyed. This means that no freedom from the subtlest forms of the *Kleśas* is possible until full Enlightenment of *Kaivalya* is attained through the practice of *Dharma-Megha-Samādhi*. This conclusion is confirmed by IV-30 according to which freedom from *Kleśas* and *Karmas* is obtained only after *Dharma-Megha-Samādhi* which precedes the attainment of *Kaivalya*.

११. ध्यानहेयास्तद्वृत्तयः ।

Dhyāna-heyās tad-vṛttayaḥ.

ध्यान (by) meditation हेयाः (*Kleśas* which are) to be avoided तद्वृत्तयः their modifications; ways of existing; activities.

11. Their active modifications are to be suppressed by meditation.

This *Sūtra* gives the method of dealing with the *Kleśas* in the preliminary stage when they have to be reduced from an active to a passive state. The means to be adopted are given in one word *Dhyāna*. It is therefore necessary to understand the meaning of this word in its full scope. The word *Dhyāna*, of course, literally means meditation or contemplation as explained elsewhere but here it obviously stands for a rather comprehensive self-discipline of which meditation is the pivot. It is easy to see that a *Sādhaka* who is under the domination of *Kleśas* in their active form will have to attack the problem from many sides at once. In fact, the whole technique of *Kriyā-Yoga* will have to be utilized for this purpose, for one of the two objects of *Kriyā-Yoga* is to attenuate the *Kleśas* and the reduction of the *Kleśas* from their active to the passive form is the first step in this attenuation. *Svādhyāya*, *Tapas* and *Īśvara-praṇidhāna*, all the three elements of *Kriyā-Yoga*, have therefore to be used in this work. But the essential part of all these three is really *Dhyāna*, the intensive concentration of the mind in order to understand the deeper problems of life and to solve them effectively for the realization of one's main objective. Even *Tapas*, the element of *Kriyā-Yoga* which outwardly seems to involve merely going through certain self-disciplinary and purificatory exercises, depends for its effectiveness to a large extent on *Dhyāna*. For, it is not the mere external performance of the act which brings about the desired result but the inner concentration of purpose and the alert mind which underlie the act. If these latter are not present the outer action will be of no avail. No success in *Yoga* is possible unless all the energies of the soul are polarized and harnessed for achieving the central purpose. So the word *Dhyāna* in II-11 implies all mental processes and exercises which may help the *Sādhaka* to reduce the active *Kleśas* to the passive condition. It may include reflection, brooding over the deeper problems of life, changing habits of thought and attitudes by means of meditation (II-33), *Tapas* as well as meditation in the ordinary sense of the term.

It is necessary to note in this connection that reducing the *Kleśas* to a latent or passive condition does not mean merely bringing them to a temporary state of quiescence. Violent disturbances of the mind and emotions which result from the activity of the *Kleśas* (*Kleśa-Vṛtti*) are not always present and we all pass through phases in which *Kleśas* like *Rāga-Dveṣa* seem to have become latent. A *Sādhaka* may retire for sometime into solitude. As long as he is cut off from all kinds of social relationships, *Rāga* and *Dveṣa* will naturally become inoperative but that does not mean that he has reduced these to a latent state. It is only their outer expression which has been suspended and the moment he resumes his social life these *Kleśas* will re-assert themselves with their usual force. Reducing the *Kleśas* to the latent state means making the tendencies so feeble that they are not easily aroused, though they have not yet been rooted out.

Another point which may be noted is that attacking one particular form or expression of a *Kleśa* is not of much avail, though in the beginning this may be done to gain some knowledge of the working of the *Kleśas* and the technique of mastering them. A *Kleśa* can assume innumerable forms of expression and if we merely suppress one of its expressions it will assume other forms. It is the general tendency which has to be tackled and it is this isolation, as it were, of this tendency and tackling it as a whole which tests the intelligence of the *Sādhaka* and determines the success of the endeavour.

१२. क्लेशमूलः कर्माशयो दृष्टादृष्टजन्मवेदनीयः ।

Kleśa-mūlaḥ karmāśayo dṛṣṭādṛṣṭa-janma-vedanīyaḥ.

क्लेशमूलः rooted in *Kleśas* कर्माशयः reservoir of *Karmas*; the vehicle of the seeds of *Karma* दृष्ट seen; present अदृष्ट unseen; future जन्म lives वेदनीयः to be known; to be experienced.

12. The reservoir of *Karmas* which are rooted in *Kleśas* brings all kinds of experiences in the present and future lives.

Sūtras 12, 13 and 14 give in a very concise and lucid manner the essential features of the twin laws of *Karma* and Reincarnation, the well-known doctrines formulating the Universal Moral Law and cycle of births and deaths underlying human life. As the students of *Yoga* are generally familiar with the broad aspects of these doctrines it is not necessary to discuss them here and we shall confine ourselves to the particular aspects referred to in these three *Sūtras*. It may be pointed out at the very outset that Patañjali has not attempted to give us a general idea concerning the Laws of *Karma* and Reincarnation. His object is merely to show the underlying cause of human misery so that we may be able to appreciate the means adopted in *Yogic* discipline for its effective removal. He, therefore, takes only those particular aspects of these laws which are needed for his argument. But, incidentally, he has given in three brief *Sūtras* the very essence of these all-embracing laws.

The first idea given in II-12 which we have to note is that *Kleśas* are the underlying cause of the *Karmas* we generate by our thoughts, desires and actions. Each human soul goes through a continuous series of incarnations reaping the fruits of thoughts, desires, and actions done in the past and generating, during the process of reaping, new causes which will bear their fruits in this or future lives. So every human life is like a flowing current in which two processes are at work simultaneously, the working out of *Karmas* made in the past and the generation of new *Karmas* which will bear fruit in the future. Each thought, desire, emotion and action produces its corresponding result with mathematical exactitude and this result is recorded naturally and automatically in our life's ledger.

What is the nature of this recording mechanism upon which depends the working out of causes and effects with mathematical precision? The answer to this question is contained only in one word, *Karmāśaya*, given in this *Sūtra*. This word means literally the reservoir or sleeping place of *Karmas*. *Karmāśaya*, obviously, refers to the vehicle in our inner constitution which serves as the receptacle of all the *Saṃskāras* or impressions made by our thoughts, desires, feelings and actions. This vehicle serves as a permanent record of all that we have thought, felt or done during the long course of evolution extending over a series of lives and provides patterns and contents of the successive lives. People who are familiar even with elementary physiology should find no difficulty in understanding and appreciating this idea because the impressions produced in our brain by our experiences on the physical plane provide an exact parallel. Everything which we have experienced through our sense-organs is recorded in the brain and can be recovered in the form of memory of those experiences. We cannot see these impressions and yet we know that they exist.

Students who are familiar with Hindu philosophical thought will find no difficulty in identifying this *Karmāśaya* with the *Kāraṇa Śarīra* or 'causal body' in the *Vedāntic* classification of our inner constitution. This is one of the subtle vehicles of consciousness which lies beyond the *Manomaya Kośa* and is so called because it is the source of all causes which will be set in motion and will mould our present and future lives. It is the receptacle into which the effects of all that we do are being constantly poured in and being transformed into causes of experiences which we shall go through in this and future lives.

Now, the important point to note here is that though this 'causal' vehicle is the immediate or effective cause of the present and future lives and from it, to a great extent, flow the experiences which constitute those lives, still, the real or ultimate cause of these experiences are the *Kleśas*. Because, it is the *Kleśas* which are responsible for the continuous generation of *Karmas* and the causal vehicle merely serves as a mechanism for adjusting the effects of these *Karmas*.

१३. सति मूले तद्विपाको जात्यायुर्भोगाः ।

Sati mūle tad-vipāko jāty-āyur-bhogāḥ.

सति मूले there being the root तद् (of) it (*Karmāśaya*) विपाकः fruition; ripening जाति class आयुः (span of) life भोगाः (and) experiences.

13. As long as the root is there it must ripen and result in lives of different class, length and experiences.

As long as the *Kleśas* are operating in the life of an individual the vehicle of *Karmas* will be continually nourished by the addition of new causal impressions and there is no possibility of the series of lives coming to an end. If the root remains intact the *Saṃskāras* in the causal vehicle will naturally continue to ripen and produce one life after another with its inevitable misery and suffering. Though the nature and content of experiences gone through by human beings in their lives is of infinite variety, Patañjali has classified these under three heads (1) class, (2) length of life, and (3) pleasant or unpleasant nature of the experiences. These are the principal features which determine the nature of a life. First, *Jāti* or class. This determines the environment of the individual and thus his opportunities and the type of life which he will be able to lead. A man born in a slum has not the same opportunities as a man born among cultured people. So the kind of life a person has is determined in the first place by *Jāti*.

The second important factor is the length of life. This naturally determines the total number of experiences. A life cut short in childhood contains a comparatively smaller number of experiences than a long life running its normal course. Of course, since the successive lives of an individual form one continuous whole, from the larger point of view, a short life intervening in this manner does not really matter very much. It is as if a person could not have a full day for work but had to go to bed early. Another day dawns when he can continue his work as usual.

The third factor is the nature of the experiences gone through as regards their pleasant or unpleasant quality. *Jāti* also determines the nature of the experiences but there we consider the experiences in relation to the opportunities for the growth of the soul. Under *Bhoga* we consider experiences in relation to their potentiality to bring pain or pleasure to the individual. There are some people who are well placed in life but have a difficult time—nothing but suffering and unhappiness from birth to death. On the other hand, we may have a life lived in comparatively poor circumstances but the experiences may be pleasant all along. The pleasures and pains which we have to bear are not entirely dependent upon our *Jāti*. There is a personal factor involved as we can ourselves see by observing the lives of people around us.

१४. ते ह्लादपरितापफलाः पुण्यापुण्यहेतुत्वात् ।

Te hlāda-paritāpa-phalāḥ puṇyāpuṇya-hetutvāt.

ते they ह्लाद joy परिताप (and) sorrow -फलाः (having for their) fruit पुण्य merit as opposed to sin or demerit अपुण्य demerit; sin (पुण्य and अपुण्य are the assets and liabilities superphysically registered in the soul) हेतुत्वात् being caused by; on account of.

14. They have joy or sorrow for their fruit according as their cause is virtue or vice.

Upon what depends the nature of the experiences we have to go through in life? Since everything in the Universe works according to a hidden and immutable law it cannot be due to mere chance that some of these experiences are joyful and others are sorrowful. What determines this pleasurable or painful quality of the experiences? II-14 gives an answer to this question. The pleasurable or painful quality of experiences which come in our life is determined by the nature of the causes which have produced them. The effect is always naturally related to the cause and its nature is determined by the cause. Now, those thoughts, feelings and actions which are 'virtuous' give rise to experiences which are pleasant while those which are 'vicious' give rise to experiences which are unpleasant. But we must not take the words 'virtuous' and 'vicious' in their narrow, orthodox religious sense but in the wider and scientific sense of living in conformity with the great Moral Law which is universal in its action and mathematical in its expression. In Nature the effect is always related to the cause and corresponds exactly to the cause which has set it in motion. If we cause a little purely physical pain to somebody it is reasonable to suppose that the fruit of our action will be some experience causing a corresponding physical pain to us. It cannot be a dreadful calamity causing terrible mental agony. This will be unjust and the Law of *Karma* is the expression of the most perfect justice that we can conceive of. Since *Karma* is a natural law and natural laws work with mathematical precision we can to a certain extent predict the *Karmic* results of our actions and thoughts by imagining their consequences. The *Karmic* result, or 'fruit' as it is generally called, of an action is related to the action as a photographic copy is related to its negative, though the compounding of several effects in one experience may make it difficult to trace the effects to their respective causes. The orthodox religious conceptions of hell and heaven, in which are provided rewards and punishments without any regard for the natural relationship of causes and effects, are sometimes absurd in the extreme though they do, in a general way, relate virtue to pleasure and vice to pain.

१५. परिणामतापसंस्कारदुःखैर्गुणवृत्तिविरोधाच्च दुःखमेव सर्वं विवेकिनः ।

Pariṇāma-tāpa-saṃskāra-duḥkhair guṇa-vṛtti-virodhāc ca duḥkham eva sarvaṃ vivekinaḥ.

परिणाम (on account of) change ताप acute anxiety; suffering संस्कार impression; stamping with a tendency दुःखैः pains (three causes mentioned above) गुण (between the three) *Guṇas* वृत्ति (and) modification (of the mind) विरोधात् on account of opposition or conflict च and दुःखम् (is) pain; misery एव only विवेकिनः to the enlightened; to the person who has developed discrimination.

15. To the people who have developed discrimination all is misery on account of the pains resulting from change, anxiety and tendencies, as also on account of the conflicts between the functioning of the *Guṇas* and the *Vṛttis* (of the mind).

If virtue and vice beget respectively pleasurable and painful experiences the question may arise 'Why not adopt the virtuous life to ensure in time an uninterrupted series of pleasurable experiences and to eliminate completely all painful experiences?'. Of course, for some time the results of vicious actions we have done in the past would continue to appear but if we persist in our efforts and make our life continuously and strictly moral, eliminating vice of every description, a time must come when the *Saṃskāras* and *Karmas* created from vicious thoughts and actions in the past would get exhausted and life thenceforth must become a continuous series of pleasant and happiness-giving experiences. This is a line of thought which will appeal especially to the aspirant who is having a nice time and is attached to the nice things of the world. The philosophy of *Kleśas* will appear to him unnecessarily harsh and pessimistic and the ideal of a completely virtuous life will seem to provide a very happy solution of the great problem of life. It will satisfy his innate moral and religious sense and ensure for him the happy and pleasant life that he really wants. The orthodox religious ideal which requires people to be good and moral so that they may have a happy life here and hereafter is really a concession to human weakness and the desire to prefer the so-called happiness in life to Enlightenment.

This idea of ensuring a happy life by means of virtue, apart from the impracticability of living a perfectly virtuous life continuously while still bound by illusion, is based on a delusion about the very nature of what the ordinary man calls happiness and II-15 explains why this is so. This is perhaps one of the most important *Sūtras*, if not the most important, bearing on the philosophy of *Kleśas* and a real grasp of the significance of the fundamental idea expounded in it is necessary not only for understanding the philosophy of *Kleśas* but the *Yogic* philosophy as a whole. Not until the aspirant has realized to some extent the illusion underlying the so-called 'happiness' which he pursues in the world can he really give up this futile pursuit and devote himself whole-heartedly to the task of transcending the Great Illusion and finding that Reality in which alone can one find true Enlightenment and Peace. Let the serious student, therefore, ponder carefully over the profound significance of this *Sūtra*.

The *Sūtra* in general means that *all* experiences are either actively or potentially full of misery to the wise person whose spiritual perception has become awakened. This is so because certain conditions like change, anxiety, habituation and conflicts between the functioning of the *Guṇas* and *Vṛttis* are inherent in life. Let us take up each of these conditions and see what it means.

Pariṇāma: means change. It should be obvious to the most unintelligent man that life as we know it is governed by a relentless law of change which is all-pervasive and applies to all things at all times. Nothing in life abides right from a Solar system to a grain of dust, and all things are in a state of flux though the change may be very slow, so slow that we may not be conscious of it. One effect of *Māyā* is to make us unconscious of the continuous changes which are taking place within and without us. People are afraid of death but they do not see the fact that death is merely an incident in the continuous series of changes in and around us. When the realization of this continuous, relentless change affecting everything in life dawns upon an individual he begins to realize what illusion means. This realization is a very definite experience and is one aspect of *Viveka*, the faculty of discrimination. The ordinary man is so immersed and completely identified with the life in which he is involved that he cannot separate himself mentally from this fast moving current. Theoretically he may recognize the law of change but he has no realization.

The first result of this realization when *Viveka* dawns is fear. The very ground from under our feet seems to have been cut away. We seem to have no foothold, nothing to which we can hold on in this fast-moving current of time and material changes. The whole Universe appears to be a swirling flux of phenomena like water running under a bridge. People and objects around us which appeared so real become mere phantoms in the panorama which is passing before us. We seem to be standing in a void and the horror of loneliness unspeakable engulfs us.

What do we do when this realization comes to us accidentally or as a result of deep and continuous pondering over the real nature of phenomenal life? We generally get alarmed, terrified and try to shut it out again by plunging more violently into the activities and interests of the worldly life, even though we theoretically continue to believe in the unreality of the things around us. But, if we do not try to smother this horrible vision, and facing it squarely, take to the self-discipline prescribed in *Yoga*, then sooner or later, beneath this fast flowing stream of phenomena, we begin, first to sense, and later to discern something which is abiding, which transcends change and gives us an eternal foothold. We begin to realize that the phenomena change but not That in which the phenomena take place. First only dimly but later in its fullness this realization of the Eternal grows within us. But we have to pass through the valley of fear before this realization comes. We must see the whole solid world of men and things disintegrate and disappear into a flux of mere phenomena before we can see the Real hidden beneath the unreal.

It is only when we have passed through this kind of experience that we see with sadness the illusion and the pathos in the life of the world, in the pursuit of little pleasures and ambitions, in the ephemeral love and happiness to which people desperately cling, in the short-lived glory of the man in power, in the effort to hold tenaciously to things which must be given up sooner or later. Viewed in this light even the most exquisite pleasures and splendid achievements of life pale into insignificance, nay assume the form of misery. It is the usual practice to ask a man under sentence of death to name any simple pleasure which he would like to indulge in before he is executed, a drink, a dish which he likes. But those who see such a man satisfying his whim for the last time are conscious of a peculiar pathos in this desire to clutch at pleasure before death snuffs out the life of the individual. To the man in whom *Viveka* has been developed the pathetic pursuit of pleasures, ambitions and the like appears in a similar light. We are all under sentence of death in a way, only we are not conscious of this fact and do not know when that sentence will be carried out. If we did, all our so-called pleasures will cease to be pleasures.

Tāpa: The second affliction which is inherent in human life is *Tāpa* or anxiety. All pleasures, indulgences and the so-called happiness are associated with anxiety, conscious or sub-conscious. For indulgence in pleasure, or dependence for our happiness on the uncertain and passing things in the outer world owing to attachment, means fear of losing those objects which give us pleasure or happiness. If we have money then there is always the fear that the money may be lost and our security may be threatened. If we love people then there is the fear that those people may die or may be taken away from us. Most of us have such fears and anxieties gnawing at our heart constantly though we may not acknowledge or be even conscious of this fact. It is only when a crisis comes in our life that these fears emerge into our consciousness but they are always present in the sub-conscious mind and secretly poison our life. We may be too dull to notice them or too ' strong ' mentally to allow them to worry us markedly but there is hardly any person not following the path of *Yoga* who is above them.

Saṃskāra: This word means impression but in the present context it can best be translated by the word ' habituation ' as we shall see presently. There is a law of Nature according to which any experience through which we pass produces an impression on all our vehicles. The impression thus produced makes a channel for the flow of a corresponding force and the channel thus becomes deeper and deeper as the experience is repeated. This results in our acquiring habits of various kinds and getting used to particular kinds of environment, modes of living and pleasures. But there is at work simultaneously, the law of change, referred to already, which is constantly changing our outer environment and places us among new surroundings, circumstances and people. The result of this simultaneous action of two natural forces is that we are constantly acquiring new habits, getting used to new circumstances and also being forced out of them. No sooner do we settle down in a new habit or a new environment than we are forced out of it, sometimes easily and gradually, at other times roughly and suddenly. This continuous necessity for adjustment in life is a source of constant discomfort and pain to every individual. Nature hardly allows us breathing time and is continuously driving us into new kinds of experiences, much as we would like to settle down in our grooves and comfortable positions which we have gained. Of course, the intelligent man accepts this necessity for adjustment and does what he can to reconcile himself to it but the fact remains that this is a major affliction of life from which everyone would like to be free.

Guṇa-Vṛtti-Virodha: The word *Vṛtti* is sometimes taken to refer to the *Guṇas* and to mean the modifications or functions of the *Guṇas*. According to this interpretation *Guṇa-Vṛtti-Virodha* would be the opposition or conflict between the functioning of the three *Guṇas* amongst themselves. As this does not make much sense it is much better to interpret *Vṛtti* as referring to the states of the mind. *Guṇa-Vṛtti-Virodha* would then mean the conflict between the natural tendencies caused by the preponderance of one of the *Guṇas* and the states of the mind which are constantly changing. Such a conflict is very common in human life and is the cause of much dissatisfaction in the life of the average individual. The following example will illustrate this conflict and show how it is one of the major causes of human misery.

There is a man who is lazy by temperament owing to the predominance of *Tamas* in his nature. He hates activity but is placed in circumstances where he has to exert himself for his living. So he desires constantly a peaceful and inactive life and the result of this strong desire entertained persistently is that in his next life his desire finds fruition in an environment where he is forced to be quite inactive (he may be born as an Eskimo or be placed in charge of a lighthouse). But in this life there may be a preponderance of *Rajas* in his nature and he therefore wants activity in an environment where not much activity is possible. He, therefore, frets and is as dissatisfied with his new lot as he was with the old. Sometimes, this conflict between the *Guṇas* prevailing at the time and the state of the mind or desire is of a temporary nature but it always has the effect of producing discontentment for the time being.

Thus, Nature, by the natural operation of its laws is bringing about constantly these oppositions between our tendencies and the states of our mind and this is why we see everywhere general discontentment. Nobody seems to be satisfied with his lot or circumstances. Everybody wants what he has not got. That is how *Guṇa-Vṛtti-Virodha* becomes one of the causes of human misery in general. The wise man sees the inevitability of all this and therefore renounces desires altogether, taking what comes to him in life without elation or resentment. What we should remember in this connection is that every set of circumstances in which we find ourselves is the outcome of our own desires, although by the time a particular desire finds fruition it may have been replaced by another desire of an opposite kind. Our desires cannot by the very nature of things find immediate fulfilment and there must be a certain time lag in their realization. During this intervening period our nature, temperament and desires may undergo considerable change and when we face the fulfilment of our own desire we may hardly believe that we ourselves desired what has now come to us.

The existence of the four kinds of afflictions mentioned above which are inherent in human life produces such conditions that nobody who has developed *Viveka* or spiritual discrimination can possibly consider the so-called happiness of ordinary life as real happiness. It is true that to the man of the world immersed in its illusory pursuits of pleasure or power life may appear to consist of a mixture of pleasures and pains, joys and sorrows but to the wise man whose spiritual faculties have become awakened *all* life must appear full of misery and its illusory happiness merely a sugar-coated pill containing only pain and suffering hidden inside. This is a statement which may appear to give a distorted view of life but let the student ponder deeply over these facts—these hard facts of life—and it is probable that he will also come to the same conclusion. Anyway, unless the aspirant for the *Yogic* life realizes the truth enshrined in this *Sūtra* he is not really fully qualified to attempt the long and difficult climb which leads to the mountain-top of Self-realization.

१६. हेयं दुःखमनागतम् ।

Heyaṃ duḥkham anāgatam.

हेयम् to be avoided दुःखम् misery अनागतम् not yet come; in future.

16. The misery which is not yet come can and is to be avoided.

The next question which naturally arises is whether it is possible to avoid this misery which has been shown to be inherent in human life in the last *Sūtra.* A large number of thoughtful people who have pondered deeply over this problem will perhaps concede that life is essentially an unalloyed misery but they will say that one has to take life as it is and to make the best of it since there is no way of getting out of it except through the gate-way of death. They may not believe like the ordinary orthodox religious man that all the sorrows and sufferings will somehow be compensated in the life after death but they do not see what can be done in the matter except to accept thankfully the little pleasures and to bear the pains with stoic indifference.

Now, it is in this respect that the philosophy of *Yoga* differs fundamentally from most of the orthodox religions of the world which offer nothing better than an uncertain and nebulous happiness in the life after death. They say in effect 'Lead a good life to ensure happiness after death, put your faith in God and hope for the best'. According to *Yogic* philosophy death no more solves your spiritual problem than night solves your economic problem. If you are poor you do not expect on going to bed that your economic problem will be automatically solved next day.

You will have to get up next day and begin where you left off the previous night. If you are poor economically you do not expect to get rich overnight and if you are poor spiritually, bound by illusions and limitations of all kinds, you cannot expect to become Enlightened in your next life, or if you do not believe in reincarnation, in the vague and unending life which is supposed to follow death.

According to the *Yogic* philosophy it is possible to rise completely above the illusions and miseries of life and to gain infinite knowledge, bliss and power through Enlightenment *here and now* while we are still living in the physical body. And if we do not attain this Enlightenment while we are still alive we will have to come back again and again into this world until we have accomplished this appointed task. So it is not a question of choosing the path of *Yoga* or rejecting it. It is a question of choosing it now or in some future life. It is a question of gaining Enlightenment as soon as possible and avoiding the suffering in the future or postponing the effort and going through further suffering which is unnecessary and avoidable. This is the meaning of II-16. No vague promise of an uncertain post-mortem happiness is this, but a definite scientific assertion of a fact verified by the experience of innumerable *Yogis*, saints and sages who have trodden the path of *Yoga* throughout the ages.

१७. द्रष्टृदृश्ययोः संयोगो हेयहेतुः ।

Draṣṭṛ-dṛśyayoḥ saṃyogo heya-hetuḥ.

द्रष्टृ (of) Seer; (*Puruṣa*) दृश्ययोः (and) Seen; *Prakṛti* संयोगः union; association हेय (of) that which is to be avoided हेतुः cause.

17. The cause of that which is to be avoided is the union of the Seer and the Seen.

Now we come to the question of means, not the actual technique of *Yoga* which has to be employed but the general principle on which the freedom from the *Kleśas* has to be worked out. It is to be noted that the objective is not a temporary and partial solution of the problem but a permanent and complete solution, not a palliative but a remedy which will root out the disease altogether. If the disease is to be rooted out we must go to the root-cause of the malady and not bother about the mere outward superficial symptoms. What is the root-cause of the misery which is caused by the *Kleśas* and which is to be avoided? The answer is given in II-17. The nature of the Seer and Seen and the reason why they are yoked together are explained in the subsequent *Sūtras* but before dealing with those questions let us try to understand the problem in a general way.

It has already been pointed out in dealing with the nature of *Asmitā* or the tendency of consciousness to identify itself with its vehicles that this process begins with the coming together of consciousness and matter as a result of the veil of *Māyā* involving it in illusion and consequent *Avidyā*. This problem which is linked with the origin of things and takes us back to the question of the initial involution of the individual consciousness in matter is really one of the ultimate problems of philosophy about which philosophers have been speculating since the beginning of time. It is like all such problems beyond the scope of the limited intellect and it is no use trying to solve it through the agency of the intellect. It can be solved—or it would perhaps be better to use the word dissolved—only in the light of the transcendent knowledge we can gain in Enlightenment. So let us not try to answer the question why the *Puruṣa* who is pure and perfect is yoked to *Prakṛti*. Let us hold our soul in patience and wait till we have transcended the intellect and its illusions and are face to face with that Reality which holds within itself the answer to this ultimate question.

But though we cannot know the answer to this fundamental question there is no difficulty in understanding that such yoking together has taken place and also that this yoking is the cause of the bondage. Yoking always means bondage even in ordinary life and that it should be the cause of bondage in the case of the *Puruṣa* is quite conceivable. But what is the nature of the bondage it is impossible to conceive beyond what is given in the philosophy of *Kleśas*. To know that in the real sense of the term would be to know the ultimate mystery of life and to have reached

Enlightenment already. Surely, that is the end—what the aspirant sets out to achieve through *Yoga*.

After pointing out the cause of bondage in II-17, namely the yoking together of the Seer and the Seen or the entanglement of pure consciousness in matter, Patañjali proceeds to explain the essential nature of the Seer and the Seen. In the two following *Sūtras*, II-18 and 19, he has put in a nutshell all the essential facts which concern the phenomenal world and thus given us a masterly analysis of the Seen.

१८. प्रकाशक्रियास्थितिशीलं भूतेन्द्रियात्मकं भोगापवर्गार्थं दृश्यम् ।

Prakāśa-kriyā-sthiti-śīlaṃ bhūtendriyāt-makaṃ bhogāpavargārthaṃ dṛśyam.

प्रकाश (of) luminosity; light; cognition; consciousness of क्रिया activity स्थिति (and) steadiness; stability शीलं having the properties or qualities भूत elements इन्द्रिय sense-organs आत्मकं being of the nature भोग experience अपवर्ग and liberation अर्थं for the sake of; with the purpose of दृश्यम् (is) the Seen (*Prakṛti*).

18. The Seen (objective side of manifestation) consists of the elements and sense-organs, is of the nature of cognition, activity and stability (*Sattva*, *Rajas* and *Tamas*) and has for its purpose (providing the *Puruṣa* with) experience and liberation.

In II-18 we see how the master minds who developed the science of *Yoga* had the capacity to go to the heart of every matter and after separating the essential from the non-essential could grasp and formulate the essential facts. In one brief *Sūtra* Patañjali has analysed and placed before us the fundamental facts concerning the essential nature of the phenomenal world and its perception and purpose. First, he gives the essential nature of all phenomena which are the objects of perception. These according to the well-known conception of Hindu philosophy are really made up of the three *Guṇas* the nature of which will be explained later on. He then points out that the perception of the phenomenal world is really the result of the interactions of the *Bhūtas* and *Indriyas*, the ' elements ' and the ' sense-organs '. And lastly, he points out the purpose and function of the phenomenal world which is twofold. Firstly, to provide experience for the *Puruṣas* who seem to be evolving in it, and secondly, through this experience to lead them gradually to emancipation and Enlightenment.

It is necessary to note that the word used for the phenomenal world is *Dṛśyam*, that which is ' seen ' or is capable of being ' seen '. The contact of *Puruṣa* and *Prakṛti* results in the emergence of a duality which in modern language may be called the subjective and objective sides of Nature. Of these the *Puruṣa* is the essence or substratum of the subjective and *Prakṛti* that of the objective side of this duality. As consciousness recedes inwards the dividing line between the subjective and objective shifts continually but the relation between the two remains the same. The *Puruṣa* with all the vehicles which have not been separated off from his consciousness constitutes the subjective part of this dual relationship and is called *Draṣṭā* or Seer. That portion of *Prakṛti* which has been separated off in this manner constitutes the objective part and is called *Dṛśyam* or Seen. Both *Draṣṭā* and *Dṛśyam* are thus necessary for the phenomenal world.

Let us first consider the essential nature of all phenomena which are the objects of perception. These, according to the present *Sūtra*, are the result of the play of the three *Guṇas* which find expression through cognition, activity and stability. The theory of *Guṇas* forms an integral part of Hindu philosophy and the whole structure of the manifested Universe, according to this philosophy, is considered to rest on these three fundamental qualities or attributes of *Prakṛti*. In fact, according to the *Sāṃkhya* doctrine even *Prakṛti* is nothing but a condition of perfect equilibrium of the three *Guṇas—Triguṇa-Sāmyāvasthā*.

Although the theory of *Guṇas* is one of the fundamental doctrines of Hindu philosophy it is surprising how little it is understood. The *Guṇas* are referred to over and over again in the

Bhagavad-gītā; there is hardly any important book in *Saṃskṛta* dealing with religion or philosophy in which the word *Triguṇa* does not occur; and yet, nobody seems to know what the three *Guṇas* really stand for. There is a vague idea that they have something to do with properties because the word *Guṇa* in *Saṃskṛta* generally means a property or attribute. That is also the general impression which the various contexts in which the word is used seem to produce. But one looks in vain for any clear exposition of the real significance of the word or what it really stands for in terms of modern thought.

It is not difficult to understand why the nature of the *Guṇas* is so difficult to comprehend. They lie at the very basis of the manifested world and even the working of the mind through which we try to comprehend their nature depends upon their interplay. Trying to comprehend the nature of the *Guṇas* with the help of the mind is like trying to catch the hand with a pair of tongs held by the hand. Not until the *Yogi* crosses the boundary of manifestation and transcends the domain of the *Guṇas* as indicated in IV-34 can he realize their true nature. But this does not mean that the student of *Yoga* cannot understand their nature at all and should remain satisfied with the vague and nebulous notions which are generally prevalent with regard to this basic doctrine. The advances which have taken place in the field of physical sciences and the light which this has thrown on the structure of matter and the nature of physical phenomena has now placed us in a position to be able to gain a faint glimpse into the essential nature of the *Guṇas*. It is true that this knowledge is connected with the superficial aspects of the *Guṇas* but the student can, by the exercise of deep thought and intuition, gain some understanding of the subject, enough to convince him that the *Guṇas* are not a mere elusive phantom of philosophy but are part of that profound mystery which surrounds the founding of a manifested Universe. This is not the place to deal exhaustively with this interesting but abstruse subject but a few ideas may be discussed to enable the student to know in which direction he should seek for more knowledge if he wants to understand the subject more fully. This discussion will involve some knowledge of modern scientific ideas though an effort will be made to keep it as free from technicalities as possible. After all, if we want to understand any problem in terms of modern scientific facts we must have at least a general knowledge of those facts.

What is the essential nature of the phenomena which we perceive through the instrumentality of the sense-organs? The first point we should note in arriving at an answer to this question is that an object of perception will be found on analysis to consist of a number of properties or *Dharmas* cognized through the sense-organs. That every object is merely a bundle of properties and our knowledge with regard to that object is confined to the direct or indirect observation of these properties is a well-known philosophical conception which every student can understand.

The second question which arises is: What is the nature of these properties or rather on what does the cognition of these properties depend? If we analyse the flux of physical phenomena around us in the light of modern scientific knowledge we shall find three principles of a fundamental character underlying these phenomena. These three principles which ultimately determine the nature of every phenomenon are all connected with motion and may be called different aspects of motion. It is very difficult to express these principles by means of single words, for no words with a sufficiently comprehensive meaning are known, but for want of better words we may call them: (1) vibration which involves rhythmic motion of particles, (2) mobility which involves non-rhythmic motion of particles with transference of energy, (3) inertia which involves relative position of particles. These principles are really the three fundamental aspects of motion and may be crudely illustrated respectively by a number of soldiers drilling on a parade ground, a number of people walking in a crowd and a number of prisoners confined in separate cells. Whatever the nature of the phenomenon, we shall find at the basis of that phenomenon these principles working in various ways and determining the *Dharmas* or properties which are manifest.

Let us take for the sake of illustration, one by one, the sensuous phenomena which are observed through the five sense-organs. The cognition of visual phenomena depends upon the presence of light vibrations which by their action on the retina of the eye give the impression of form and colour. Auditory phenomena depend upon sound vibrations which acting upon the drum of the ear produce the sensation of sound. The sensation of heat, etc., depends upon the impact of moving atoms and molecules on the skin. The sensations of taste and smell depend upon the action of chemical substances on the membranes of the palate and nose, the nature of the chemical substance (which is determined by the relative position and the nature of the atoms in the molecules) determining the sensation which is experienced. In every case we find vibration or rhythmic motion, mobility or irregular motion, inertia or relative position at work and determining the nature of the senuous phenomenon.

Up to this time we have assumed the presence of particles which by their motion determine the phenomenon. But what are these particles? Science tells us that these particles are also nothing but combinations of protons, neutrons and electrons, the electrons whirling round the nucleus of protons and neutrons at tremendous speeds and determining the properties of the atoms. In view of the discovery of the equivalence and interconvertibility of mass and energy it will probably be found ultimately that the nucleus of the atom is also an expression of energy and that the ultimate basis of the manifested physical universe is nothing but motion or energy. The day this is proved conclusively materialism of the orthodox type will be buried for ever and the philosophy of *Yoga* will be fully vindicated.

We see, therefore, that all properties can be reduced to their simplest elements—wave motion (*Prakāśa*), action (*Kriyā*) and position (*Sthiti*) at least as far as the physical universe is concerned and since these are also the ideas associated with the nature of the three *Guṇas*, Science has to a certain extent corroborated the theory of *Guṇas*. It is true that the *Guṇas* underlie the whole manifested Universe and not only the physical world, and so we cannot comprehend their true nature by simply taking into account their physical manifestations. But a study of their interplay in the physical world may help the student to gain a faint glimpse into their real nature and the truth underlying IV-13.

There is one other important point we have to understand in relation to the *Guṇas* if we would grasp the significance of ideas given in III-56 and IV-34. This point is connected with the relation of the three *Guṇas* to one another. Every student of elementary Science knows that wave motion or vibration is a harmonious combination of mobility and inertia. And if the three *Guṇas* are connected as we have seen with these three aspects of motion it follows that *Sattva* is merely a harmonious combination of *Rajas* and *Tamas* and is not anything apart from *Rajas* and *Tamas*. So the development of *Sattva* is not really the creation of something new but the harmonization of the existing *Rajas* and *Tamas*. This fact is very important because it serves to throw some light on the relation of the *Puruṣa* and *Sattva*. When the *Puruṣa* comes in contact with *Prakṛti* at the beginning of the evolutionary cycle his contact disturbs the equilibrium of the three *Guṇas* and gradually brings into play the forces of *Prakṛti*. Through this disturbed atmosphere the *Puruṣa* cannot see his *Svarūpa* because this *Svarūpa* can be expressed or reflected only through a sufficiently purified *Sattva Guṇa*. In the early stages of evolution this question does not arise. The vehicles of consciousness are slowly being organized and the powers latent in *Prakṛti* are being unfolded. But after evolution has reached a sufficiently advanced stage and the desire for Self-realization is born within the soul *Rajas* and *Tamas* have to be replaced gradually by *Sattva*. So the object in *Yoga* is to harmonize *Rajas* and *Tamas* into *Sattva*. And as it is the harmonization of two opposites a perfect harmonization means really the virtual disappearance of the opposites and the attainment of a condition which is free from the opposites.

The question now arises ' Is the *Triguṇa-Sāmyāvasthā* before the *Puruṣa* came in contact with *Prakṛti* exactly the same as the condition of pure *Sattva* developed after going through the evolutionary cycle and attaining *Kaivalya*? ' The answer to this question must be in the negative. Because, if the two conditions were the same the whole purpose of evolution as outlined in II-23 would be defeated. It would really amount to supposing that the *Puruṣa* descends into matter, goes through the long and tedious evolutionary cycle and then again lapses into the condition from which he started.

If the two conditions are not identical, what is the difference between them? This is not the place to enter into this highly philosophical question but an analogy from the field of Science may serve to throw some light on the nature of the difference. A condition of equilibrium may be of two kinds which we may for the sake of convenience call static and dynamic. In static equilibrium two equal and opposite things combine in such a manner that the combination is a dead thing. You cannot get anything out of the combination because it does not contain potentially any power. If we mix together equivalent quantities of an acid and a base—two opposites—we get a neutral salt from which we cannot get anything else. On the other hand it is possible to produce a harmonious equilibrium of two equal and opposite things which is dynamic and contains potential power. Take a storage battery. In it lie two opposite kinds of electricity combined equally and harmoniously. Outwardly, the battery also appears a dead or inert thing. But only outwardly. We have only to connect the two poles to see the difference.

Now, the equilibrium of *Sattva* is something analogous to this equilibrium in a storage battery. It contains potentially the power to produce any combination of the *Guṇas* as required and yet reverting instantaneously to the original condition when the power is not needed. It is in this sense that the recession of the *Guṇas* to their origin in IV-34 should be understood. The *Guṇas* do not cease to function permanently for the Self-realized *Puruṣa*. They cease to function when he withdraws into himself and come into play as soon as he projects his consciousness outwards. In short, they lose their independent activity and become merely his instruments.

This conception of the *Guṇātīta* state not only imparts a new significance to the evolutionary cycle but is also in accordance with facts as known to Occultism. The mighty Adepts of *Yoga* who emerge as *Jīvanmuktas* from the evolutionary cycle do not merge into God and become indistinguishable from Him by losing their identity for ever. They become free from the domination of the *Guṇas* and the illusion of *Prakṛti* and yet retain all the knowledge and powers which they have acquired through evolution. Of all the misconceptions and partially understood truths of Hindu philosophy perhaps none is more absurd and a travesty of the real facts than this idea of *Puruṣa* merging completely with God and being lost in Him for ever. If a human being were to erect a house and then demolish it as soon as it was completed we should consider him mad. But we attribute to God a worse kind of irrationality in believing that on the attainment of *Jīvanmukti*, *Jīvātmā* merges with the *Paramātmā* and is lost for ever.

Having considered the nature of the material basis of the phenomenal world let us now pass on to the second generalization contained in the *Sūtra* which gives the *modus operandi* of the perception of this world. How is this world which is the result of the interplay of the *Guṇas* perceived? What are the basic elements involved in this perception? The answer to this question again is contained in a generalization which is a masterpiece of analytic technique. According to *Yogic* philosophy there are only two factors involved in perception—the *Bhūtas* and the *Indriyas*. What these *Bhūtas* and *Indriyas* are and how, by their interaction, they produce an awareness of the external world in the consciousness of the *Puruṣa* has been explained to some extent in discussing III-45 and III-48. We need not therefore enter into this question here but there is one important fact which may be pointed out before we pass on to the third generalization of the *Sūtra*. The words *Bhūtas* and *Indriyas* are used in the widest sense of these terms and have reference to the physical as well as the superphysical planes. The mechanism through which consciousness becomes aware of objects differs from plane to plane, but the *modus operandi* of this mechanism on every plane is essentially the same, namely the interaction of the *Bhūtas* and the *Indriyas*. Not only is the *modus operandi* the same on all the planes but the five states of the *Bhūtas* and *Indriyas* referred to in III-45 and III-48 are also the same on all the planes. *Saṃyama* on these states will therefore lead to the mastery of the *Bhūtas* and the *Indriyas* on all the planes.

The third generalization in this *Sūtra* gives the purpose of the phenomenal world. This is to provide experience and ultimately liberation for the *Puruṣa*. It is in some way, which is not quite comprehensible to the intellect, necessary for the *Puruṣa* to descend into matter and pass through the evolutionary process before he can become perfect and free from the domination of matter. The phenomenal world provides for him the necessary experiences through which alone evolution of his vehicles and unfolding of his consciousness can take place. As the seed after being sown absorbs the necessary nourishment from its environment and gradually develops into a full-grown tree after the likeness of its progenitor, in the same way, the germ of Divine Life when it is put in the phenomenal world is acted upon by all kinds of stimuli and influences and gradually unfolds the Divine Life and powers which are hidden within it. As this idea has been discussed fully later, in connection with II-23, we shall not consider it here.

The *Yogic* idea that the phenomenal world definitely exists for the growth and perfection of the individual centres of consciousness is in refreshing contrast to the bleak and vain speculations of modern Science on the origin and purpose of this manifested Universe. The idea that this wonderfully and beautifully designed Universe in which we live has no purpose, is really an insult to human intelligence and yet it is tacitly accepted by the large majority of modern scientists or the so-called intellectuals. If you ask the average scientist what he has to say about the purpose behind the Universe he will most probably show his impatience and reply that he does not know and does not care to know. He has very conveniently put aside the question of 'why' of the Universe so that he may be able to devote himself to the 'how' without being pestered by any uncomfortable doubts with regard to the utility of what he is doing. The most convenient way of avoiding your pursuers is to shut your eyes and forget about them.

१९. विशेषाविशेषलिङ्गमात्रालिङ्गानि गुणपर्वाणि ।

Viśeṣāviśeṣa-liṅgamātrāliṅgāni guṇa-parvāṇi.

विशेष particular; specific अविशेष non-specific; archetypal; universal लिङ्गमात्र a mere mark अलिङ्गानि (and) without mark or differentiating characteristic गुण (of) the *Guṇas* पर्वाणि stages of development; states.

19. The stages of the *Guṇas* are the particular, the universal, the differentiated and the undifferentiated.

The nature of the three *Guṇas* which was indicated in the last *Sūtra* is further elaborated in this *Sūtra*. The *Guṇas*, according to this *Sūtra*, have four states or stages of development corresponding to the four stages of *Saṃprajñāta Samādhi* mentioned in I-17. As consciousness and matter work together in the phenomenal world it is to be expected that the expression of the deeper layers of consciousness should require a subtler form of the three *Guṇas*. The essential nature of the *Guṇas* remains the same but they undergo a kind of subtilization, matching, as it were, each of these deeper or finer states of consciousness and enabling these to be expressed through matter. An illustration from the field of Science will perhaps enable the student to understand this relation between the states of consciousness and the stages of the *Guṇas*. Sound can be transmitted through a comparatively heavy medium like air but light, which is a much finer vibration, requires for its transmission a subtler medium like the ether.

As the states of consciousness which the *Yogi* has to pass through in *Samādhi* before he is released from the domination of the *Guṇas* are four, there should naturally be four stages of the *Guṇas*. While it is easy to understand why there should be four stages, still, when we come to the nature of these stages as defined in the present *Sūtra*, we find some difficulty in grasping the subtle significance of the words used for these stages. Since these stages correspond to the four stages of the unfoldment of consciousness in *Samādhi*, let us see whether we can find some help in studying these correspondences.

The characteristics of the four states of consciousness, the stages of the *Guṇas* and the vehicles through which these states of consciousness find expression are shown in the following table:

Characteristics of the states of consciousness	Stages of the Guṇas	Vehicle for expression in Vedāntic terminology
Vitarka	Viśeṣa	Manomaya Kośa
Vicāra	Aviśeṣa	Vijñānamaya Kośa
Ānanda	Liṅga	Ānandamaya Kośa
Asmitā	Aliṅga	Ātmā

The four stages of *Samprajñāta Samādhi* have already been discussed in dealing with I-17 and it has been shown that these stages correspond to the functioning of consciousness through the four vehicles as shown above. When the stages of the *Guṇas* are studied in the light of these correspondences the meanings of the words which are used to denote these stages become clear to some extent though it is impossible to grasp their full significance on account of the limitations of the intellect and the physical brain. Let us do the best we can under our present limitations.

The word *Viśeṣa* means particular and the *Viśeṣa* stage of the *Guṇas* obviously refers to the stage of the lower mind which sees all objects only as particular things with names and forms. To the lower mind every object seems to have a separate and independent existence and a separate identity. It is isolated, seen apart from its archetype and from the Divine consciousness of which it is a part and in which it is embedded, as it were. This stage of the *Guṇas* corresponds to the *Vitarka* stage of *Samādhi* because while consciousness is functioning through the lower mind *Vitarka* is its most important and essential function. *Vitarka* is that activity of the lower mind through which it differentiates a particular object from all others. How do we differentiate a particular dog, for example, from all other objects in the phenomenal world? The mental process may be illustrated by the following line of reasoning. A particular dog, say Bonzo, is a living animal. This differentiates it from all inanimate objects. Bonzo is an animal of the canine species. This differentiates it from all other species. Bonzo is a fox-terrier. This differentiates it from dogs of other breeds. We can in this way narrow down the range of objects from which Bonzo has still to be differentiated until we come down to the last stage when the object has been completely isolated in the mind and stands apart as a particular object in the Universe different and distinguishable from all other objects. This isolation or differentiation of a particular object which is illustrated by the crude example given above is called *Vitarka* and it is through such a process that the first stage of *Samādhi* is reached. The student will also see from the above the significance of the word *Viśeṣa*, particular, in indicating the first or crudest stage of the *Guṇas*.

Then we come to the next stage *Aviśeṣa* which means universal or non-specific. This corresponds to the activity of the higher mind whose function is to deal with universals, archetypes and principles which underlie the world of names and forms. The lower mind deals with particular objects with names and forms, the higher mind with abstract ideas and archetypes. Reverting to the previous illustration we saw that Bonzo was a particular dog of a particular breed. But what is this thing 'dog' of which Bonzo is a particular representative? The word 'dog' stands for an abstract idea. From observation of a large number of dogs we isolate all the characteristics which constitute their 'doghood' and combine them in a single concept which we denote by the word 'dog'. Every common noun is such an abstraction although we are hardly aware of this fact when we use such words. The mental process whereby these qualities are isolated from particular objects and combined in a single abstract concept is called *Vicāra*. The function of the higher mind is to form such universal concepts and to grasp their inner significance. It should be noted here that while *Vitarka* isolates a particular object from all the rest *Vicāra* isolates a particular concept, archetype, law, or universal principle from all such *Sūkṣma Viṣayas* referred to in I-44. This stage in which consciousness is functioning through the higher mind corresponds to the *Vicāra* stage of *Saṃprajñāta Samādhi* and the *Aviśeṣa* stage of the *Guṇas*. The justification for using the word *Aviśeṣa*, universal, for this second stage of the *Guṇas* will be seen, to a certain extent, from what has been said above.

It may be pointed out here that the simple mental process of *Vitarka* or *Vicāra* which we may engage in during the course of our studies and thinking should not be considered equivalent to the corresponding mental processes as they take place in the state of *Samādhi*. In the state of *Samādhi* the mind is completely isolated from the outer world, is fused, as it were, with the object in a state of abstraction. It is in a peculiar and to the ordinary man incomprehensible state. And so, concrete and abstract thinking are merely faint reflections, qualitative representations of the extremely subtle mental processes which take place in *Samādhi*. The reason why words like *Vitarka* and *Vicāra* are used to indicate these subtle mental processes lies in the fact that the ordinary reasoning processes are familiar to the student and it is only in this way that he can get some idea of the subtler processes. From the known to the unknown is always the right method of advancing in the realm of the mind.

Then we come to the next stage of the *Guṇas—Liṅga.* This word means a mark which serves to identify, and in the present context *Liṅga-mātra* means a state of consciousness in which particular objects and even principles are mere marks or signs which serve to distinguish them from other objects. This stage of the *Guṇas* corresponds to the supra-mental consciousness which transcends the intellect and is expressed through *Buddhi* or intuition. The corresponding stage in *Samādhi* is accompanied by *Ānanda* which confirms the conclusion that this stage of the *Guṇas* corresponds to the functioning of consciousness through the *Buddhic* vehicle or *Ānandamaya Kośa* as it is called in *Vedāntic* terminology.

But why is this stage of the *Guṇas* called *Liṅga*? Because in the corresponding state of consciousness all objects and universal principles become part of a universal consciousness. They are seen, embedded as it were, in one consciousness, as parts of an indivisible whole. But they still have their identity, are still distinguishable or recognizable. Each object is itself and yet part of a whole. It is a condition of unity in diversity.

The next and the last stage of the *Guṇas* is called *Aliṅga* or without mark or differentiating characteristic. In this stage the objects and principles lose their separate identity. Consciousness becomes so predominant that they go out of focus, as it were. According to the highest conceptions of the Hindu philosophy all objects, archetypes, everything in the manifested Universe is a modification of consciousness—*Brahma-Vṛtti.* In the *Liṅga* stage awareness of objects exists side by side with the awareness of consciousness. In the *Aliṅga* stage the former go out of focus and only awareness of the Divine consciousness of which they are modifications remains. A concrete example may perhaps help the student to understand the significance of the different stages of the *Guṇas.* Suppose we have a number of objects made of gold—a ring, a bracelet and a necklace, placed on a table. We may see them merely as separate objects, as a child would see them. This corresponds to the *Viśeṣa* stage. We may see them as ornaments with a common function of serving to adorn the human body, as a woman would see them. This is the *Aviśeṣa* stage. We may see them as objects with a common decorative function but we may also be interested in the fact that they are made of gold, i.e., we see their common substratum and their separate identity simultaneously, as a goldsmith would see them. This corresponds to the *Liṅga* stage. And lastly, we may see only the gold and may hardly be conscious of their separate identities or common function, as a thief would see them. This is analogous to the *Aliṅga* stage. In this stage the *Yogi* is conscious, chiefly of the substratum of all phenomenal objects, particular or universal. He is aware predominantly of the Divine consciousness in which they are merely *Vṛttis* or modifications. The objects as separate entities do exist but they have ceased to have any meaning for him. This stage of the *Guṇas* corresponds to the last stage of *Saṃprajñāta Samādhi* of which *Asmitā* is the predominant characteristic. The consciousness of pure existence which is denoted by *Asmitā* swallows up the consciousness of objects.

The progressive expansion of consciousness which takes place when it passes through the different stages of *Samādhi* does not mean that these states of consciousness are separated from each other by water-tight compartments and the lower aspects of object disappear when the higher come into view. Many students feel confused because they suffer from a common misconception about the functioning of consciousness in the higher worlds. They think, for example, that when the *Yogi* passes into the world of the higher mind he lives solely in a world of abstract ideas, archetypes and principles with no objects having names and forms with which he has been familiar. Such a world of pure abstractions would be an impossible world to live in and does not exist anywhere as the experiences of all mystics and occultists testify. The higher always includes and enriches the lower though it also enables the lower to be seen in its correct perspective. What was considered important may now appear unimportant or what was considered insignificant may now assume tremendous significance, and *vice versa*, but everything is there within the expanded consciousness, and the *Yogi* does not therefore feel he has entered into a strange and incomprehensible world. On the other hand, every expansion of consciousness makes him see greater richness, beauty and significance in everything which is within the range of his perception. Expansion of consciousness means inclusion of more and more and exclusion of nothing. This fact is quite clear from what is stated in III-50 III-55 and IV-31.

It will be seen that the four stages of the *Guṇas* are denoted by the predominant nature of the mental perception and activity which characterize those stages. We are told how the changes in the *Guṇas* affect the expression of consciousness through them but we are not given any indication as to the nature of the changes in the *Guṇas* themselves. This kind of classification which is based upon the secondary effects of the changes in the *Guṇas* does not, therefore, throw much further light on the nature of the *Guṇas* themselves. Since the *Guṇas* lie at the very basis of the manifested Universe and their roots are embedded in the deepest layers of consciousness their subtle nature can be realized only in *Samādhi* (III-45). The intellect can, at best, enable us to gain only a general idea with regard to their nature and their gross expressions on the lowest plane.

२०. द्रष्टा दृशिमात्रः शुद्धोऽपि प्रत्ययानुपश्यः ।

Draṣṭā dṛśimātraḥ śuddho 'pi pratyayā-
nupaśyaḥ.

द्रष्टा the Seer; *Puruṣa* दृशिमात्रः pure consciousness only; pure awareness only शुद्ध pure अपि though प्रत्यय concept; content of the mind अनुपश्यः appears to see along with.

20. The Seer is pure consciousness but though pure, appears to see through the mind.

After dealing with *Dṛśyam* or the objective side of the phenomenal world in II-18 and 19, Patañjali now tries to give us some idea with regard to the *Draṣṭā* or the Seer who is the basis of the subjective side of the phenomenal world. This is a comparatively more difficult task because the *Puruṣa* according to the *Yogic* philosophy is the ultimate Reality hidden behind the phenomenal world in its subjective aspect. Although it is through him that the *Prakṛti* is galvanized into life and cognition takes place, he always eludes us, because he is always behind the veil, the hidden witness of the objective through the subjective. If we take a powerful electric light and cover it up with a number of concentric semi-transparent and coloured globes, one within the other, the outermost globe will be illuminated in some measure by the light of the electric lamp. But though this illumination will be derived from the light of the electric lamp we will not be able to see the light of the electric lamp as it is, but only as it comes out after being filtered and dimmed by all the intervening globes. If we remove the outermost globe the next globe comes into view and the light becomes stronger and purer. But do we now see the light of the electric lamp? No! It is still hidden behind the remaining globes. As we remove globe after globe, the light becomes stronger and purer but we never see it in its purity and fullness as long as any globe remains covering the electric lamp. It is only when the last globe is removed that the pure light of the electric lamp in its total brilliance comes into view. Can the man who has never seen an electric lamp know by observing the outermost globe what the light of the electric lamp is like? Not until he has removed all the globes, one by one.

The relation of the *Puruṣa* to the vehicles through which he manifests is similar. The light of his consciousness comes streaming through the complete set of vehicles, each vehicle removing, as it were, some of the constituents and decreasing its intensity, until in the physical body it is at its dullest and encumbered with the largest number of limitations. The only way to see the light of his pure consciousness is to separate off all the vehicles and see that light in its purity without the obscuration even of the subtlest vehicle as pointed out in IV-22. This is the isolation of pure consciousness (*Kaivalya*) involved in the attainment of *Kaivalya*, the ultimate goal of *Yogic* life.

The first point we should note in this *Sūtra* is that the Seer who is the subjective element in the phenomenal world is pure consciousness and nothing else. The word *Mātraḥ* of course means 'only' and is used to emphasize the necessity of not mistaking the Seer for any partial manifestation of his consciousness through a subtler vehicle. When consciousness withdraws, step by step, from the lower worlds in *Samādhi* and begins to function in the higher realms of the Spirit the change is so tremendous and the sudden influx of power, knowledge and bliss, on the progressive removal of limitations, is so overwhelming that one is apt to mistake this partial manifestation for the ultimate Reality. But the fact is that the consciousness is still encumbered by veils of matter, thin veils it is true, but veils all the same which impose certain limitations and illusions. Not until the last vehicle has been transcended can consciousness be known in its purity. That is the *Puruṣa*, the real *Draṣṭa*.

The second point to be noted is that though the Seer is pure consciousness, and not consciousness as modified by the vehicles, still, when he manifests through a vehicle he *seems* to be lost in the *Pratyaya* which is present at the moment in the mind. Just as a mirror reflects or assumes the form of anything placed before it and *seems* to be that thing, in the same way the pure consciousness assumes, as it were, the form of the *Pratyaya* and appears indistinguishable from the *Pratyaya*. Or, to take another example, when the pure light from the electric bulb in a cinematograph falls on the screen it assumes the form of the picture being projected, though in itself it is pure and quite distinct from the picture. *Pratyaya*, of course, as has been explained elsewhere, is the content of the mind when consciousness comes in contact with any vehicle and differs from vehicle to vehicle.

Not only is the *Pratyaya* indistinguishable from consciousness but as a result of this mixing up of the two, the functions of the vehicles appear to be performed by the *Puruṣa*. Thus when abstract thinking is done through the higher mind is it the *Puruṣa* who does the thinking? No! The thinking is the function of the vehicle. The contact of consciousness with the vehicle sets it in motion and enables it to perform its respective function. When a magnet is thrust into a coil of wire a current of electricity is produced in the wire. To a person who is ignorant of the facts the magnet appears to produce the current. As a matter of fact the magnet does not directly produce the current though it is in a mysterious manner connected with the production of the current. If the whole mechanism for the production of the current is there and all the necessary conditions are provided then only the insertion of the magnet will make the mechanism work to produce the current. How the mere contact of *Puruṣa* with *Prakṛti* galvanizes it into life and makes it perform its highly intelligent function is a problem which has been much debated by philosophers. To the practical student of *Yoga* this question is not of much importance. He knows that all such theoretical questions can be solved only by direct knowledge.

२१. तदर्थ एव दृश्यस्यात्मा ।

Tad-artha eva dṛśyasyātmā.

तद्+अर्थः(intended) for the sake of that (the Seer) एव alone दृश्यस्य of the Seen (*Prakṛti*) आत्मा (being); nature.

21. The very being of the Seen is for his sake (i.e. *Prakṛti* exists only for his sake).

In the previous *Sūtras* the essential natures of the Seer and Seen have been pointed out, and it has been shown that even when they seem to be blended completely in their intimate relationship they are really quite distinct and separate from each other like oil and water in an emulsion. This *Sūtra* points out that in this close association of *Puruṣa* and *Prakṛti*, the latter plays a subordinate role, that of merely serving the *Puruṣa*. The purpose of the Seen has already been given in II-18, namely providing experience and means of emancipation for the *Puruṣa*. The *Sūtra* under discussion further clarifies this point and emphasizes that *Prakṛti* exists only for subserving the purposes of the *Puruṣa*. It has no purpose of its own. The whole drama of creation is being played in order to provide experience for the growth and Self-realization of the *Puruṣas* who are involved in the show.

२२. कृतार्थं प्रति नष्टमप्यनष्टं तदन्यसाधारणत्वात् ।

Kṛtārthaṃ prati naṣṭam apy anaṣṭaṃ
tad-anya-sādhāraṇatvāt.

कृतार्थं (one) whose purpose has been fulfilled प्रति for; to नष्टम् destroyed; non-existent अपि although अनष्टम् not destroyed; existent तत् (than) that अन्य to others साधारणत्वात् on account of being common.

22. Although it becomes non-existent for him whose purpose has been fulfilled it continues to exist for others on account of being common to others (besides him).

This *Sūtra* again deals with a purely theoretical problem of philosophy connected with the relationship existing between *Puruṣa* and *Prakṛti*. If the purpose of *Prakṛti* is to enable the *Puruṣa* to obtain Self-realization what happens to it when that purpose has been fulfilled? The answer given is that *Prakṛti* ceases to exist as far as that *Puruṣa* is concerned. But what does this mean? Does *Prakṛti* cease to exist altogether? Obviously not, because the other *Puruṣas* who have not attained *Kaivalya* still remain under its influence and continue to work for their emancipation.

If *Prakṛti* ceases to exist only for the Self-realized *Puruṣa*, then is it purely subjective in its nature or has it an independent existence of its own? The answer to this fundamental question differs according to different schools of thought which have tried to speculate about it. According to *Vedānta* even *Prakṛti*, the substratum of the phenomenal world, is a purely subjective thing, the product of *Māyā*. According to *Sāṃkhya* which provides to a great extent the theoretical basis of the *Yogic* philosophy *Prakṛti* has an independent existence of its own. *Puruṣa* and *Prakṛti* are the two ultimate, eternal and independent principles in existence. *Puruṣas* are many, *Prakṛti* is one. The *Puruṣas* get involved in matter, go through the cycle of evolution under the fostering care of *Prakṛti*, attain Self-realization and then pass out of the illusion and influence of *Prakṛti* altogether. But *Prakṛti* always remains the same. It will be seen that there is no real contradiction involved in these two views. *Vedānta* merely carries the process of idealization to a further stage which alone can be the ultimate stage. In it the multiplicity of the *Puruṣas* on the one hand, and the duality of the *Puruṣas* and the *Prakṛti* on the other, are integrated into a higher conception of the One Reality.

It may be pointed out here that a system of philosophy however lofty and true it may be should not be expected to give us an absolutely correct picture of the transcendent truths as they really exist. Because philosophy works through the medium of the intellect and the intellect has its inherent limitations, it cannot understand or formulate truths which are beyond its scope. So, in dealing in its own way with these realities of the spiritual life it can give us only partial and distorted interpretations of those realities. Contradictions, paradoxes and inconsistencies are inevitable when we try to see and interpret these realities through the instrumentality of the intellect. We have to accept these limitations when we use the intellect as an instrument for understanding and discovering these truths in the initial stages. It is no use throwing away this instrument, poor and imperfect though it is, because it gives us at least some help in organizing our effort to know the truth in the only way in which it can be known—by Self-realization. If we want to know any country the only way to do it is to go and see it with our own eyes. But that does not mean that we should throw away the maps and plans which are meant to give us a rough idea with regard to the country. These do not give us true knowledge with regard to the country but they do help us in finding the country and seeing it directly with our own eyes. Philosophy, at its best, serves only this kind of purpose. Those who are content to take it as a substitute for the real truth blunder. Those who ignore it completely also make a mistake because they throw away a thing which might be usefully utilized in the attainment of their objective. The wise student of *Yoga* takes the various doctrines of philosophy and religion lightly, as tentative explanations and interpretations of truths beyond the realm of the intellect, but uses them as best as he can in his direct discovery of those truths. *Yoga* is an essentially practical science and the truths and experiences which it deals with are not dependent upon the particular philosophy or philosophies which are put forward to provide a rational picture of the objective and the various processes which lead to it. We do not know really the nature of electricity. There are many theories. But that does not prevent us from utilizing this force for gaining our physical ends in a thousand and one ways. In the same way the philosophy which provides the theoretical background of *Yoga* and its inadequacies does not affect materially the results which can be obtained by the practice of *Yoga*. Let us give philosophy its proper place in the study of *Yoga* and not mix it up with the practical and scientific part of the subject.

२३. स्वस्वामिशक्त्योः स्वरूपोपलब्धिहेतुः संयोगः ।

Sva-svāmi-śaktyoḥ svarūpopalabdhi-hetuḥ saṃyogaḥ.

स्व (of) it (*Prakṛti*) स्वामि (and) of the master (*Puruṣa*) शक्त्योः of the (two) powers स्वरूप own form; real or essential nature उपलब्धि experiencing; knowledge हेतुः cause; reason; purpose संयोगः union; coming together.

23. The purpose of the coming together of the *Puruṣa* and *Prakṛti* is gaining by the *Puruṣa* of the awareness of his true nature and the unfoldment of powers inherent in him and *Prakṛti*.

It is generally thought that the idea of evolution is an entirely new contribution made by Science to modern civilization, and Darwin is considered to be the father of this idea. But as we often say there is nothing new under the Sun and the idea of evolution has come down to us in one form or another from the earliest times. It would be really surprising if the master minds who lived in the past and who had such a wonderful grasp of the essential realities of life had missed this important and all-pervading Law underlying the manifestation of life. It is perhaps true that this Law was not studied and presented in the detailed form as we have it now but then nothing pertaining to the phenomenal world which was not essential for real human happiness was studied by them in great detail. It was thought sufficient to have a general idea of the fundamental principles. They never lost sight of the limitations of the intellect and probably did not consider it worth while wasting their time and energy on the accumulation of unnecessary details with regard to the general principles which at best could be understood very imperfectly through the medium of the illusion-bound intellect. It was thought that the energy which would be needed for gaining knowledge of the non-essential details had better be employed in unravelling the Great Mystery of Life itself, for when that mystery was unravelled all the problems of life were understood automatically and simultaneously and in a way they could never be understood by a process of intellectual analysis and reasoning.

But while these adepts in the Science of Life did not think it worth their while descending to non-essential details with regard to the facts of the phenomenal worlds they tried and managed to get a wonderfully complete and true picture of the fundamental principles. It is this clear and firm grasp of the fundamental principles and laws which enabled them to put these principles and generalizations in the form of *Sūtras*. What a modern writer would take a chapter or book to convey was condensed in a masterly manner in a single *Sūtra*. There are many examples of such condensed knowledge in the *Yoga-Sūtras*, and II-23 which we shall now consider is a striking instance of this nature. In one *Sūtra* Patañjali has put the essential and fundamental idea underlying the theory of Evolution and also managed to bring into his generalization the most important aspect of evolution which unfortunately is missing in the modern scientific theory. So absorbed are most of our modern scientists with details, so full of their own achievements, so obsessed by their materialistic outlook that they often miss the most important aspects of their researches, aspects which are under their very noses and which they could not fail to recognize if they were at all open-minded. The theory of Evolution which we are now considering is a case in point.

According to the modern theory, considered in a very general way, there is an evolutionary trend discernible in the bodies of plants and animals, and the bodies in their effort to adapt themselves to their environment develop new powers and capacities.

Putting the idea in a different way we may say that the study of the form side of living creatures shows that these forms are steadily, though slowly, becoming more and more complex and capable of expressing the powers which are inherent in life. Life and form are always found together. The forms are found to evolve. What about the life? Modern Science does not know and what is more surprising does not care to know. For the idea that life evolves side by side with form is well known and is really complementary to the idea of the evolution of forms, which has been developed by Science. It is by combining this idea of the evolution of life with that of the evolution of forms that the theory of evolution becomes intelligible and its beauty and significance are revealed. The forms evolve to provide better vehicles for the evolving life. The mere evolution of forms would be a meaningless process in a Universe in which all natural phenomena appear to be guided by intelligence and design. And yet modern Science is pursuing this idea of the evolution of forms and refusing to combine it with its complementary idea. No wonder it got bogged in a plethora of details in this field and missed the discovery of some basic facts of general and vital interest to humanity.

II-23 answers the question 'Why is *Puruṣa* brought into contact with *Prakṛti*?' The answer is: To unfold the powers latent in *Prakṛti* and himself and to enable him to gain Self-realization. That is the complete idea of evolution in a nutshell. But it is necessary to elaborate this idea to understand its full implications. Let us first see what are the powers of *Puruṣa* and *Prakṛti* referred to in this *Sūtra*. In order to understand this we have only to recall how total evolution leads to the gradual unfoldment of consciousness on the one hand and *pari passu* to the increase in the efficiency of the vehicles on the other. Leaving out of account the mineral kingdom in which the unfoldment of consciousness is so rudimentary as to be hardly perceptible we find on studying the vegetable, animal and human kingdoms that consciousness in these kingdoms shows a remarkable increase in the degree of unfoldment as we pass from one kingdom to another. And side by side with the unfoldment of consciousness we find that the vehicle also becomes more and more complex and efficient for the expression of the unfolding consciousness. Not only do we find a remarkable increase in this dual evolution of life and form as we pass from one kingdom to another but taking any one kingdom by itself we can trace the steady evolution from one step to another, so that we can see the whole ladder of life as far as it can be seen with our limitations, stretching from the mineral kingdom to the civilized stage of the human kingdom with hardly any rungs missing.

What do we mean by the powers of *Prakṛti* referred to in this *Sūtra*? Obviously, these are not the general powers which are inherent in Nature and which are independent, as it were, of the dual evolution of life and form which is taking place around us. The powers of *Prakṛti* to which reference is made here are undoubtedly the capacities which develop in the vehicles as they evolve in association with consciousness. Compare the brain of a snail with that of a monkey and this again with that of a highly civilized man and you see the tremendous change which has taken place as regards the capacity of the vehicle to express the powers which are latent in consciousness. And the mental and spiritual powers which are exhibited by the highly civilized and intellectual men and women of today are as nothing compared to the powers which are developed by the advanced *Yogi* and which are in store for every child of man when he undertakes his higher evolution. A study of the various *Siddhis* or occult powers which are dealt with in Section III of the *Yoga-sūtras* will give the student some idea of the latent capacities which are lying hidden within each one of us, capacities which can be developed by the technique outlined in this book.

It is necessary to distinguish between the powers of *Prakṛti* and *Puruṣa* although the two are generally exercised in conjunction. The power of *Prakṛti* is obviously the capacity of the vehicle to respond to the demands of consciousness. A particular vehicle of consciousness is a certain combination of matter on a particular plane integrated and held together by various forces and its efficiency depends upon how far it can respond to the powers of consciousness. The brain of an idiot is made of the same substance as the brain of a highly intellectual man but there is a world of difference between the capacities of the two to respond to thought vibrations. It is in the increasing peculiarity and complexity of the vehicle that the secret of its greater responsiveness and efficiency lies and this is what evolution of the vehicle really means.

If the response to consciousness determines the evolution of the vehicle what is meant by the unfoldment of the powers of consciousness or *Puruṣa*? According to *Yogic* philosophy consciousness itself does not evolve. It is in some way which is incomprehensible to the intellect perfect, complete, eternal. When we refer to the powers of the *Puruṣa* in this joint development of the powers of the two what is meant is the power of consciousness to function through and in collaboration with the vehicle. As *Puruṣa* is pure consciousness and consciousness is eternal, there cannot be an evolution of his powers in the sense in which we take the word evolution. But we may suppose that he has to acquire the capacity to use those in association with the matter of the different planes. So that, as evolution proceeds his consciousness is able to express itself more and more fully on these planes and to manipulate and control his vehicles with increasing freedom and efficiency. What a tremendous task this is can be grasped only when we study in detail the long process of evolution through the different kingdoms of Nature and the total constitution of man which is involved in the process. As long as we confine ourselves to the phenomena of the physical plane we can never have an adequate idea of the magnitude and nature of the task, even though on the physical plane also the different phases of this long process present a stupendous spectacle. It is in the invisible realms of the mind and the Spirit that evolution produces its most magnificent results and the powers of the *Puruṣa* find their chief expression.

Perhaps some idea of the necessity and manner of this development may be obtained from a simile. The music which a great musician can produce depends upon the quality and the efficiency of his instrument. Place an instrument in his hand which he has never used and he will feel helpless till he has mastered that instrument. The poor quality of the instrument will handicap him enormously. The quality of the music which can be produced depends upon three factors, the capacity of the musician, the efficiency of the instrument and the co-ordination of the two. Even though the *Puruṣa* has all the powers potentially unless he is provided with an efficient set of vehicles and learns to control and use these vehicles he may remain a helpless spectator of the world drama which is being played around him. It is in some such way that we can visualize through the intellect the gradual unfoldment of the powers of the *Puruṣa* along with the powers of *Prakṛti*, though fundamentally, this question is an ultimate question connected with the 'why' of manifestation and thus beyond the scope of the intellect.

The simultaneous development of the vehicles on all the planes of manifestation and the capacity to use them is not the only purpose of bringing together *Puruṣa* and *Prakṛti*. The *Puruṣa* has not only to master these vehicles but has also to transcend them. For, until and unless he can do this he will remain under the limitations of the planes to which he is confined and be subject to their illusions. He is destined to be above the limitations and illusions of those planes as well as to be a master of those planes. This is what Self-realization or *Svarūpopalabdhi* means to accomplish. These are not to be considered as two independent objectives. The complete mastery of the lower planes and their transcendence are really two aspects of the same problem because complete mastery on these planes is not possible until the *Puruṣa* passes out of the control of *Prakṛti*. The last step in the mastery of anything generally consists in transcending it or going beyond its influence and control. Then only we can know it fully and control it completely.

२४. तस्य हेतुरविद्या।

Tasya hetur avidyā.

तस्य its (of the union) हेतुः (effective) cause अविद्या ignorance; lack of awareness of his Real nature.

24 Its cause is the lack of awareness of his Real nature.

After giving the purpose of the union of *Puruṣa* and *Prakṛti* in the last *Sūtra* Patañjali gives in this *Sūtra* the effective cause of the union or the means whereby the union is brought about. It should be noted that the word *Hetuḥ* is used both in the sense of object as well as effective cause and it is used in the latter sense in this *Sūtra.* The *Puruṣa* by his very nature is eternal, omniscient and free and his involution in matter which involves tremendous limitations is brought about by his being made to lose the awareness of his Real nature. The power which deprives him of this knowledge or rather awareness of his Real nature is called *Māyā* or Illusion in Hindu philosophy and the result of this privation of knowledge is called *Avidyā* or ignorance. It is obvious that the words illusion and ignorance are used in their highest philosophical sense and we can barely get a glimpse into the real significance of these words. To understand *Māyā* and *Avidyā* in the real sense is to solve the Great Mystery of Life and to be free from their domination. This is the end and not the starting point of the search.

How *Avidyā* brings about in its train the other *Kleśas* and lies at the root of all miseries to which embodied life is subject has been dealt with already in explaining the nature of *Kleśas,* but there is one aspect of this union of *Puruṣa* and *Prakṛti* which must be pointed out if we are to understand the meaning of this travail and suffering which evolution undoubtedly involves. We have seen already that there appears to be a mighty purpose hidden behind the working of the Universe though the nature of this purpose may be beyond our comprehension. One part of this purpose which we can see and understand is the gradual evolution of life culminating in the perfection and emancipation of the individual units of consciousness who are called *Puruṣas.* We have been sent down into the lower worlds in order that we may attain perfection through the experiences of these worlds. It is a tremendously long and tedious discipline but it is worthwhile as anybody will see who understands what this perfection means and knows those in whom this perfection is embodied. Anyway, whether we like this process or not we are in it and have to go through it and it is no use behaving like children who try to avoid going to school and have to be sent there against their will. The best way of freeing ourselves from this necessity is to acquire perfection as quickly as we can. Then there will be no necessity of our being forced to remain in this school and our freedom will come automatically.

It is very necessary to point out this aspect of our bondage because there are a large number of aspirants, especially in India, who have a rather strange notion with regard to the cause and nature of the bondage in which they find themselves. They do not take life on the lower planes as a kind of school in which they have to learn certain things but rather as a prison from which they have to escape as soon as possible. They hardly realize the implications of this attitude which really means that they consider God as a heartless Being who sends His children into the lower worlds just for the fun of seeing them go through all this pain and suffering. If life in the lower worlds is taken as a school then we shall not only feel no resentment against the severe discipline to which we are subjected but will also adopt the right means for getting out of the miseries and sufferings which are incidental to this life. The right means obviously is that we should learn the necessary lessons as thoroughly and as quickly as possible instead of merely devising means of escape which are bound to prove ineffective in the long run. Seen in this light *Yogic* discipline is merely the last phase of our training whereby our education is completed and rounded off before we are allowed to lead a free and independent life.

२५. तदभावात् संयोगाभावो हानं तद् दृशेः कैवल्यम् ।

Tad-abhāvāt saṃyogābhāvo hānaṃ tad dṛśeḥ kaivalyam.

तद् (of) that (*Avidyā*) अभावात् from absence or elimination संयोग (of) union; association अभाव: disappearance हानं (is) avoidance; remedy तत् that दृशेः of the Seer कैवल्यम् (is) isolation; separation from everything (Liberation).

25. The dissociation of *Puruṣa* and *Prakṛti* brought about by the dispersion of *Avidyā* is the real remedy and that is the Liberation of the Seer.

If the union of *Puruṣa* and *Prakṛti* has been brought about by *Māyā* or *Avidyā* and leads through the development of the *Kleśas* to the misery and sufferings of embodied existence it follows logically that the removal of these latter is possible only when the union is dissolved by the destruction of *Avidyā*. The union is the sole cause of bondage. Its dissolution must therefore be the only means available for Emancipation or *Kaivalya* of the Seer. The bondage is maintained by the *Puruṣa* identifying himself with his vehicles right from the *Ātmic* to the physical plane. The release is brought about by his disentangling himself *in consciousness* from his vehicles one after another until he stands free from them, even though using them merely as instruments.

It should be clearly understood that the dissociation of consciousness from a particular vehicle is not merely a matter of understanding brought about by a process of reasoning and intellectual analysis; though such efforts can help us to a certain extent in relation to our lower vehicles. The illusion is destroyed completely and in the real sense only when the *Yogi* is able to leave the vehicle at will in *Samādhi* and to look down upon it, as it were, from a higher plane. Then he realizes definitely that he is different from that particular vehicle and can never, after such an experience, identify himself with that vehicle as has been explained in dealing with II-6. The process of separating off the vehicle and disentangling consciousness from it is repeated over and over again on the superphysical planes until the last vehicle—the *Ātmic*—is transcended in *Nirbīja Samādhi* and the *Puruṣa* stands free (*Svarūpe'vasthānam*) 'in his own-form'. It will be seen, therefore, that the discarding of the successive vehicles of consciousness on the subtler planes, which can be done through the practice of *Samādhi*, is the only way of destroying *Asmitā* and *Avidyā* and people who think that by merely repeating mentally formulas like *Ahaṃ Brahmāsmi* (I am Brahman) or by trying to imagine themselves separate from their vehicles they can gain Self-realization do not really know the nature of the task which they are trying to accomplish. It is really amazing to what extent people can over-simplify problems and hypnotize themselves into believing that their generally trivial experiences mean realization of the Ultimate Truth.

२६. विवेकख्यातिरविप्लवा हानोपायः।

Viveka-khyātir aviplavā hānopāyaḥ.

विवेकख्याति: discriminative cognition; awareness of the distinction between the Self and the not-Self; awareness of Reality अविप्लवा unbroken; unfluctuating; unfailing; incessant हानोपाय: the means of avoidance; the means of abolition; remedy; the means of dispersion.

26. The uninterrupted practice of the awareness of the Real is the means of dispersion (of *Avidyā*).

Having given in the previous *Sūtra* the general principle underlying the destruction of *Avidyā* the author gives in this *Sūtra* the practical method which has to be adopted to bring this about. The method prescribed is the practice of uninterrupted *Viveka-Khyāti*. What is this *Viveka-Khyāti?* *Viveka* means, of course, discrimination between the Real and the unreal and the general idea underlying this word is familiar to students of *Yogic* philosophy. *Khyāti* is usually translated as knowledge or consciousness. So *Viveka-Khyāti* means knowledge of the discrimination between the Real and the unreal. As this does not make much sense let us examine the two words *Viveka* and *Khyāti* more fully.

Viveka is generally used for that state of the mind in which it is aware of the great problems of life and the illusions which are inherent in ordinary human life. In the state of *Aviveka* we take everything as a matter of course. The great problems of life do not exist for us, or if they do, they are of mere academic interest. There is no desire to question life, to see beyond its ordinary illusions, to discriminate between the things of real and permanent value and those of passing interest. When the light of *Viveka* dawns on the mind all this changes. We become very much alive to the fundamental problems of life, begin to question life's values and detach ourselves from the current of ordinary thoughts and desires, and above all, we want to find that Reality which is hidden behind the flux of phenomena. This is not a mere process of thinking but an illuminated state of the mind. It may come temporarily as a result of some shock in life or may grow naturally and become a permanent feature of our outlook on life.

When it is a normal feature of our life it is really the harbinger of the spiritual development which is to follow. The soul is awakening from its long spiritual sleep and now wants to find itself. It has reached maturity and wants to come into its Divine heritage. Ordinary *Viveka* is merely a symptom of these changes which are taking place in the recesses of the soul.

Now, the point to be noted here is that this kind of *Viveka* is only a reflection of the spiritual consciousness into the lower mind, a sensing, as it were, of the Reality hidden within us. It is not an actual *awareness* of Reality. *Viveka-Khyāti* is an actual awareness of Reality, a direct, immediate contact with the innermost spiritual consciousness, *Pratyakṣa* knowledge of Reality. What the sense of touch is to the sense of sight that is *Viveka* to *Viveka-Khyāti.* In the case of the former we merely sense the Reality within us more or less dimly. In the case of the latter we are in direct contact with it though in different degrees.

The awareness of Reality or *Viveka-Khyāti* is the opposite of *Avidyā*—lack of awareness of Reality, the two being related to each other as light and darkness. When the *Puruṣa* is fully aware of Reality he is out of the dominion of *Avidyā.* When he loses this awareness he relapses into *Avidyā* and the other *Kleśas.* It will be seen that real discrimination between the Real and the unreal is possible only when we have experienced Reality and know both the Real and the unreal. When a beginner is asked to discriminate between the Real and the unreal what is really meant is that he should learn to discriminate between the things of permanent value in life and those which are transitory.

In the light of what has been said above the meaning of the *Sūtra* we are dealing with should become clear. Since *Avidyā* can be overcome only by the awareness of Reality the cultivation of the latter obviously is the only means whereby release from bondage can be achieved. The significance of the word *Aviplavā* is, of course, apparent. The awareness must be continuous, undisturbed. It is only then that *Kaivalya* may be considered to be attained. A mere glimpse of Reality does not constitute

Kaivalya although it certainly shows that the goal is near. The *Puruṣa* must have reached the stage where this awareness can no longer be obscured even temporarily by *Avidyā*. This point is developed more fully in the last Section.

२७. तस्य सप्तधा प्रान्तभूमिः प्रज्ञा ।

Taṣya saptadhā prānta-bhūmiḥ prajñā.

तस्य His (*Puruṣa's*) सप्तधा sevenfold प्रान्तभूमिः a definite stage; step; layer; 'bordering' province प्रज्ञा the cognitive consciousness.

27. In his case the highest stage of Enlightenment is reached by seven stages.

This *Sūtra* merely points out that the state of uninterrupted awareness of Reality is attained through seven stages. After the *Yogi* has obtained his first glimpse of Reality he has to pass through seven stages of increasing awareness before he reaches the final goal of *Kaivalya*. The word *Prānta-bhūmiḥ* is used to indicate that progress through these stages does not take place by sudden jumps, as it were, but by gradual transition from one stage to another like traversing a country divided into seven adjacent provinces.

A good deal of rigmarole has been written in explaining this *Sūtra* by some commentators. It is quite natural that the process of attaining full Enlightenment should be gradual and should be attained by stages. But to identify these transcendent changes in consciousness with ordinary processes of thinking as has been done by some commentators is really absurd. It is better to leave the problem as it is, as a matter of transcendent experiences which cannot be interpreted in terms of the thinking processes.

२८. योगाङ्गानुष्ठानादशुद्धिक्षये ज्ञानदीप्तिरा विवेकख्यातेः ।

Yogāṅgānuṣṭhānād aśuddhi-kṣaye jñāna-dīptir ā viveka-khyāteḥ.

योगाङ्ग (of) component parts of *Yoga*; (exercises) or steps of *Yoga* अनुष्ठानात् by practice or following अशुद्धि of impurity क्षये on the destruction (the idea is of gradual diminishing) ज्ञान knowledge (spiritual knowledge) दीप्तिः shining forth; radiance आ विवेकख्यातेः till awareness of Reality or discriminative knowledge (arises).

28. From the practice of the component exercises of *Yoga*, on the destruction of impurity, arises spiritual illumination which develops into awareness of Reality.

II-28 deals with the problem of guidance needed on the path of *Yoga*. It has been said already that ordinary *Viveka* is an expression of the spiritual consciousness hidden behind the mind. If it is real it gives a sufficiently strong urge to the aspirant to take to the path of *Yoga* and adopt its discipline. But it is not sufficiently definite to lead him on the path of *Yoga* and to provide him with the necessary guidance in the mysterious realm of the Unknown. Where is this guidance to come from? According to this *Sūtra* guidance on the path of *Yoga* comes from within in the form of spiritual illumination. This light of spiritual consciousness which is akin to intuition but more definite in its working appears only when the impurities of the mind have been destroyed to a great extent as result of practising *Yogic* discipline. This inner light of wisdom has been given many beautiful and suggestive names such as 'The Voice of the Silence', 'Light on the Path' and perhaps the most graphic and illuminative description of its nature and mode of expression is found in the little book *Light on the Path* by Mabel Collins.

There are two points which the *Sādhaka* must note with regard to this *Jñāna-dīpti*. The first is that this light comes from within and makes him, to a great extent, independent of external guidance. The more we penetrate into the deeper recesses of our consciousness the more we have to rely upon our own inner resources since nothing outside can help us. In a way, a *Sādhaka* becomes really qualified to tread the path of *Yoga* only after this inner light appears within his mind. All preliminary training in *Yoga* is meant to provide him with this inner source of illumination.

All teachers who help him in the early stages have this as their main objective so that he may be able to stand on his own legs.

The second point to note in this connection is that this inner light of wisdom continues to grow and provide guidance until the stage of *Viveka-Khyāti* is reached. That is the significance of the word *Ā* preceding the word *Viveka-Khyāti* in the *Sūtra.* The light grows stronger and stronger as the *Sādhaka* makes progress on the Path and draws near to his goal, until he gains his first experience of Reality. Then, of course, the light of spiritual wisdom becomes unnecessary as far as he is concerned because he is now in the primary source of inner Illumination, the Enlightenment of Reality itself. It will be seen that ordinary *Viveka*, *Jñāna-dīpti*, *Viveka-Khyāti* are manifestations in different degrees of the same Light which shines in its fullest and uninterrupted splendour in *Kaivalya*. *Viveka* enables the *Sādhaka* to enter the path of *Yoga*, *Jñāna-dīpti* enables him to tread it safely and steadily, *Viveka-Khyāti* gives him the experience of Reality and *Kaivalya* sees him established in that Reality permanently.

The philosophy of *Kleśas* which has been expounded by Patañjali in such a masterly manner in the first portion of Section II deals with the great problem of human life completely and effectively. It goes to the root-cause of human bondage and suffering and prescribes a remedy which is not only effective but brings about a permanent cure. This philosophy should therefore be considered not as a mere accessory but an integral part of *Yogic* philosophy, upon which alone a stable structure of *Yogic* life can be built. Those who come to *Yoga* out of curiosity drop out sooner or later unable to bear its ceaseless strain and the ruthless stripping of the personality which is involved. Some come driven by vulgar ambition and a spirit of self-aggrandizement. Their career, if it is not cut short in some way, generally ends in disaster or leads them to the Left-hand path, which is worse. A few come to *Yoga* because they find that it is the only means of securing release from the limitations and illusions of human life and its miseries. They have understood thoroughly the philosophy of *Kleśas* and even *Siddhis* or other attractions of the *Yogic* life have no power to hold them back or make them tarry in the illusions of the higher realms. They are the only people who are really qualified to tread this path.

२९. यमनियमासनप्राणायामप्रत्याहारधारणाध्यानसमाधयोऽष्टावङ्गानि ।

Yama-niyamāsana-prāṇāyāma-pratyāhāra-dhāraṇā-dhyāna-samādhayo'ṣṭāv aṅgāni.

यम Self-restraints; vows of abstention नियम fixed observances; binding rules which must be observed आसन posture प्राणायाम regulation of breath प्रत्याहार abstraction धारणा concentration; holding on to one idea or object in the mind or by the mind ध्यान meditation; contemplation ('con-templa-tion' which means working out an area, a templum for observation fits in with the difinition of धारणा in the text and con-centra-tion which means confining to a centre fits in with the definition of ध्यान as given in the text. Yet, on the whole, considering the conventional uses of the two words it seems best to render धारणा by concentration and ध्यान by contemplation) समाधयः (and) trance अष्टौ (are) the eight अङ्गानि limbs; constituent parts.

29. Self-restraints, fixed observances, posture, regulation of breath, abstraction, concentration, contemplation, trance are the eight parts (of the self discipline of *Yoga*).

The system of *Yoga* put forward by Patañjali has eight parts and is therefore called *Aṣṭāṅga Yoga*. Other systems which are based on a different technique naturally adopt other classifications and have therefore a different number of *Aṅgas*. This *Sūtra* merely enumerates the eight constituent parts of this system of *Yoga*.

The only point which is worth considering in this *Sūtra* is whether the eight *Aṅgas* in this system are to be taken as independent parts or as stages which follow each other in natural sequence. The use of the word *Aṅgas* which means limbs implies that they are to be taken as related but non-sequential parts, but the manner in which Patañjali has dealt with them in the text shows that they have a certain sequential relationship. Anyone who examines carefully the nature of these parts cannot fail to see that they are related to one another in a definite manner and follow one another in a natural manner in the order in which they are given above. In systematic practice of higher *Yoga*, therefore, they have to be taken in the sense of stages and the order in which they are given has to be adhered to, as far as possible. But, as a *Sādhaka* can take up for practice any of the *Aṅgas* without adhering to this sequence these parts may be considered independent also to some extent.

३०. अहिंसासत्यास्तेयब्रह्मचर्यापरिग्रहा यमाः ।

Ahiṃsā-satyāsteya-brahmacaryāparigrahā yamāḥ.

अहिंसा non-violence; harmlessness सत्य truthfulness अस्तेय honesty; non-misappropriativeness ब्रह्मचर्य sexual continence अपरिग्रहा (and) non-possessiveness; non-acquisitiveness यमाः (are) self-restraints; vows of abstention.

30. Vows of self-restraint comprise abstention from violence, falsehood, theft, incontinence and acquisitiveness.

Yama and *Niyama* the first two *Aṅgas* of *Yoga* are meant to provide an adequate moral foundation for the *Yogic* training. The very fact that they are placed before the other *Aṅgas* shows their basic character. Before dealing with the moral qualities and general mode of life which are implied in *Yama-Niyama* it is necessary to explain a few things about the place of morality in the *Yogic* life.

Incredible as it may sound, morality of a high order is not always necessary for the practice of *Yoga*. There are two kinds of *Yoga*—lower and higher. The lower has for its object the development of certain psychic faculties and supernormal powers and for this the transcendent morality implied in *Yama-Niyama* is not at all necessary; in fact, it acts as a hindrance because it causes inner conflict and prevents the *Yogi* from going ahead with his pursuit of personal power and ambitions. There are a large number of *Yogis* scattered throughout India, Tibet and other countries who undoubtedly possess supernormal powers and faculties but who are not distinguishable from the ordinary man of the world by any special moral or spiritual traits of character. Some of these men are good people, self-centred or vain but harmless. Others, of another class, cannot be considered innocent and harmless. They are prone to take part in questionable activities and under provocation can cause injury to those who cross their path. There is a third class of *Yogis* who definitely tread the Left-hand path and are called Brothers of the Shadow. They have powers of various kinds developed to a high degree, and unscrupulous and dangerous, though outwardly they may adopt a mode of life which makes them appear religious. But anyone in whom intuition is developed can spot these people and distinguish them from the followers of the Right-hand path by their tendency to cruelty, unscrupulousness and conceit.

The higher *Yoga* which is expounded in the *Yoga-sūtras* should be distinguished very carefully from the lower *Yoga* referred to above. It has for its objective not the development of powers which can be used for self-aggrandizement or satisfaction of conceit but Enlightenment and consequent freedom from the illusions and limitations of the lower life. Since in gaining this Enlightenment the *Sādhaka* has to undergo certain physical and mental disciplines which are the same as those adopted by the followers of the Left-hand path, the two paths seem to run parallel for some distance. But the time comes at an early stage when the paths begin to diverge rapidly. One leads to an ever-increasing concentration of power in the individual and his isolation from the One Life, the other to the progressive merging of the individual consciousness in the One Consciousness and freedom from bondage and illusion. The hope of the former is naturally very limited and confined to the realm of the intellect while there is no limit to the achievement of the *Yogi* on the other.

On the path of higher *Yoga* morality of a high order is essential and it is a morality not of the conventional type, not even of ordinary religious type. It is a transcendent morality based on the higher laws of Nature and organized with a view to bring about the liberation of the individual from the bonds of illusion and ignorance. Its object is not to achieve limited happiness within the illusions of the lower life but to gain true and lasting happiness or Peace by transcending those illusions. This is a point which must be clearly understood because to many students of *Yogic* philosophy *Yogic* morality appears to be unnecessarily harsh and forbidding. They cannot understand why it should not be possible to practise a morality which will allow us to have reasonable enjoyments of the worldly life as well as the peace and knowledge of the higher, the best of both the worlds as we say. According to some, *Brahmacarya* should be compatible with moderate sexual indulgence. *Ahiṃsā* should allow one to defend oneself against attacks from others. Such compromises with the demands of *Yogic* morality seem quite reasonable from the worldly standpoint, but anyone who studies the philosophy of *Yoga* carefully will see the utter futility of trying to keep a hold on this world while trying to conquer the Great Illusion. Not that it is not possible to practise *Yoga* at all without giving up these things entirely but the progress of the *Sādhaka* is bound to stop at one stage or another if he tries to make these compromises.

Another important point to understand with regard to *Yogic* morality is that the virtues which are prescribed have a much wider scope and deeper significance than what appears on the surface. Each virtue included in *Yama*, for example, is a typical representative of a class of virtues which have to be practised to a high degree of perfection. The injunction against killing, stealing, lying, etc., under *Yama* does not seem to represent a very high standard of morality even from ordinary standards. Any decent and good individual is expected to abstain from such anti-social conduct. Where is then the high standard of morality which is demanded by higher *Yoga*? In order to remove this doubt it is necessary to remember, as has been pointed out above, that each virtue is more comprehensive in its meaning than what it is generally considered to be. Thus

Ahiṃsā does not mean merely abstaining from murder but not wilfully inflicting any injury, suffering or pain on any living creature, by word, thought or action. *Ahiṃsā* thus stands for the highest degree of harmlessness which is found only among saints and sages and any ordinary person trying to practise it seriously in his life will soon begin to feel that perfect harmlessness is an unrealizable ideal. The same holds true in the case of the other virtues comprised in *Yama*. To what degree of perfection these virtues can be developed is shown in the eleven *Sūtras*, II (35-45).

It should thus be clear that the morality enjoined in *Yama-Niyama*, though apparently simple, represents a very drastic ethical code and is designed to serve as a sufficiently strong foundation for the life of higher *Yoga*. It does not deal with the superficial aberrations and failings of human nature nor is its purpose to make a good, social, law-abiding individual. It goes to the very bedrock of human nature and lays the foundation of the *Yogic* life there, so that it may be able to bear the enormous weight of the sky-scraper which *Yogic* life really is.

The main object of this relentless ethical code is to eliminate completely all mental and emotional disturbances which characterize the life of an ordinary human being. Anyone who is familiar with the working of the human mind should not find it difficult to understand that no freedom from emotional and mental disturbances is possible until the tendencies dealt with under *Yama-Niyama* have been rooted out or, at least, mastered to a sufficient degree. Hatred, dishonesty, deception, sensuality, possessiveness are some of the common and ingrained vices of the human race and as long as a human being is subject to these vices in their crude or subtle forms so long will his mind remain a prey to violent or hardly perceptible emotional disturbances which have their ultimate source in these vices. And, as long as these disturbances continue to affect the mind it is useless to undertake the more systematic and advanced practice of *Yoga*.

After this general consideration of *Yama-Niyama* let us discuss briefly the significance of the five moral qualities given in II-30 under *Yama*. Since this is a matter which is of the greatest importance to the beginner it may be discussed in some detail

Ahiṃsā: *Ahiṃsā* really denotes an attitude and mode of behaviour towards all living creatures based on the recognition of the underlying unity of life. As *Yogic* philosophy is based on the doctrine of the One Life it is easy to see why our outer behaviour should be made to conform to this all-embracing Law of Life. If we understand this principle thoroughly the application of the ideal in our life will become much easier.

There are many people who, without making any earnest effort to practise *Ahiṃsā*, start raising imaginary problems and enter into academic discussions as to what *Ahiṃsā* really is and how far it is practicable in life. This is essentially a wrong approach to the problem because no hard and fast rules can be laid down in this as in other matters related to our conduct. Each situation in life is unique and requires a fresh and vital approach. What is right under a particular set of circumstances cannot be determined in a mechanical fashion by weighing all the facts and striking a balance. The correct insight into right action under every set of circumstances is the result of a developed and purified *Buddhi* or discriminative faculty and this function of *Buddhi*, unhindered by the complexes in our mind, is possible only after prolonged training in doing the right thing at all costs. It is only by doing the right that we get added strength to do right in the future and also acquire the capacity to see what is right. There is no other way. So the *Sādhaka* who wishes to perfect himself in the practice of *Ahiṃsā* leaves all academic considerations aside, keeps a strict watch over his mind, emotions, words and actions and starts regulating them in accordance with his ideal. Slowly, as he succeeds in putting his ideal into practice, the cruelties and injustices involved in his thoughts, actions and words will gradually reveal themselves, his vision will clear up and the right course of conduct under every set of circumstances will become known intuitively. And gradually, this seemingly negative ideal of harmlessness will transform itself into the positive and dynamic life of love both in its aspect of tender compassion towards all living creatures and its practical form, service.

Satya: The second moral quality denoted by the word *Satya* has also to be taken in a far more comprehensive sense than mere truthfulness. It means strict avoidance of all exaggerations, equivocation, pretence and similar faults which are involved in saying or doing things which are not in strict accordance with what we know as true. Downright lying is considered bad in civilized society but there are many variants of untruthfulness in speech and action which are not regarded as reprehensible in our conventional life. But all these must be completely eliminated from the life of the *Sādhaka*.

Why is truthfulness essential for the *Yogic* life? Firstly, because untruthfulness in all its various forms creates all kinds of unnecessary complications in our life and so is a constant source of disturbance to the mind. To the foolish man whose intuition has become clouded lying is one of the simplest and easiest means of getting out of an undesirable situation or difficulty. He is unable to see that in avoiding one difficulty in this manner he creates many others of a more serious nature. Anyone who decides to keep a watchful eye on his thoughts and actions will notice that usually one lie requires a number of other lies for its support and in spite of all his efforts, in most cases, circumstances take such an unexpected turn that the lie is exposed sooner or later. This effort to keep up falsehoods and false appearances causes a peculiar strain in our sub-conscious mind and provides a congenial soil for all kinds of emotional disturbances. Of course, these things are not noticed by the ordinary man living a life of conventional falsehoods. It is only when he begins to practise truthfulness that the subtler forms of untruthfulness begin to reveal themselves to his eye. It is a law of Nature that we become aware of the subtler forms of any vice when we have eliminated its grosser forms.

Apart from the considerations given above, truthfulness has to be practised by the *Sādhaka* because it is absolutely necessary for the unfoldment of *Buddhi* or intuition. The *Yogi* has to face many problems, the solution of which cannot be found either in reference books or conclusions based on correct thinking. The only means at his disposal to solve such problems is an unclouded or pure *Buddhi* or intuition. Now, there is nothing which clouds the intuition and practically stops its functioning in this manner as untruthfulness in all its forms. A person who starts practising *Yoga* without first acquiring the virtue of utter truthfulness is like a man going for exploration into a jungle at night without any light. He has nothing to guide him in his difficulties and the illusions created by the Brothers of the Shadow are sure to lead him astray. That is why the *Yogi* must first put on the armour of perfect truthfulness in thought, word and deed, for no illusions can pierce such an armour.

Leaving these utilitarian considerations aside the absolute necessity of leading a perfectly straightforward life for the *Yogi* follows from the very nature of the Reality upon which the Universe and our life are based. This Reality in its essential nature is Love and Truth and expresses itself through the great fundamental laws of Love and Truth which ultimately conquer everything. The outer and inner life of the *Yogi* who is seeking this Reality must, therefore, conform strictly to these basic laws of Nature if his efforts are to be crowned with success. Anything which is against the law of Love puts us out of harmony with this law and we are pulled back sooner or later at the cost of much suffering to ourselves—that is why *Ahiṃsā* is enjoined. Similarly, untruthfulness in any form puts us out of harmony with the fundamental law of Truth and creates a kind of mental and emotional strain which prevents us from harmonizing and tranquillizing our mind.

Asteya: *Asteya* literally means abstaining from stealing. Here also we have to take the word in a very comprehensive sense and not merely interpret it in terms of the penal code. Few people who have developed some moral sense will go to the length of actual stealing but there are very few who can be considered quite guiltless from the strictly moral point of view. This is so because many indirect and subtle forms of misappropriation are connived at in our conventional life and our rather insensitive conscience does not feel appreciably disturbed when we take part in these shady transactions. The so-called civilized man will not allow himself to put a silver spoon in his pocket when he goes out to a public dinner but his conscience may not prick him adequately when he gives or receives gratification for doing his duty.

Asteya should really not be interpreted as abstaining from stealing but abstaining from misappropriation of all kinds. The would-be *Yogi* cannot allow himself to take anything which does not properly belong to him, not only in the way of money or goods but even such intangible and yet highly prized things as credit for things he has not done or privileges which do not properly belong to him. It is only when a person succeeds in eliminating to a certain extent this tendency towards misappropriation in its cruder forms that he begins to discover the subtler forms of dishonesty which are woven in our life and of which we are hardly conscious. The aspirant who intends to tread the path of higher *Yoga* has to proceed systematically in the gradual elimination of these undesirable tendencies until their last traces have been removed and the mind rendered pure and in consequence tranquil. He should practise these prescribed virtues as a fine art aiming at greater and greater refinement in the application of the moral principles to the problems of his daily life.

Brahmacarya: Of all the virtues enjoined in *Yama-Niyama* this appears to be the most forbidding and many earnest students who are deeply interested in *Yogic* philosophy fight shy of its practical application in their life because they are afraid they will have to give up the pleasures of sex-indulgence. Many Western writers have tried to solve the problem by suggesting a liberal interpretation of *Brahmacarya* and taking it to mean not complete abstinence but regulated moderate indulgence within lawful wedlock. The Eastern student who is more familiar with the traditions and actual conditions of *Yogic* practice does not make this mistake. He knows that the real *Yogic* life cannot be combined with the self-indulgence and waste of vital force which is involved in the pleasures of sex life and he has to choose between the two. He may not be required to give up sex life all at once but he has to give it up completely before he can start the serious practice of higher *Yoga* as distinguished from mere theoretical study or even *Yogic* practices of a preparatory nature.

To the serious and advanced student this desire to combine the enjoyments of the worldly life with the peace and transcendent knowledge of the higher life seems rather pathetic and shows the absence of a true sense of values with regard to the realities of the *Yogic* life and therefore unfitness for leading this life. Those who can equate or even consider comparable sensual enjoyments with the peace and bliss of the higher life for which the *Yogi* strives and can consequently hesitate in giving up the former, have yet to develop the strong intuition which tells them unequivocally that they have to sacrifice a mere shadow for the real thing, a passing sensation for life's greatest gift. Let the student who feels hesitation in giving up such enjoyments of the senses or seeks a compromise, honestly ask himself whether he believes that a person who is a slave of his passions is really fit to embark on this divine adventure and the answer that he will get from within will be clear and unequivocal.

So this is the first thing which must be clearly understood with regard to *Brahmacarya*. The practice of higher *Yoga* requires complete abstinence from sex life and no compromise on this point is possible. Of course, there are many *Aṅgas* of *Yoga* which the would-be *Yogi* can practise, to some extent, by way of preparation, but he must definitely and systematically prepare to give up completely not only physical indulgence but even thoughts and emotions connected with the pleasures of sex.

The second point to note in this connection is that *Brahmacarya* in its wider sense stands not only for abstinence from sexual indulgence but freedom from craving for all kinds of sensual enjoyments. The pursuit of sensual pleasures is so much a part of our life and we depend to such an extent on these for our happiness that it is considered quite natural and blameless for anybody to indulge in these enjoyments within the limits of moderation and social obligations. The use of scents, indulgence in the pleasures of the palate, wearing furs and similar pleasures of the senses are so common that no blame attaches to the pursuit of such enjoyments even where they involve terrible suffering to countless living creatures. It is all taken as a matter of course and very few people ever give even a passing thought to these things. And for the man who is leading the ordinary life in the world moderate enjoyments of a kind which do not involve any suffering to other creatures do not really matter. They are a part of the normal life at his stage of evolution. But for the would-be *Yogi* these seemingly innocent enjoyments are harmful, not because there is anything 'sinful' about them, but because they carry with them the potentiality for constant mental and emotional disturbances. No one who allows himself to be attracted by the 'objects of the senses' can hope to be free from the worries and anxieties which characterize the life of the worldly man. Besides being a source of constant mental disturbance the pursuit of sensual enjoyments tends to undermine the will and to keep up an attitude of mind which militates against a whole-hearted pursuit of the *Yogic* ideal.

It is, however, necessary to understand what is really to be aimed at in giving up sensual enjoyments. As long as we are living in the world and moving among all kinds of objects which affect the sense-organs we cannot avoid feeling sensuous pleasures of various kinds. When we eat tasty food we cannot help feeling a certain amount of sensuous pleasure—it is the natural result of the food coming in contact with the taste-buds and arousing particular sensations. Has the *Yogi* then to attempt the impossible task of shutting out all pleasurable sensations? No! not at all. The trouble lies not in feeling the sensation which is quite natural and in itself harmless but in the craving for the repetition of the experiences which involve pleasurable sensations. It is that which has to be guarded against and rooted out because it is the desire (*Kāma*) which disturbs the mind and creates *Saṃskāras* and not the actual sensation. The *Yogi* moves among all kinds of objects as anybody else but his mind is not attached to objects which give pleasure or repelled from objects which give pain. He is, therefore, unaffected by the presence or absence of different kinds of objects. The contact with an object produces a particular sensation but the matter ends there.

But this condition of non-attachment can be attained only after a very prolonged and severe self-discipline and renunciation of all kinds of objects which give pleasure, though in the case of some exceptional *Sādhakas* who bring powerful *Saṃskāras* from past lives it comes naturally and easily. There are some people who allow themselves to remain under the self-deception that they are unattached to enjoyments of the senses even though they continue outwardly to indulge in them. It will help these people to destroy this self-deception if they ask themselves seriously why they continue to indulge in those pleasures if they have really outgrown them. The fact is that for the ordinary *Sādhaka* it is only by renouncing pleasures of the senses that indifference towards them can be developed and tested. Austerity is thus a necessary part of the *Yogic* discipline. Those who allow themselves to lead the soft life of sensual pleasures under the illusion that 'these things do not touch them' are merely postponing the effort for the earnest pursuit of the *Yogic* ideal. To the worldly-minded this austerity appears forbidding if not meaningless and they frequently wonder what the *Yogi* really lives for. But to the *Yogi* this freedom from attachment brings an undefinable peace of mind and inner strength beside which the enjoyments of the senses appear intolerable.

Aparigraha: *Aparigraha* is sometimes translated as absence of greediness but non-possessiveness perhaps gives the underlying idea better. In order to understand why it is essential for the would-be *Yogi* to eliminate this tendency in his life we have only to consider the tremendous bias which it gives to our life. The tendency to accumulate worldly goods is so strong that it may be considered almost a basic instinct in human life. Of course, as long as we live in the physical world we have to have a few things which are essential for the maintenance of the body, although essential and non-essential are relative terms and there seems to be no limit to the cutting down of even what are considered the necessities of life. But we are not satisfied with the necessities of life. We must have things which may be classed as luxuries. These are not necessary for keeping body and soul together but are meant to increase our comforts and enjoyments. We do not, however, stop even at luxuries. When we have at our disposal all the means that can ensure all possible comforts and enjoyments for the rest of our life we are still not satisfied and continue to amass wealth and things. One would think that a palace should suffice for the real needs of a human being but one who has a palace is not satisfied and wants to build a few more. Of course, these extra things do not serve any purpose except that of satisfying our childish vanity and desire to appear superior to our fellow men. There is no limit to our desire for wealth and the material things which we like to have around us and obviously, therefore, we are dealing here with an instinct which has no relation with reason or commonsense.

Apart from the complications which this human instinct causes in the world in the social and economic fields which we need not discuss here, its effect on the life of the individual is of a nature which makes its elimination for the would-be *Yogi* an absolute necessity. Let us consider a few of the factors which are involved. First, you have to spend time and energy in the accumulation of things which you do not really need. Then you have to spend time and energy in maintaining and guarding the things which you have accumulated, the worries and anxieties of life increasing proportionately with the increase in the accumulations. Then consider the constant fear of losing the things, the pain and anguish of actually losing some of them every now and then and the regret of leaving them behind when you ultimately bid goodbye to this world. Now add up all these things and see what a colossal waste of time, energy and mental force all this involves. No one who is at all serious about the solution of the deeper problems of life can afford to squander his limited resources in this manner. So the would-be *Yogi* cuts down his possessions and requirements to the minimum and eliminates from his life all these unnecessary accumulations and activities which fritter away his energies and are a source of constant disturbance to the mind. He remains satisfied with what comes to him in the natural course of the working of the law of *Karma*.

It may be pointed out, however, that it is really not the quantity of things by which we are surrounded but our attitude towards them which matters. For there may be only a few things in our possession and yet the instinct of possessiveness may be very strong. On the other hand, we may be rolling in wealth and yet be free from any sense of possession. Many interesting stories are told in the Hindu scriptures to illustrate this point, the story of Janaka who lived in a palace and the hermit who lived in a hut being well known. It is possible to live in the most luxurious circumstances with no feeling of possession and readiness to part with everything without the slightest hesitation. But though this is possible it is not easy and the would-be *Yogi* would do well to cut out all unnecessary things, for it is only in this way he can learn to live the simple and austere life. Even if he is not attached to his possessions he will have to spend time and energy in maintaining the paraphernalia and this he cannot afford to do.

But it must be clearly understood that the necessity for cultivating this virtue lies chiefly in ensuring a state of mind which is free from attachments. The additional advantages which have been referred to above, though important, are of a subsidiary nature.

३१. जातिदेशकालसमयानवच्छिन्नाः सार्वभौमा महाव्रतम्।

Jāti-deśa-kāla-samayānavacchinnāḥ sārvabhaumā mahā-vratam.

जाति (by) class; birth-type देश place काल time समय (and) occasion; circumstance; condition अनवच्छिन्नाः not-limited, qualified or conditioned सार्वभौमाः extending or applying to all stages; महाव्रतम् the Great Vow.

31. These (the five vows), not conditioned by class, place, time or occasion and extending to all stages constitute the Great Vow.

After giving the five basic virtues which have to be practised by the would-be *Yogi* in II-30, Patañjali lays down another principle in the next *Sūtra* the importance of which is not generally realized. In the practising of any virtue there are occasions when doubts arise whether it is feasible or advisable to practise that particular virtue in the particular situation which has arisen. Considerations of class, place, time or occasion may be involved in these situations and the *Sādhaka* may find it difficult to decide what should be done under those circumstances. Take for illustration the following hypothetical situations. A friend of yours whom you know to be innocent is going to be hanged but can be saved if you tell a lie. Should you tell that lie? (occasion). Accumulation of wealth and its proper distribution is the *Dharma* of a *Vaiśya* according to Hindu *Varṇāśrama Dharma*. Should a *Vaiśya* who aspires to be a *Yogi*, therefore, relax his vow with regard to *Aparigraha*, and continue to amass wealth? (class). Your country is at war with another. Should you join the army and agree to kill the nationals of the enemy as you are required to do? (time). You have to go to the Arctic region where it is necessary to kill animals for food. Are you free to modify your vow with regard to *Ahiṃsā* in the peculiar circumstances in which you are placed? (place). Hundreds of such questions are bound to arise in the life of the would-be *Yogi* and he may sometimes be in doubt whether the five vows are to be practised strictly or exceptions can be made under special circumstances. This *Sūtra* sets at rest all such doubts by making it absolutely clear that no exceptions can be allowed in the practice of the Great Vow as the five vows are called collectively. He may be put to great inconvenience, he may have to pay great penalties in the observance of these vows—even the extreme penalty of death—but none of these vows may be broken under any conditions. Even if life has to be sacrificed in the observance of his vow he should go through the ordeal cheerfully in the firm conviction that the tremendous influx of spiritual power which is bound to take place under these conditions will far outweigh the loss of a single life. He who is out to unravel the Ultimate Mystery of life has to risk his life in doing the right on many occasions, and considering the tremendous nature of the achievement which is at stake the loss of one or two lives does not matter. Besides, he should know that in a Universe governed by Law and based on Justice no real harm can come to a person who tries to do the right. When he has to suffer under these circumstances it is usually due to past *Karma* and it is therefore better to go through the unpleasant experience and have done with the *Kārmic* obligation for good. Usually, the problems which arise are meant only to test us to the utmost and when we show our determination to do the right thing at any cost they are resolved in the most unexpected manner.

While, in one way, this uncompromising adherence to one's principles makes the observance of the Great Vow not an easy matter and may involve great hardships on occasions, in another way, it simplifies the problem of our life and conduct to a very great extent. It eliminates completely the difficulty of deciding what has to be done under all kinds of situations in which the *Sādhaka* may find himself. The universality of the Vow leaves no loop-holes through which his mind may tempt him to escape and his course of action on most occasions will be quite clear. He can follow the right path unhesitatingly, knowing that there is no other path open to him.

It should be noted, however, that though there is insistence on doing the right, the interpretation of what is right is always left to his discretion. He has to do what he thinks to be right, not what others tell him. If he does wrong, thinking it to be right, nature will teach him through suffering but the will do to the right at any cost will progressively clear his vision and lead him to the stage where he can see the right unerringly. Seeing the right depends upon doing the right. Hence the tremendous importance of righteousness in the life of the *Yogi*.

३२. शौचसंतोषतपःस्वाध्यायेश्वरप्रणिधानानि नियमाः ।

Śauca-saṃtoṣa-tapaḥ-svādhyāyeśvara-
praṇidhānāni niyamāḥ.

शौच purity; cleanliness संतोष contentment तपः austerity स्वाध्याय self-study; study which leads to knowledge of the Self ईश्वरप्रणिधानानि (and) self-surrender; resignation to God नियमाः (fixed) observances.

32. Purity, contentment, austerity, self-study and self-surrender constitute observances.

We now come to *Niyama*, the second *Aṅga* of *Yogic* discipline which serves to lay the foundation of the *Yogic* life. Before we deal with the five elements of *Niyama* enumerated in this *Sūtra* it is necessary to consider the distinction between *Yama* and *Niyama*. Superficially examined, *Yama* and *Niyama* both seem to have a common purpose—the transmutation of the lower nature so that it may serve properly as a vehicle of the *Yogic* life. But a closer study of the elements included under the two heads will reveal at once the difference in the general nature of the practices enjoined for bringing about the necessary changes in the character of the

Sādhaka. The practices included in *Yama* are, in a general way, moral and prohibitive while those in *Niyama* are disciplinal and constructive. The former aim at laying the ethical foundation of the *Yogic* life and the latter at organizing the life of the *Sādhaka* for the highly strenuous *Yogic* discipline which is to follow.

This difference in the general purpose of *Yama* and *Niyama* involves a corresponding difference in the nature of the practices themselves. In the observance of the Great Vow connected with *Yama* the *Sādhaka* is not required to do anything. Day after day, he is required to react to the incidents and events in his life in a well-defined manner, but the number and character of the occasions which will arise in his life requiring the exercise of the five virtues will naturally depend upon his circumstances. If, for example, he goes and lives alone in a jungle as an ascetic there will hardly arise any occasion for putting the virtues into practice. The Great Vow will be binding on him always, but if we may say so, will remain inoperative for want of opportunities for its practice.

Not so in the case of *Niyama* which involves practices which have to be gone through regularly, day after day, whatever the circumstances in which the *Sādhaka* is placed. Even if he is living alone completely isolated from all social relationships the necessity for going through these practices will remain as great as when he was living in the busy haunts of men.

Śauca: The first element of *Niyama* is *Śauca* or purity. Before we can understand how the problem of purifying our nature is to be tackled we should clarify our ideas with regard to purity. What is purity? According to the *Yogic* philosophy the whole of the Universe, seen or unseen, is a manifestation of the Divine Life and pervaded by the Divine Consciousness. To the Enlightened sage or saint who has had the Divine vision everything from an atom to the *Īśvara* of a *Brahmāṇḍa* is a vehicle of the Divine Life and therefore pure and sacred. From this higher point of view nothing can therefore be considered impure in the absolute sense. So, when we use the words pure and impure in relation to our life we obviously use them in a relative sense. The word purity is used in relation to our vehicles, not only the body which we can cognize with our physical senses but also the superphysical vehicles which serve as the instruments of emotion, thought and other spiritual faculties. A thing is pure in relation to a vehicle if it enables or helps the vehicle to serve efficiently as an instrument of the Divine Life expressing through it at the particular stage of evolution. It is impure if it hinders the full expression of that life or offers impediments in the exercise of the vehicle's functions. Purity is, therefore, nothing absolute, only functional and related to the next stage of evolution which life is seeking to attain. Purification, therefore, means elimination from the vehicles belonging to an individual of all those elements and conditions which prevent them from exercising their proper functions and attaining the goal in view. For the *Yogi* this goal is Self-realization through the merging of his individual consciousness with the Consciousness of the Supreme or the attainment of *Kaivalya* in terms of the *Yoga-sūtra*. Purification for the *Yogi*, therefore, means specifically the maintenance and transformation of the vehicle in such a manner that they can serve increasingly to bring about this unification.

Purity, though it is functional, depends to a great extent upon the quality of the material of which a particular vehicle of consciousness is composed. The functional efficiency of the vehicle depends not only upon its structural organization but also upon the nature of the material incorporated in it. The expression of consciousness through a vehicle may be compared to the production of different kinds of sounds by a piece of stretched metallic wire. We know that the sound which is produced depends upon three factors, the nature of the metal, the structure (diameter and length) of the wire and the tension to which it is subjected. In the same way the capacity of a vehicle to respond to different states of consciousness depends upon its material, its structural complexity which increases as a result of evolution, and its sensitiveness.

The reason why the material of the vehicle determines to a certain extent its vibrational capacity lies in the fact that quality of material and vibrational capacity are indissolubly linked in nature, each kind of material responding to a limited range of vibrations. So, if we want to bring down into the lower vehicles the high and subtle vibrations corresponding to the deeper layers of human consciousness we must provide in them the right and corresponding type of material.

All the lower vehicles of a *Jīvātmā* are constantly changing and purification consists in gradually and systematically replacing the comparatively coarse material of the bodies by a more refined type of material. In the case of the physical body purification is a comparatively simple matter and may be brought about by supplying to the body the right kind of material in the form of food and drink. According to the Hindu system of *Yogic* culture foods and drinks are divided into three classes—*Tāmasic*, *Rājasic* and *Sāttvic* and only those which are considered *Sāttvic* are allowed to the *Yogi* who is building a pure and refined physical vehicle. Meat, alcohol and so many other accessories of a modern diet make the physical body utterly useless for the *Yogic* life and if the aspirant has been coarsening the body through the use of these he will have to go through a prolonged period of careful dieting to get rid of the undesirable material and make the body sufficiently refined.

The purification of the subtler vehicles which serve as instruments for the expression of thoughts and emotions is brought about by a different and more difficult process. In their case the vibrational tendencies are gradually changed by excluding all undesirable thoughts and emotions from the mind and replacing these constantly and persistently by thoughts and emotions of a higher and subtler nature. As the vibrational tendencies of these bodies change the matter of the bodies also changes *pari passu* and after some time, if the effort is continued long enough, the vehicles are adequately purified. The test of real purification is provided by the normal vibrational tendencies which one finds in the vehicle. A pure mind easily and naturally thinks pure thoughts and feels pure emotions and it becomes difficult for it to entertain undesirable thoughts and emotions in the same way as it is difficult for an impure mind to entertain high and noble thoughts and emotions.

Another device recommended in the Hindu system of spiritual culture for the purification of the subtler vehicles is the constant use of *Mantras* and prayers. These make the vehicles vibrate frequently at very high rates of frequency, bring about an influx of spiritual forces from the planes above and the agitation thus set in motion, day after day, gradually washes out, as it were, all the undesirable elements from the different vehicles. It will be seen, therefore, that purification or *Śauca* is a positive practice. It does not take place of itself. One has to go through purificatory exercises, day after day, for long periods of time. That is why it has been included in *Niyama*.

Saṃtoṣa: The second element of *Niyama* is *Saṃtoṣa* which is generally translated as contentment. It is necessary for the aspirant for the *Yogic* life to cultivate contentment of the highest order because without it there is no possibility of keeping the mind in a condition of equilibrium. The ordinary man living in the world is subjected all day long to all kinds of impacts, and he reacts to these impacts according to his habits, prejudices, training or mood of the moment, according to his nature as we say. These reactions involve in most cases greater or lesser disturbances of the mind, there being hardly any reaction which is not accompanied by a ruffling of the feeling or the mind. The disturbance from one impact has hardly had time to subside before another impact throws it out of equilibrium again. The mind seems to be apparently calm sometimes but this calmness is only superficial. Beneath the surface there is an undercurrent of disturbance like the swell in a superficially calm sea.

This condition of mind which need not necessarily be unpleasant and which is taken as natural by most people is not at all conducive to one-pointedness and as long as it lasts must result in *Vikṣepa*, the strong tendency of the mind to be outward-turned. So the *Sādhaka* has to change this state of constant disturbance into a state of constant equilibrium and stillness by a deliberate exercise of the will, meditation and other means that may be available. He aims at attaining a condition in which he remains perfectly calm and serene whatever may happen in the outer world or even in the inner world of his mind. His aim is not merely to acquire the power to quell a mental disturbance if and when it arises but the more rare power to prevent any disturbance taking place at all. He knows that once a disturbance has been allowed to occur it takes far more energy to overcome it completely and, even though outwardly it may disappear quickly, the inner sub-conscious disturbance persists for a long time.

This kind of equanimity can be built only on the foundations of perfect contentment, the capacity to remain satisfied whatever may happen to the *Sādhaka*. It is an extremely positive and dynamic condition of the mind which has nothing in common with that negative mentality which is based on laziness and lack of initiative and which is rightly held in profound contempt by people in the world. It is based on perfect indifference to all those personal enjoyments, comforts and other considerations which sway mankind. Its object is the attainment of that Peace which takes one completely beyond the realm of illusion and misery.

The cultivation of this supreme contentment and consequent tranquillity of the mind is the result of prolonged self-discipline and going through many experiences which involve pain and suffering. It cannot be acquired by a mere assertion of the will once for all. Habits stronger than nature and habits developed through innumerable lives cannot be changed all at once. That is why constant alertness and training of the mind in maintaining the right attitude is necessary and that is also why this virtue is placed under *Niyama*.

Tapas and the next two elements of *Niyama* have already been referred to in II-1 and the reason why they together are called *Kriyā-Yoga* has been given in dealing with that *Sūtra*. *Tapas* is a very comprehensive term and has really no exact English equivalent. It combines in itself the significations of a number of English words: purification, self-discipline, austerity. The word stands for a class of various practices the object of which is to purify and discipline the lower nature and to bring the vehicles of the *Jīvātmā* under the control of an iron will. The meaning of the word is probably derived from the process of subjecting alloyed gold to strong 'heating' whereby all the dross is burnt off and pure gold is left behind. In a way the whole science of character-building whereby we purify and bring under control our lower vehicles may be considered as a practice of *Tapas* but in the orthodox sense the word *Tapas* is used particularly for some specific exercises adopted for the purification and control of the physical body and the development of will-power. These include such practices as fasting, observing vows of various kinds,

Prāṇāyāma etc. Some misguided people take the most extraordinary vows in practising *Tapas* such as holding up the hand and keeping it in that position for a number of years even though it withers. But such foolish practices are considered highly reprehensible in the enlightened schools of *Yoga* and are called *Āsuric*, demoniacal.

The systematic practice of *Tapas* generally begins with simple and easy exercises which require the exertion of will-power and is continued by progressive stages with more difficult exercises, the object of which is to bring about the dissociation of the vehicle from consciousness. In the case of the ordinary man the consciousness is to a great extent identified with the vehicle through which it works. The practice of *Tapas* gradually loosens up this association, enables the consciousness to be partially separated from the vehicle and this progressive awareness of the vehicle as part of the 'not-Self' means attenuation of '*Asmitā*' or 'I am this' consciousness. It is only when this power to dissociate consciousness from the vehicles has been acquired to some extent that the *Sādhaka* can effectively purify and control the vehicles and use them for the purposes of *Yoga*.

Svādhyāya: The word *Svādhyāya* is sometimes used in a limited sense for the study of the sacred scriptures. But this is only a part of the work which has to be done—the first step. The student has naturally first to make himself thoroughly familiar with all the essential literature bearing on the different aspects of *Yoga* just as he does in the study of any science. In this way he acquires the necessary knowledge of the theoretical principles and practices which are involved in the pursuit of the *Yogic* ideal. He also gets an idea of the relative values of the different methods and a correct perspective with regard to all matters connected with *Yogic* practices.

While this study is only theoretical and does not take him very far on the road to Self-realization it is none the less of great value to the student. Many people who set out on this quest have a very vague and confused intellectual background and lack that clear and broad grasp of the subject which is so necessary for steady progress. Being insufficiently equipped with the necessary knowledge concerning the various problems which are involved they are apt to over-simplify these problems and to expect impossible results. Sooner or later they become disheartened and frustrated or fall a prey to those unscrupulous people who pose as great *Yogis* and promise all kinds of fantastic things to entice people into their fold. A broad and general intellectual background is necessary for achieving success in any sphere of scientific endeavour and since *Yoga* is a science *par excellence* it is true of this science also.

But though a thorough and detailed study of *Yogic* literature is a necessary part of *Svādhyāya* it is only the first step. The next is constant brooding and reflection over the deeper problems which have been studied in their intellectual aspect through books, etc. This constant reflection prepares the mind for the reception of real knowledge from within. It produces a sort of suctorial action and draws the breath of intuition into the mind. The student thus begins to get a deeper insight into the problems of *Yogic* life. The clearer the insight into these problems the keener becomes the desire for the real solution, or gaining that transcendent knowledge in the light of which all doubts are completely resolved and the Peace of the Eternal is attained. This brooding and reflection on the great and fundamental truths of life gradually and imperceptibly begins to take the form of meditation in the ordinary sense of the term, that is, the mind becomes increasingly engrossed in the object of the search. This object need not necessarily be an abstract truth of a philosophical nature. It may be an object of devotion with whom the *Sādhaka* wants to commune and become united. The nature of the object will differ according to the temperament of the individual but the condition of the mind—a state of deep absorption and intense desire to know—will be the same, more or less.

In bringing about this one-pointed state of absorption the use of *Mantras* is very helpful. The *Sādhaka* may use the *Mantra* of his *Iṣṭa-Devatā* or any of the well-known *Mantras* like *Gāyatri* or *Praṇava*. These *Mantras*, as has been shown already, harmonize the lower vehicles of consciousness, make them sensitive to the subtler vibrations and ultimately bring about a partial fusion of the lower and higher consciousness. So, it will be seen that though *Svādhyāya* begins with intellectual study it must be carried through the progressive stages of reflection, meditation, *Tapas* etc. to the point where the *Sādhaka* is able to gain all knowledge or devotion from within, by his own efforts. That is the significance of the prefix *Sva* in *Svādhyāya*. He leaves all external aids such as books, discourses, etc. and dives into his own mind for everything he needs in his quest.

Īśvara-praṇidhāna: This is usually translated as resignation to *Īśvara* or God but in view of the fact that the advanced practice of *Īśvara-praṇidhāna* is able to bring about *Samādhi*, it is obvious that the word is used in a far deeper sense than the superficial mental effort of the ordinary religious man to resign himself to the will of God. When such a man makes a mental assertion of this kind what he really means is that the will of God is supreme in the world over which He rules and he submits to that will gladly, although the experience which has evoked that assertion may not be a pleasant one. This attitude is not unlike the attitude of a loyal subject to the fiat of his king.

It is clear, however, that though this attitude of the pious individual is superior to the common attitude of resentment towards the inevitable calamities and sufferings of life and conduces to a peaceful state of mind, it cannot by itself take him very far along the path of spiritual unfoldment and realization which culminates in *Samādhi*. The fact that the progressive practice of *Īśvara-praṇidhāna* can ultimately lead to *Samādhi* shows definitely that it signifies a much deeper process of transformation in the *Sādhaka* than a mere acceptance of whatever experiences and ordeals come to him in the course of his life.

To understand the significance and technique of *Īśvara-praṇidhāna* it is necessary to recall how the *Puruṣa* gets involved in *Prakṛti* through *Avidyā* which results in his becoming subject to illusion and consequent sufferings and miseries of life. As this question has been discussed thoroughly in dealing with the theory of *Kleśas* it is not necessary to go into its details here, but there is one central idea bearing on the problem under consideration which may be briefly referred to in this connection. According to the philosophy upon which the Science of *Yoga* is based, the Reality within us is free from the fundamental illusion which is responsible for the limitations and miseries of our life. The individual consciousness or *Puruṣa* is a manifestation of that Reality.

How does he then become subject to the Great Illusion and the consequent sufferings of the lower life? By the imposition of the 'I' consciousness which makes him identify himself with his vehicles and with the environment in which his consciousness is immersed. As long as this veil of *Asmitā* or 'I'-ness covers his true nature—*Svarūpa*—he remains bound by the limitations and illusions of life and the only way in which he can regain his freedom from them is by removing this covering of 'I' consciousness. This is the basic idea underlying the whole philosophy of *Yoga* and all systems of *Yoga* aim at the destruction of this 'I' consciousness directly or indirectly, by one means or another. The practice of *Īśvara-praṇidhāna* is one of such means. It has for its object the dissolution of *Asmitā* by the systematic and progressive merging of the individual will with the Will of *Īśvara* and thus destroying the very root of the *Kleśas*.

The practice of *Īśvara-praṇidhāna* therefore begins with the mental assertion "Not my will but Thy Will be done", but it does not end there. There is a steady effort to bring about a continuous recession of consciousness from the level of the personality which is the seat of 'I' consciousness into the consciousness of the Supreme whose will is working out in the manifested world. This effort may take many forms according to the temperament and previous *Saṃskāras* of the *Sādhaka*. There may be an earnest desire to become a conscious instrument of the Supreme Will which is finding expression in the unfolding of the manifested Universe. This Will finds obstruction in its expression at the human level owing to the limitations of the personality, the greater the egoism the greater the obscuration and the consequent obstruction. Such a *Sādhaka* who is trying to practise *Īśvara-praṇidhāna* tries to remove this obstruction of the personality by doing *Niṣkāma-Karma*, so that his personality may become a willing and conscious instrument of the Divine Will. It is needless to say that this is a gradual process and for a long time the *Sādhaka* has to work, as it were, in the dark, trying to do scrupulously what he thinks to be right without having any conscious knowledge of the Divine Will. It is, however, not necessary to know the Divine Will until the personality has been brought under control, for even if that Will were known the wayward and uncontrolled personality will not allow it to be expressed freely and fully. But as in all processes of this nature the effort to realize an ideal gradually removes the obstructions in the way of realization and if the *Sādhaka* pursues his ideal with perseverance he succeeds in becoming a conscious agent of the Divine. His false lower ' I ' disappears and the Divine Will can work freely through the ' I '-less centre of his consciousness. This is real *Karma-Yoga.*

The practice of *Īśvara-praṇidhāna* takes a different form if the *Sādhaka* is a person with a highly emotional temperament and is treading the path of *Bhakti.* Here the emphasis is not on the merging of the individual will in the Divine Will but on the union with the Beloved through love. But as love naturally expresses itself in self-abnegation and subordination of personal desires to the Will of the Beloved the path of *Bhakti* also leads indirectly to the dissolution of the ' I ' or *Asmitā.* Here it is love which is the driving force and which brings about the destruction of egoism and fusion of consciousness, and *Samādhi* is the result.

The careful student will be able to see in *Īśvara-praṇidhāna* the essence of *Bhakti-Yoga.* It is thought by many students of the system of *Yoga* outlined in the *Yoga-Sūtras* that there is not much of a place for a *Bhakta* in this system, and *Bhakti* has not been given the weight it deserves considering its importance in spiritual culture. It is true that the manner in which the subject has been dealt with by Patañjali does give that impression, but does not *Īśvara-praṇidhāna* contain in a nutshell the whole essential technique of *Bhakti-Yoga*? *Navadhā-Bhakti* which comprises the practical side of *Bhakti-Yoga* is merely of a preparatory nature and it is meant to lead the *Sādhaka* to the stage where he is able to renounce all external aids and to surrender himself completely to the Will of the Lord and depend upon Him completely for everything. Surely, this advanced technique of spiritual culture and ultimate union with the Beloved in *Samādhi* is nothing but *Īśvara-praṇidhāna.*

३३. वितर्कबाधने प्रतिपक्षभावनम् ।

Vitarka-bādhane-pratipakṣa-bhāvanaṃ.

वितर्क evil thoughts; evil passions बाधने on oppression by; on disturbance by प्रतिपक्ष the opposites भावनम् dwelling (in mind) on; (constant) pondering over.

33. When the mind is disturbed by improper thoughts constant pondering over the opposites (is the remedy).

In dealing with the subject of *Yama-Niyama*, Patañjali has given two *Sūtras* which are of great help to the practical student of *Yoga*. The first of these which is being considered gives an effective method of dealing with the habits and tendencies which interfere with the practice of *Yama-Niyama*. The student who tries to practise *Yama-Niyama* brings with him the momentum of all kinds of tendencies from previous lives, and in spite of his resolve, the undesirable habits and tendencies in which he has indulged assert themselves strongly and force him to act, feel and think in ways which go against his ideals. What is he to do under these circumstances? He should ponder constantly over the opposites of the undesirable tendencies when these latter trouble him. In this *Sūtra* the author has given one of the most important laws of character-building, a law which modern psychology recognizes and recommends in dealing with problems of self-culture.

The rationale of this technique for overcoming bad habits and undesirable tendencies, whether they relate to action, feeling or thinking lies in the fact that all evil tendencies are rooted in wrong habits of thought and attitudes and, therefore, the only effective means of removing them completely and permanently is to attack the trouble at its source and alter the thoughts and attitudes which underlie the undesirable manifestations.

As is well known, an undesirable mental habit can be changed only by replacing it by a mental habit of an exactly opposite kind—hatred by love, dishonesty by uprightness. New and desirable mental channels are created by the new thoughts in which mental energy begins to flow in ever increasing measure, starving and gradually replacing the undesirable habits of thoughts and the wrong attitudes which are derived from them. The amount of mental energy required and the time taken will depend naturally upon the strength of the undesirable habit and the will-power of the *Sādhaka*, but if he puts his heart into the work and perseveres the thing can be done.

३४. वितर्का हिंसादयः कृतकारितानुमोदिता लोभक्रोधमोहपूर्वका मृदुमध्याधिमात्रा दुःखाज्ञानानन्तफला इति प्रतिपक्षभावनम् ।

Vitarkā hiṃsādayaḥ kṛta-kāritānumoditā lobha-krodha-moha-pūrvakā mṛdu-madhyādhimātrā duḥkhājñānānanta-phalā iti pratipakṣa-bhāvanam.

वितर्का evil or improper thoughts and emotions हिंसादयः (of) violence, etc. कृत done by self कारित done through others अनुमोदिताः (and) abetted; approved लोभ greed; avarice क्रोध anger मोह confusion; delusion पूर्वकाः preceded by; caused by मृदु mild मध्य medium अधिमात्राः (and) intense दुःख pain; misery अज्ञान ignorance अनन्त endless फलाः fruit; result इति thus; so; in this way प्रतिपक्ष (on) the opposites भावनम् dwelling in mind.

34. As improper thoughts, emotions (and actions) such as those of violence, etc. whether they are done (indulged in), caused to be done or abetted, whether caused by greed, anger or delusion, whether present in mild, medium or intense degree, result in endless pain and ignorance; so there is the necessity of pondering over the opposites.

In this *Sūtra* Patañjali has given a brilliant analysis of the factors which are involved in this gradual transformation of undesirable into desirable tendencies and modern psychology should incorporate the many valuable ideas given in this *Sūtra* in its system of ethics. This *Sūtra* is a typical example of the vast and varied information which can be condensed in the few words of a *Sūtra* and made readily available to the practical student. The first factor we have to deal with in relation to the evil tendencies which are sought to be overcome by *Yama-Niyama*, is the question of instrumentality.

Instrumentality: Evil action may be (*a*) done directly, (*b*) caused to be done through the agency of another, (*c*) be connived at or approved. Common law takes cognizance of and recognizes responsibility in case of (*a*) and (*b*) but not in (*c*). But according to the ethics of *Yoga*, blame attaches to all three types of evil actions, there being only a question of degree. The man who sees a thief breaking into a house but does not do anything to prevent the crime is partly responsible for the crime and will to that extent have to bear the *Kārmic* result and degradation of character.

It is desirable to have clear ideas with regard to this question because a very large number of people—good, honest people—manage to deceive themselves and ease their conscience by supposing that if they have not taken a direct part in an evil action they are quite free from blame. Thus, for example, in India many people would shrink with horror if they were asked to slaughter a goat and yet they allow themselves to believe that they incur no *Kārmic* responsibility in taking meat because it is the butcher who kills the goat. This illustrates incidentally the enormous capacity for self-deception in the case of human beings where their prejudices come in or where their self-indulgences are at stake.

But more noteworthy than this doing of evil action indirectly is perhaps the third way of participating in it. We sometimes witness a crime but owing to callousness or desire to avoid getting into trouble do nothing about it or may even silently approve of it. We assume that because we have not taken any part—direct or indirect—in the crime we are quite free from blame. But it is not so according to the *Yogic* ethics embodied in *Yama-Niyama*. According to the more stringent rules of *Yogic* morality a man who connives at or is indifferent to a crime being done in his presence in which, from common humaneness he should have interfered is partly guilty of the crime. 'Inaction in a deed of mercy is action in a deadly sin' as the Buddha warned. If, for example, we see a person being lynched or a child or animal being treated very cruelly it is our duty to interfere whatever the consequences to ourselves. And if we save our skin by remaining indifferent or inactive we incur responsibility and invite *Kārmic* retribution. Of course, this does not mean that we have to become a nuisance and like a busy-body interfere constantly in the lives of other people with the object of getting wrongs redressed. *Yogic* life does not mean bidding good-bye to reason and commonsense.

Cause: The next factor we have to consider is the cause of the evil tendencies which hinder us in the practice of *Yama-Niyama.* Patañjali has given three causes—greed, anger and delusion. It should be noted that these three are conditions of mind which precede wrong thoughts, feelings and actions. This is indicated by the word *Pūrvaka. Lobha* is the condition of the mind which produces the desire to grasp things for ourselves. *Krodha* is the agitation of the mind produced when any person or thing stands in the way of fulfilment of our desire. *Moha* is the conditioning of the mind which results when we are attached to any person or thing. All these conditions of the mind bring about a clouding of *Buddhi* which renders a person incapable of judging right and wrong. It is this confused and unenlightened state of the mind which provides the necessary soil for wrong thoughts, feelings and actions. That is why pondering over the opposites and thus clearing up the confusion has been prescribed as the remedy in the previous *Sūtra.* What has to be remembered is that we have to go to the root of the evil and tackle it there.

Degree: The next question to be considered in regard to *Vitarka* is that of degree. In the Hindu philosophical systems the usual method of classifying a number of things which differ in degree or intensity is to consider them under three broad sub-heads—mild, medium and intense. This method of sub-division is simple and elastic though naturally it suffers from lack of definiteness. But as the *Sādhaka* has to free himself completely from these evil tendencies this lack of definiteness in the division is not of any practical importance.

The importance of sub-dividing the degree or intensity of *Vitarka* does not lie in providing a scientific method of classification.

Its real object is to bring home to the *Sādhaka* the importance of attending to the minor faults in his thinking and conduct which he is likely to overlook or ignore. The *Sādhaka* has to develop a high degree of scrupulousness with regard to his thoughts, feelings and actions which is generally lacking in people who strive to lead a moral life. It is, in fact, this meticulous attention to our inner and outer life which produces moral perfection and brings about those results which are mentioned in the eleven *Sūtras* beginning with II-35.

It should be borne in mind that the subtler forms of an evil tendency do not reveal themselves to us unless and until the grosser ones have been eliminated. So, this complete elimination of any particular kind of *Vitarka* will seem to be continually receding and it may appear to the aspirant that he can never acquire the perfection for which he is striving. But far better this never-get-done feeling than the easy complacence which is fatal for the man who is treading the path of *Yoga*. The results in which the practice of different elements of *Yama-Niyama* culminate (II-35-45), can always enable the *Sādhaka* to check his progress and to know definitely whether he has completed the task of developing any particular trait.

Result: The last point dealt with in this *Sūtra* is the result of the tendencies which are sought to be eradicated by practising *Yama-Niyama*. The two inevitable consequences of an undisciplined and unrighteous life are *Duḥkha* and *Ajñāna*, pain and ignorance—both words being used not only in their ordinary sense but also in their more comprehensive philosophical sense. The word *Duḥkha* is used in *Yogic* philosophy not only for the ordinary pains and sufferings which are the Kārmic results of evil thoughts and deeds but also for that general unhappiness which pervades all human life and which really poisons even the best and happiest periods of our existence. This point has been discussed thoroughly in II-15 and we need not go into it again here. In the same way *Ajñāna* means not only the confusion of mind and lack of wisdom which result from our evil tendencies but also the lack of that fundamental knowledge of our true Divine nature which is responsible for our bondage and suffering in human life.

Duḥkha and *Ajñāna* are thus the two general and inevitable results of a life which is not fashioned according to the ideals embodied in *Yama-Niyama.* All the undesirable tendencies in our character produce an endless (*Ananta*) series of causes and effects which keep the soul in bondage and consequently in misery. The only method of escape from this vicious circle of causes and effects which is available to a human being is, first to discipline his lower nature according to the ideals of *Yama-Niyama* and then, treading the further stages of the path of *Yoga,* to gain Enlightenment. That is the real reason why *Yama-Niyama* should be practised to perfection and all *Vitarka* should be removed by 'pondering over the opposites'.

It may be worth while mentioning here that although the ten elements included in *Yama-Niyama* have been mentioned specifically and have to be practised separately we should not forget the unity underlying human nature. Our nature, though it seems to have different facets, is essentially one. We cannot, therefore, divide life in water-tight compartments and practise the different elements of *Yama-Niyama* one by one as if each had an independent existence and could be isolated from the others. The fact is that all these elements are closely inter-related and the qualities which they are meant to develop are the different aspects of our inner life. How far we are able to develop one of the qualities will depend to a great extent upon the general tone of our life. No one can practise *Ahiṃsā,* for example, even if he tries his best, if he neglects the other elements of *Yama-Niyama,* so closely is one part of our nature bound up with the other parts. All parts of our nature hang together and we rise and fall as a whole, to a very great extent. So, it is the general quality of our life and moral nature which has to be improved, step by step, though we may concentrate on different qualities for some time. The value of a diamond depends upon the quality of the stone as a whole and not upon the polish of one facet. But in order to produce a finished gem we have to take up the different facets one by one.

It may also be interesting to enquire why the word *Vitarka* is used for those improper thoughts which are sought to be excluded from the mind in the practice of *Yama-Niyama.* The word

Vitarka is used to indicate a state of mind in which it passes from one alternative to another as shown in dealing with I-42. This state is also present in the earlier stages when a person tries to live according to an ideal. There is always vacillation and struggle and the mind hovers between two alternative courses. It is only when the *Sādhaka* is well established in righteousness by doing the right under all circumstances that this *Vitarka* ceases and he invariably does the right thing unhesitatingly. The student will thus see the appropriateness of the use of the word *Vitarka* in the present context.

३५. अहिंसाप्रतिष्ठायां तत्संनिधौ वैरत्यागः ।

Ahiṃsā-pratiṣṭhāyāṃ tat-saṃnidhau vaira-tyāgaḥ.

अहिंसा (in) non-violence प्रतिष्ठायाम् on being firmly established तत्-सन्निधौ in his (*Yogi's*) vicinity वैर of hostility त्यागः abandonment.

35. On being firmly established in non-violence there is abandonment of hostility in (his) presence.

In this and the subsequent ten *Sūtras* Patañjali gives the specific results of practising the ten elements of *Yama-Niyama*. The purpose of pointing out these accomplishments which mark the culmination of the practise of *Yama-Niyama*, is two-fold. In the first place, it serves to emphasize that the virtue has to be developed or the practice has to be carried on to a high degree of perfection. Too many people begin to imagine they have acquired perfection in the development of a particular virtue while they are still at the initial stage. In the second place, by indicating the nature of the developments which take place when the virtue has been acquired in perfection, the author provides a measuring rod for the *Sādhaka* by which he can judge his progress and know definitely when he has succeeded in accomplishing that particular task. It need hardly be pointed out that these extraordinary developments are not based on pious hopes but strict, scientific laws verified by innumerable *Yogis* and saints. The results follow as surely though not so easily as the production of fruit from a sapling planted in the ground and nurtured carefully. But, of course, as in all scientific experiments, the correct conditions must be provided if the desired results are to be obtained. Whether it is necessary for the *Sādhaka* to develop each quality to the degree indicated in the *Sūtras* is another question, but there should be no doubt that the thing can be done.

The student of *Yogic* philosophy will see in these unusual developments which take place on practising *Yama-Niyama* the tremendous possibilities which lie hidden in the apparently simple things of life. It appears that one has only to penetrate deeply into any manifestation of life to encounter the most fascinating mysteries and sources of power. Physical science which deals with the crudest manifestation of life touches the mere fringe of these mysteries and the results which it has achieved are little short of miraculous. There is, therefore, nothing to be surprised at in the fact that the *Yogi* who dives into the far subtler phenomena of mind and consciousness finds still deeper mysteries and extraordinary powers. This point will be made clearer when we deal with the question of *Siddhis*.

II-35 gives the specific result of developing *Ahiṃsā*. This is what should be expected if *Ahiṃsā* is a positive and dynamic quality of universal love and not a mere negative attitude to harmlessness. An individual who has developed *Ahiṃsā* carries about him an invisible aura surcharged with love and compassion even though these may not be expressed at the emotional level. Also, because love is the power which binds together in a spiritual union all the separated fragments of the One Life, any individual who is imbued with such love is inwardly attuned to all living creatures and automatically inspires confidence and love in them. That is how the violent and hateful vibrations of those who come near the *Yogi* are for the time being over-powered by the much stronger vibrations of love and kindness emanating from him and even beasts of prey become harmless and docile for the time being. Of course, when a creature goes out of the immediate influence of such a *Yogi* its normal nature is bound to assert itself but even this brief contact is likely to leave a permanent mark on it and uplift it a little.

३६. सत्यप्रतिष्ठायां क्रियाफलाश्रयत्वम् ।

Satya-pratiṣṭhāyāṃ kriyā-phalāśrayatvam.

सत्य (in) truthfulness प्रतिष्ठायाम् on being firmly established क्रिया (of) action फल fruit; result आश्रयत्वम् state of being a substratum.

36. On being firmly established in truthfulness fruit (of action) rests on action (of the *Yogi*) only.

This *Sūtra*, giving the result of acquiring perfect truthfulness, requires some explanation. The apparent meaning of the *Sūtra* is that in the case of a *Yogi* who has acquired this virtue in perfection the fruit of any action that he may do follows unfailingly. For example, if he says something concerning the future then the event predicted must take place according to his prediction. This has been interpreted by many commentators in a rather absurd manner and all the laws of Nature are supposed to be capable of being violated to uphold the fiats of such a person. For example, if he says that the Sun will not set in the evening then the movement of the earth will stop to make his words effective. Stories in the *Purāṇas* which in most cases are mere allegories are taken in a literal sense in support of such a view.

It is, however, not necessary to push the meaning of this *Sūtra* to the logical and absurd conclusion in this manner provided we understand its underlying significance. Let us see.

When an ordinary man says or does anything with the object of achieving any definite result, the thing aimed at may or may not materialize. Of course, any intelligent person with full knowledge of all the relevant conditions can predict the result to a great extent, but no one can be quite sure because there are many unforeseen circumstances in the future which may affect the course of events. Only he can predict the result with certainty whose *Buddhi* is developed and purified sufficiently to reflect the Universal Mind in which the past, present and future can be seen to a great extent. Now, as has been said already, the practice of truthfulness develops and purifies *Buddhi* in a remarkable manner and the mind of a person who has acquired perfection in this virtue becomes like a mirror reflecting the Divine Mind to some extent. He has become, as it were, a mirror of Truth and whatever he says or does reflects at least partially that Truth. Naturally, whatever such a person says will come true; whatever he attempts to accomplish will be accomplished. But why 'the fruit rests on action' in the case of such a person is not due to the fact that God changes the course of events and allows violation of natural laws in order to fulfil his words and resolutions, but because the words and actions of such a man merely reflect God's will and anticipate what is to happen in the future. Taken in this light the meaning of the *Sūtra* becomes quite intelligible and it is possible to avoid the absurd assumption that the Divine Order in the Cosmos can be upset by the whims and decisions of a perfectly truthful person. It is contended that if such a person says something even by mistake that thing must materialize at any cost. This idea is based upon the assumption that such a person can be careless and irresponsible like ordinary people of the world. One who has developed truthfulness to such a high degee must have acquired previously the capacity to weigh every word that comes out of his mouth and to say whatever he has to say deliberately and of set purpose.

३७. अस्तेयप्रतिष्ठायां सर्वरत्नोपस्थानम् ।

Asteya-pratiṣṭhāyāṃ sarva-ratnopasthānam.

अस्तेय (in) honesty; non-misappropriativeness प्रतिष्ठायां on being firmly established सर्व (of) all रत्न gems; precious things उपस्थानम् self-presentation; coming up.

37. On being firmly established in honesty all kinds of gems present themselves (before the *Yogi*).

'All kinds of gems present themselves' does not mean that precious stones begin to fly through the air and fall at his feet. It is a way of saying that he becomes aware of all kinds of treasures in his vicinity. For example, if he is passing through a jungle he becomes cognizant of any treasure buried in the neighbourhood or any mine of precious gems which may be present underground. This cognizance may be of the nature of clairvoyance or mere intuitional awareness like the one possessed by water-diviners.

As long as we have in us the tendency to misappropriate or grasp things which do not belong to us we are governed by the ordinary laws of Nature. When we have risen above this tendency completely and would not even think of taking anything even if a treasure were to fall within our grasp, then we rise, as it were, above the law which confines us strictly to the limited means allotted to us by our *Karma*. Then people around us offer their wealth at our feet, we become mysteriously aware of all kinds of hidden treasures and mines of precious stones hidden within the bowels of the earth. But all this is useless now, for us. We can take nothing for ourselves. When we are bound by the ordinary desires for wealth etc. we have to earn everything by adopting the ordinary means. When we have conquered those desires the ordinary laws are no longer binding on us.

३८. ब्रह्मचर्यप्रतिष्ठायां वीर्यलाभः ।

Brahmacarya-pratiṣṭhāyāṃ vīrya-lābhaḥ.

ब्रह्मचर्य (in) sexual continence प्रतिष्ठायाम् on being firmly established वीर्य (of) vigour; energy लाभः gain.

38. On being firmly established in sexual continence vigour (is) gained.

Vīrya which is translated as vigour does not mean merely physical vigour which no doubt results from the conservation of sexual energy. *Vīrya* is connected with our whole constitution and refers to that vitality which makes all its parts vibrant, so that all weakness, laxity and inadequacy disappear and are replaced by extraordinary resilience, strength and energy. It appears as if there is an influx of tremendous vitality from the higher planes imparting vigour and strength to every vehicle which it touches.

It is worth while referring here to one interesting fact in connection with the conservation of sexual energy which is involved in *Brahmacarya*. It is a well-known doctrine of *Yogic* philosophy that there is a very intimate relation between sexual energy and the energy which is required for bringing about the mental, moral and spiritual regeneration aimed at in *Yogic* discipline. In fact the sexual energy may be considered to be only a gross form of this subtler energy which is called *Ojas*. As long as the sex life continues much of this special kind of available energy in the body is used up in this manner. But after *Brahmacarya* has been well established the possibility opens for the utilization of the conserved energy for the various changes which the *Sādhaka* is trying to bring about in his body and mind. The current of energy which had previously been kept directed to the sexual regions and was being exhausted in sexual indulgence can now be utilized for the purposes mentioned above. But this sublimation and diversion of this energy is possible only for those who have obtained a complete mastery of their sexual instincts and not merely abstained from indulgence for some time. Such people who are able to conserve, transmute and direct this energy continuously towards the cerebrum are called *Ūrdhva-retās*, *Ūrdhva* meaning upwards and *Retas* meaning sexual energy.

This complete control of sexual energy is acquired not merely by abstention from the sex act but also by a very strict and rigid control of thoughts and desires so that not the slightest thought or desire connected with sex or suggesting sex ever enters the mind of the *Sādhaka*. For this current of energy referred to above is extremely susceptible to thought and the slightest thoughts connected with sexual desires immediately stir up and direct the current to the sex organs. *Brahmacarya*, therefore, is not so much a matter of abstention from the sex act as a control of thoughts so complete that not the slightest stirring of our sex instincts is possible at any time. It is only under such conditions that the grosser energies of the body can be sublimated to serve the higher purposes of the soul. And the earlier in life we begin this self-discipline the easier it is to acquire this control.

३९. अपरिग्रहस्थैर्ये जन्मकथंतासंबोधः ।

Aparigraha-sthairye janma-kathaṃtā-saṃbodhaḥ.

अपरिग्रह (in) non-possessiveness स्थैर्ये on becoming steady or confirmed जन्म (of) birth कथंता (of) the 'how' and 'wherefore' संबोधः knowledge.

39. Non-possessiveness being confirmed there arises knowledge of the 'how' and 'wherefore' of existence.

When perfection in *Aparigraha* is attained the *Yogi* acquires the capacity to know the 'how and wherefore' of birth and death. Though there is no ambiguity with regard to the literal meaning of the *Sūtra* and *Janma-Kathaṃtā* is taken to mean knowledge of our previous births it is difficult to understand the underlying significance of this *Sūtra*. Why should knowledge of his previous births arise in the case of a *Yogi* who has conquered the instinct of possessiveness? To understand this enigma we have to recall the relation between the transitory personality which is formed anew with every incarnation and the permanent individuality which is the root of every personality and which persists through the succession of incarnations. Now, the personality works in the lowest three worlds with a new set of bodies which are formed with each successive incarnation. Since these bodies perish one after another at the end of each incarnation and have not passed through the experiences of previous lives, there are no impressions (*Saṃskāras*) in them relating to these experiences. And since memory depends upon the existence of impressions relating to an experience, naturally, there is no memory of those experiences and the whole of the long past stretching through hundreds of lives is a perfect blank to the personality. But, as has been pointed out already, the individuality wears 'immortal' bodies which have passed through all those experiences and carry with them their corresponding impressions. So the *Jīvātmā* or individuality having a permanent record of experiences in the subtler vehicles has a detailed memory of all the experiences.

It should be easy to understand that if somehow these impressions can be contacted and the corresponding memories brought down in the lower vehicles of the present personality, knowledge of experiences gone through in previous lives should become available to the personality. This is what happens when *Aparigraha* is developed to a high degree of perfection. The essence of the personality is the 'I' consciousness which in its turn is the result of the identification by consciousness with the things in our environment and with our lower vehicles including the physical body. The development of non-possessiveness frees us to a very great extent from this habit of identifying ourselves with our bodies and the things with which they are surrounded and thus *loosens the bonds of the personality*. The natural result of this loosening is that the centre of consciousness gradually shifts into the higher vehicles of the *Jīvātmā* and the knowledge present in those vehicles is reflected more and more into the lower vehicles. So, although the lower vehicles have not gone through the experiences of the previous lives, this gradual fusion of the personality and the individuality results in the filtering down of some of this knowledge into the lower vehicles and thus enables the personality to share all this knowledge. That is how the practice of *Aparigraha* enables the *Yogi* to have knowledge of previous births.

The development of such an extraordinary power from the intensive practice of *Aparigraha* shows the importance of doing things with intensity. The secret of discovering the hidden and mysterious facts of life seems to lie in intensity of effort. We meet the phenomena of life superficially and so naturally do not get from them anything more than ordinary experiences. But the moment we do anything with great intensity and try to penetrate into the deeper recesses of life we come across the most extraordinary results and experiences. The extraordinary results achieved by Science in the field of atomic research should have brought home to us this great truth but we believe only in matter and consider the phenomena connected with the mind and consciousness as something intangible and therefore unreal. The truth of the matter, however, is that the mysteries, which are hidden in the realm of matter, are as nothing compared to the mysteries which are related to mind and consciousness. This is what the Science of *Yoga* has proved. To the *Yogi* who has obtained even a faint glimpse of these mysteries the remarkable achievements of Science in the realm of matter and force pale into insignificance and seem hardly worth bothering about.

४०. शौचात् स्वाङ्गजुगुप्सा परैरसंसर्गः ।

Śaucāt svāṅga-jugupsā parair asaṃsargaḥ.

शौचात् from purity स्वाङ्ग (with) one 's limbs, i e. body जुगुप्सा disgust परैः with others असंसर्गः non-contact; non-intercourse.

40. From physical purity (arises) disgust for one's own body and disinclination to come in physical contact with others.

The results of developing purity are given in two *Sūtras*, one relating to the purity of the physical body, the other to the purity of the mind. The two results which follow when the physical body is made quite pure are such as can hardly be expected.

The physical body is essentially a dirty object as a little knowledge of physiology will convince anyone. Physical beauty is proverbially skin deep and beneath this skin there is nothing but a mass of flesh, bones and all kinds of secretions and waste products which arouse disgust in our mind when they come out of the body. It requires only a little effort of the imagination to see the body as it really is inside, but so complete is our identification with it that in spite of our detailed knowledge of its contents we not only feel no disgust for it but regard it as our most loved possession. And most of us go even to the length of thinking that we are the physical body!

With the ordinary purification of the physical body we become more sensitive and begin to see things in their true light. Cleanliness is mostly a matter of sensitiveness. What is intolerably disgusting to a person of refined nature and habits is hardly noticed by another person whose nature is coarse and insensitive. So this feeling of disgust towards one's own body which develops on its purification means nothing more than that we have become sensitive enough to see things as they really are. Of course, the purity meant here is of the more superficial character which is brought about by ordinary external processes such as bathing and *Yogic Kriyās* such as *Neti*, *Dhauti* etc. Purity of a different and more fundamental character is developed by *Tapas* as pointed out in II-43.

The second result which follows on attaining purity of the physical body is naturally related to the first. A person who feels disgust for his own body is not likely to feel any attraction towards the bodies of others which are likely to be comparatively less clean. The disinclination to come in physical contact with others is thus natural and to be expected and this is perhaps one of the reasons why highly advanced *Yogis* seek seclusion and avoid external contact with the world. But it should be noted that this does not mean any feeling of repulsion towards others, for that would be positively reprehensible and against the fundamental law of Love. A positive love towards the owner of the vehicle is quite compatible with a lack of desire to come in contact with the vehicle itself when a person has the capacity to distinguish between the two.

४१. सत्त्वशुद्धिसौमनस्यैकाग्र्येन्द्रियजयात्मदर्शनयोग्यत्वानि च ।

Sattvaśuddhi-saumanasyaikāgryendriya-
jayātma-darśana-yogyatvāni ca.

सत्त्वशुद्धि purity of *Sattva*; purity of *Antaḥ-karaṇa* सौमनस्य cheerful-mindedness ऐकाग्र्य one-pointedness; fixity of attention इन्द्रियजय control of the senses आत्मदर्शन vision of the Self or *Ātmā* -योग्यत्वानि (and) fitness for च and; also (follow).

shows that the path of *Īśvara-Praṇidhāna* is practically an alternate and independent path of achieving the goal which is attained by following the *Aṣṭāṅga-Yoga* with its eight stages or parts. We have seen previously in other cases that extraordinary results can be achieved by pushing the development of a virtue or quality to the extreme limit, but perhaps the attainment of *Samādhi* through *Īśvara-Praṇidhāna* alone is the most remarkable instance of such an achievement. That, by refining and intensifying progressively and systematically an attitude of self-surrender to God, we can by stages attain the supreme Enlightenment is something which should make us pause and marvel at the wonderful mysteries hidden beneath the common things of life. The rationale of this unique accomplishment has been explained to a certain extent in II-32 but it may be worth while summarizing here the main points in the chain of reasoning.

The bondage of the *Puruṣa* in matter is maintained through the obscuring power of the *Citta-Vṛttis* which prevent his seeing the fundamental truth of his existence and knowing himself as he truly is in his Divine nature. These *Citta-Vṛttis* are caused and maintained by the 'I' consciousness which gives rise to innumerable desires and keeps the mind in a state of constant agitation in order to satisfy those desires. If, somehow, this driving force which keeps the mind in a state of perpetual motion and change can be annihilated the mind will come automatically to a state of rest (*Citta-Vṛtti-Nirodha*) just as a car comes to a stop gradually when the gas is shut off. It is not even necessary to apply the brakes though this will no doubt hasten the process of coming to a halt. How can this driving force which keeps the mind in a state of constant agitation and is ultimately responsible for the *Citta-Vṛttis* be annihilated? Obviously, by destroying the desires of the personality which provide the driving force for the mind, or to put it in other words, by dissolving the 'I'. This, as we have seen already, is exactly what is sought to be accomplished through the practice of *Īśvara-Praṇidhāna*. *Īśvara-Praṇidhāna* develops *Para-Vairāgya*, breaks the bonds of the heart, eliminates the desires of the personality and thus naturally and inevitably reduces the mind to a state of *Citta-Vṛtti-Nirodha* which is nothing but *Samādhi*.

It was mentioned in dealing with II-43 that the word *Siddhi* is used in two senses, that of perfection and occult power. It is also used in the sense of accomplishment. In the *Sūtra* under discussion it is used in two senses, that of accomplishment and perfection. Not only can *Samādhi* be attained through the practice of *Īśvara-praṇidhāna* but also perfected by the same technique. This will also be clear from IV-29 in which the technique of *Dharma-Megha Samādhi* is given. This condition will be seen by the student as the highest stage of *Īśvara-praṇidhāna*.

४६. स्थिरसुखमासनम् ।

Sthira-sukham āsanam.

स्थिर steady सुखम् (and) comfortable आसनम् posture

46. Posture (should be) steady and comfortable.

The students of *Yoga* are generally familiar with the practices which are denoted by the word *Āsana*. In fact, many people who do not know anything about *Yoga* confuse it with these physical exercises. It is, however, necessary even for the student of *Yogic* philosophy to understand clearly the place and purpose of *Āsanas* in *Rāja-Yoga*, for in *Haṭha-Yoga* and certain systems of physical culture their purpose is very different. In *Haṭha-Yoga* the subject of *Āsanas* is treated at great length and there are at least 84 *Āsanas* which are described in detail, very specific and sometimes exaggerated results being attributed to many of them. There is no doubt that many of these *Āsanas*, by affecting the endocrine glands and *Prāṇic* currents, tend to bring about very marked changes in the body and if practised correctly and for a sufficiently long time, promote health in a remarkable manner. *Haṭha-Yoga* is based on the principle that changes in consciousness can be brought about by setting in motion currents of certain kinds of subtler forces (*Prāṇa*, *Kuṇḍalinī*) in the physical body. The first step in contacting the deeper levels of consciousness is, therefore, to make the physical body perfectly healthy and fit for the influx and manipulation of these forces. That is why such a strong emphasis is laid on the preparation of the physical body and the *Sādhaka* is required to go through different kinds of physical exercises which are dealt with in treatises on *Haṭha-Yoga.*

In *Rāja-Yoga,* however, the method adopted for bringing about changes in consciousness is based essentially on the control of the mind by the Will and the gradual suppression of the *Citta-Vṛttis.* The technique of *Rāja-Yoga* is, therefore, directed towards the elimination of all sources of disturbance to the mind, whether these sources are external or internal. Now, one of the important sources of disturbance to the mind is the physical body. Even modern psychology recognizes the close connection between the mind and the body and how they act and react on each other all the time. So the *Yogi* must eliminate completely the disturbances which arise from the physical body before he tries to tackle the problem of the mind itself. This is achieved through the practice of *Āsana.* The physical body is fixed in one particular posture and it is found that when it can be kept like this for a long time it ceases to be a source of disturbance to the mind.

Patañjali gives only three *Sūtras* regarding the technique of *Āsanas* but in these he has condensed all the essential knowledge concerning the subject. The first of these given above points out the two essential requirements in the practice of *Āsana.* It should be steady and comfortable. The *Yogi* has to choose any one of the well-known *Āsanas* suitable for the practice of meditation such as *Padmāsana* or *Siddhāsana* and then practise remaining in that posture until he can maintain it for long periods of time without the slightest inclination to make any movement. Sitting in any *Āsana* becomes uncomfortable after a few minutes and the beginner will find that he cannot maintain it for any considerable time without feeling minor discomforts in various parts of the body. If, however, the *Āsana* is correctly chosen and practised in the right way, steady and persistent practice will gradually eliminate all these minor discomforts which cause constant distractions to the mind. The *Yogi* is then able to maintain his body in the correct posture indefinitely and to forget it altogether. If, in spite of prolonged practice and good health, one always feels discomfort in maintaining the posture for long periods there is something wrong either with one's choice of the *Āsana* or method of practising it and it is advisable to seek expert advice.

It is also necessary to understand thoroughly the implication of the word 'steady'. Steadiness does not mean merely the capacity to remain more or less in the same position with freedom to make minor movements and adjustments from time to time. It means a certain degree of immovability which practically amounts to fixing the body in one position and eliminating all movements of any kind. In trying to maintain this immovable position the beginner is apt to introduce a certain amount of rigidity which makes the body tense. This is definitely wrong and will react adversely on the health of the body. What should be aimed at is the ideal combination of immovability with relaxation. It is only then that it is possible to forget the body altogether.

A particular *Āsana* is considered to be mastered when the *Sādhaka* can maintain it steadily and easily for four hours and twenty minutes. This period of time as given in some books on *Haṭha-Yoga* has really no important significance and gives merely an approximate idea of the length of time for which practice may be undertaken for gaining mastery. Once the habit has been acquired the posture can be maintained for any length of time while the *Yogi's* attention is focussed on his mind.

४७. प्रयत्नशैथिल्यानन्तसमापत्तिभ्याम् ।

Prayatna-śaithilyānanta-samāpattibhyām.

प्रयत्न (of) effort शैथिल्य (by) relaxation अनन्त (on) the 'Endless' समापत्तिभ्याम् (and) by meditation.

47. By relaxation of effort and meditation on the 'Endless' (posture is mastered).

For acquiring mastery of an *Āsana* Patañjali gives two helpful suggestions. One is the gradual slackening of effort. The keeping of the physical body in an immovable position for long periods of time requires great effort of the will and the mind has to be directed constantly to the body in order to maintain it in the fixed position. But it is quite obvious that this state of the mind is the opposite of what is aimed at. The mind has to be freed from the consciousness of the body, not tied down to it in the effort to keep it in a particular posture. So the *Sādhaka* is advised to slacken the effort gradually and transfer the control of the body from the conscious to the sub-conscious mind. The conscious mind can thus be withdrawn from the body without affecting the fixed condition of the body in any manner. This is a gradual process but a definite effort has to be made to break this connection between the mind and the body, so that the latter can remain in the prescribed position without requiring any attention from the former.

The other means recommended for acquiring this steadiness is meditation on *Ananta*, the great Serpent which, according to Hindu mythology, upholds the earth. To the modern educated man this direction will appear quite meaningless but if he understands the underlying significance he will see that it is quite reasonable. What is this Serpent which is called *Ananta*? It is the symbolic representation of the force which maintains the equilibrium of the earth and keeps it in its orbit round the Sun. This force, we can see at once, must be similar to the one which works in a gyroscope, a well-known instrument which is utilized in many ways for maintaining an object in a position of equilibrium. Whenever we have to deal with a body which is liable to move from side to side or in some other manner and has to be brought back and kept in a position of equilibrium automatically the principle of the gyroscope is utilized invariably in devising the necessary machinery. Now, the problem of the person who is sitting in a particular *Āsana* for the purpose of meditation is very similar. The body tends to deviate from a fixed position and it has to acquire the tendency to come back to its position of stability automatically. So meditation on *Ananta* the Serpent which symbolizes this particular kind of force is prescribed. The reason why this force is symbolized by a serpent will be apparent to anyone who has seen a gyroscope which reminds one of a coiled snake with its head raised as shown below:

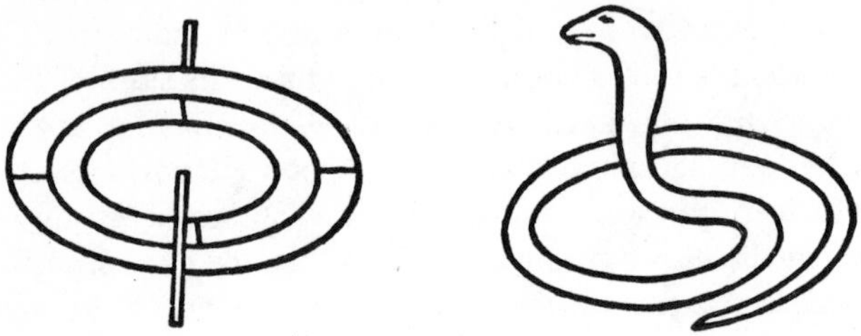

FIG. 7

In Hindu symbolism a thing is generally symbolized by an object or animal which it resembles most closely in outer appearance.

How does meditation on this force help the *Sādhaka* to acquire the stability of the physical posture which he wants to maintain? It is not necessary here to do more than refer to the well-known law of Nature according to which meditation or deep pondering over any idea or principle tends to bring down the corresponding force gradually in our life. In fact, the whole science of acquiring *Siddhis* or occult powers as expounded in Section III of the *Yoga-Sūtras* is based on this axiomatic truth of *Yogic* philosophy. It should be noted that the word used is *Samāpattibhyām* which means ' fusing the mind with '. This is really what happens when we ponder deeply or meditate on an idea and open up a channel for the influx of its corresponding power.

४८. ततो द्वन्द्वानभिघातः ।

Tato dvandvānabhighātaḥ.

ततः from that (mastery of posture) द्वन्द्व (from) pairs of opposites अनभिघातः no assaults.

48. From that no assaults from the pairs of opposites.

The third *Sūtra* hints at the most important result of attaining perfection in the practice of *Āsana*—resistance to the pairs of opposites. These pairs of opposites or *Dvandvas* as they are called in *Saṃskṛta* are the well-known opposite conditions in our outer or inner environment between which our life continually oscillates. These *Dvandvas* are of many kinds, some related to our physical nature, others to our mind. Thus heat and cold are a pair of opposites which affect primarily the physical body. Joy and sorrow are a pair which affect the mind. Now, all these conditions, related to the mind or body which are constantly changing keep the consciousness drawn to the external environment and hinder the mind in going within. They produce *Vikṣepa* or distraction and the *Sādhaka* has to acquire the capacity of rising above them if his mind is to be freed to pursue the more difficult task of suppressing its own internal disturbances and modifications. One important result of gaining perfection in the practice of *Āsana* is freedom from these disturbing reactions to changes in the external world. It is obvious that the *Dvandvas* referred to in this *Sūtra* are those which affect the physical body, such as heat and cold, humidity and dryness and not others which are related to the mind.

Patañjali has given in this *Sūtra* only one result of practising *Āsana*, a result with which the *Sādhaka* is directly concerned in the practice of *Yoga*. But there are also other important benefits which accrue from this practice. Some of these subsidiary results of practising *Āsana* are:

(1) Making the body perfectly healthy and resistant to fatigue and strain.

(2) Acquiring fitness for the practice of *Prāṇāyāma* as a result of proper regulation of *Prāṇic* currents in the body. In fact, those who become proficient in the practice of *Āsana* find that the movements of the breath begin naturally to conform to the requirements of *Prāṇāyāma* and it becomes possible to take to the practice of *Prāṇāyāma* with the greatest ease.

(3) Development of will-power. The physical body is directly and in some mysterious manner related to the *Ātmā*, the source of spiritual power. Gaining control over the physical body which mastery of *Āsana* implies brings about an extraordinary influx of that spiritual force which expresses itself in outer life as will-power.

४९. तस्मिन् सति श्वासप्रश्वासयोर्गतिविच्छेदः प्राणायामः ।

Tasmin sati śvāsa-praśvāsayor gati-
vicchedaḥ prāṇāyāmaḥ.

तस्मिन् on this (perfection of *Āsana*) सति having been (accomplished) श्वासप्रश्वासयोः of in-breathing and out-breathing; of inspiration and expiration गति (of) movement विच्छेदः cessation or break प्राणायामः (is) regulation of breath (fourth constituent part of *Yoga*).

49. This having been (accomplished) *Prāṇāyāma* which is cessation of inspiration and expiration (follows).

The reason why *Prāṇāyāma* plays such an important part in the technique of *Yoga* lies in the close relation existing between *Prāṇa* and mind. *Prāṇa* which exists on all the planes of manifestation is the connecting link between matter and energy on the one hand and consciousness and mind on the other. Consciousness expressing itself through the mind cannot come into touch with matter and function through it without the intermediate presence of *Prāṇa*. Matter in association with energy cannot affect consciousness except through the agency of *Prāṇa*. That is why *Prāṇa* is found on all the planes. It is necessary for the vitalization and functioning of all vehicles of consciousness, physical or superphysical. This capacity to act as intermediary depends upon its peculiar constitution. It combines in itself in some mysterious manner the essential qualities of both matter and consciousness and is thus able to serve as an instrument for their actions and reactions on each other.

This intimate relation existing between *Prāṇa* and mind is utilized in different schools of *Yoga* in different ways. In *Haṭha-Yoga* manipulation of *Prāṇic* currents is utilized for bringing about control of *Citta-Vṛttis* and changes in consciousness. In *Rāja-Yoga*, *Citta-Vṛttis* are controlled by consciousness through the will and *Prāṇa* thus comes under the control of the mind. Patañjali has included both the techniques in his system in order to make it as comprehensive and effective as possible. Thus *Prāṇāyāma* is utilized for preparing the mind for *Dhāraṇā*, *Dhyāna* and *Samādhi* on the one hand and *Saṃyama* on various objects or principles used for acquiring *Siddhis* on the other.

Although students of *Yogic* philosophy are generally familiar with the theory of *Prāṇāyāma* and a fairly extensive literature exists on the subject it would be worthwhile discussing here very briefly some fundamental facts in this connection. This will clear the ground for understanding the inner significance of the five *Sūtras* in which Patañjali has dealt with the subject.

Many people who have not studied the subject or studied it very superficially have the notion that *Prāṇayāma* is merely a regulation of breathing. How it is possible by merely regulating breathing which is a normal physiological process in the body, to bring about the extraordinary results attributed to *Prāṇāyāma* does not occur to them. The nature of *Prāṇāyāma* is indicated by the two words which constitute the compound word, namely *Prāṇa* and *Āyāma* (restraint). It is the regulation of *Prāṇa*. But what is *Prāṇā*? It is not the breath but the vital force which keeps up the activities of the physical body. This vital force is not something vague and mysterious which medical science believes exists within the body maintaining its equilibrium and guarding it against disease and death. It is a real, highly specialized kind of composite energy with a material basis which is entirely different from the other kinds of energies working in the body. The vehicle of this *Prāṇa* is not the dense physical body with which physiologists are familiar but the *Prāṇamaya Kośa*, a somewhat subtler vehicle interpenetrating the dense physical body and working in conjunction with it. In this subtler vehicle which is practically a counterpart of the dense physical body run currents of *Prāṇa*, flowing along well-marked channels into every organ and part of the body and vitalizing them in different ways. For, *Prāṇa* though it is a general vitalizing force, has also specific functions to perform in different organs and parts of the body and is then called by different names which are well known. It is the control of this *Prāṇa* which is aimed at in *Prāṇāyāma* and not breathing which is only one of the many manifestations of its action in the physical body.

But though *Prāṇa* is different from breath as the electric current is different from the movement of the blades in an electric fan, still, there is a close connection between the two, a connection which enables us to manipulate the currents of *Prāṇa* by manipulating breathing. This close connection between breathing and *Prāṇa* is, no doubt, responsible for the confusion between the two but it is necessary for the student to keep this distinction clearly in his mind.

The methods adopted in controlling and manipulating *Prāṇa* by regulation of the breath are a closely guarded secret which can be obtained only from a competent teacher. Those who take up these practices after merely reading books are sure to ruin their health and even risk insanity or death. So, no one should dabble in *Prāṇāyāma* for the sake of fun or for gaining supernormal powers of various kinds or even for hastening his spiritual progress. These forces are very real though not known as yet to modern Science, and many people have ruined their lives by rashly starting practices given in spurious *Yogic* literature or under the advice of immature and over-confident ' *Yogīs* '. The practice of *Prāṇāyāma* can be taken up safely and profitably only as a part of the full *Yogic* discipline and when adequately prepared for by the practice of the other accessories of *Yoga* such as *Yama-Niyama*, *Āsana* etc. and under the supervision of a competent *Guru*.

But while abstaining strictly from the ill-advised practice of *Prāṇāyāma* proper there is no harm in trying to understand its rationale and the limit to which one can go with safety in the manipulation of breathing for the sake of promoting physical and mental health. The essential knowledge with regard to this aspect of the subject may be summarized as follows:

(1) Deep breathing has nothing to do with *Prāṇāyāma* and may be practised as an exercise for promoting health to any reasonable extent. Its beneficial effects depend chiefly upon the increased intake of oxygen and a somewhat greater influx of *Prāṇa* into the body. As it does not affect the *Prāṇic* currents in the body its practice is not attended by any risks.

(2) Breathing alternately through the two nostrils begins at once to affect the *Prāṇic* currents to a certain extent and

tends to remove the congestion from the channels in which *Prāṇa* flows normally. It has been pointed out already that there is a close relation between breathing and the flow of *Prāṇic* currents in the *Prāṇamaya Kośa.* When we breathe normally the *Prāṇic* currents follow their natural course. When we breathe alternately through the two nostrils their normal flow is disturbed in some way. The effect may be likened to the flow of water in a pipe. When the water is flowing in one direction placidly, silt and other things may be deposited at the bottom and are not disturbed to any marked extent by the water. But try to force the water in opposite directions alternately and you at once disturb the deposit and if the process is continued long enough the pipe gets cleaned ultimately. This is how breathing alternately through the two nostrils may be supposed to clean the *Prāṇic* channels or to 'purify the *Nādīs*' as we say. Now, this purification of the *Nādīs* is a preparatory exercise and all those who intend to practise *Prāṇāyāma* have to go through a long course extending over several months or years. It is similar to the preliminary exercise suggested by Patañjali in I-34 and produces the same condition in the nervous system, namely absence of irritation and tranquillity. This exercise is not attended with any risk and can be adopted with caution by those who live a well-regulated and clean life and are not given to excesses of any kind. But since the *Prāṇic* currents are affected in the process, caution and moderation are necessary and it is advisable to work under the supervision of an expert.

(3) Real *Prāṇāyāma* begins when the breath is stopped for some time between inhalation and exhalation. While breathing alternately through the two nostrils the breath may be stopped for some time, the period being increased gradually and cautiously. The retention of breath, called technically *Kumbhaka,* affects the flow of *Prāṇic* currents in a very marked and fundamental manner and enables the *Yogi* to gain increasing control over these

currents so that they can be directed in any manner desired.

(4) *Prāṇāyāma* has to be practised with *Pūraka* and *Recaka* (inspiration and expiration) for a long time, the period of *Kumbhaka* being slowly increased over long periods of time. Such a *Kumbhaka* which is accompanied by *Pūraka* and *Recaka* is called *Sahita Kumbhaka*. But after prolonged practice it is possible to dispense with *Pūraka* and *Recaka* and practise *Kumbhaka* alone. Such *Prāṇāyāma*, called *Kevala Kumbhaka*, gives complete control over *Prāṇa* and enables the *Yogi* to perform not only all kinds of physical feats but also to arouse and direct *Kuṇḍalinī* towards different centres in the body. This science is a strictly guarded secret and can be learnt only by a properly qualified *Celā* from a properly qualified *Guru*.

The important point to keep in mind is this. Not only is *Kumbhaka* the essential element of real *Prāṇāyāma* but it is also the source of danger in the practice of *Prāṇāyāma*. The moment one starts retaining the breath, especially inside, in any abnormal manner the danger begins and one can never know what it will lead to, unless there is a practical and competent teacher at hand to guide and correct the flow of these forces if necessary. If all the requisite conditions are present and *Kumbhaka* is practised under the guidance of a competent teacher it unlocks the doors of unexpected experiences and powers. If it is taken up without the necessary preparation and guidance it is sure to lead to disaster and may be death, as many rash and foolish people have found to their cost.

The significance of the words *Tasmin Sati* in the beginning of the *Sūtra* should be kept in mind. As this *Sūtra* comes after the three *Sūtras* dealing with *Āsanas* these words obviously mean that the practice of *Prāṇāyāma* involving *Kumbhaka* cannot be undertaken until and unless one of the *Āsanas* has been mastered. The practice of *Āsana* definitely but slowly prepares the body for *Prāṇāyāma*. It is the common experience of practical students of *Yoga* that the body begins naturally to assume more and more the condition necessary for the practice of *Prāṇāyāma* as perfection in the practice of *Āsana* is gained. The breath begins to move slowly and rhythmically and even *Kumbhaka* occurs for short periods in a natural way.

In fact, it is not only necessary to master *Āsana* but also to acquire some proficiency in the practice of *Yama-Niyama* before beginning the practice of *Prāṇāyāma*. The advanced practice of *Prāṇāyāma* arouses the *Kuṇḍalinī* sooner or later. This can be done safely only after the desire for sex gratification has been completely mastered and eliminated. Unless, therefore, the *Sādhaka* has practised *Brahmacarya* and other elements of *Yama-Niyama* for a long time and has acquired conscious and real mastery over his desires and propensities it would be disastrous for him to engage in the practice of *Prāṇāyāma*. It must be clearly understood that these things are not meant for people who are leading the ordinary life of the world with all its desires and indulgences and who naively want the peace and bliss of the inner life as an addition to their multitudinous enjoyments in the outer world. The door on the enjoyments and comforts of the lower life has to be shut completely and once for all before one can hope to make any real progress on the path of *Yoga*.

The different elements of *Āṣṭāṅga Yoga* are not merely eight essential but quite independent parts of *Yoga* which can be practised irrespective of one another. They should be taken in the light of progressive stages, each stage preparing for the succeeding ones and requiring an adequate degree of perfection in the preceding ones. The whole treatment of *Āṣṭāṅga Yoga* by Patañjali and the experience of *Sādhakas* lends support to this view.

It is also necessary to note the difference in the words used in I-34 and II-49 in relation to breathing. In the former *Sūtra* the words used are 'expiration and retention' while in the latter the words are 'cessation of inspiration and expiration'. It is not due to any looseness of expression that different words are used to describe the regulation of breathing at different places. Not a word in the *Yoga-Sūtras* is without its significance and necessity although we may not be able to see these clearly. The obvious intention of the author is to indicate that the practice of *Prāṇāyāma* which comes after *Yama-Niyama* and *Āsana* and which prepares the mind for the further stages of *Dhāraṇa*, *Dhyāna* and *Samādhi* is essentially the practice of *Kumbhaka* even though this practice must be preceded by a long course of *Prāṇāyāma* in which *Pūraka* and *Recaka* also play a part.

५०. बाह्याभ्यन्तरस्तम्भवृत्तिर्देशकालसंख्याभिः परिदृष्टो दीर्घसूक्ष्मः ।

Bāhyābhyantara-stambha-vṛttir deśakāla-saṃkhyābhiḥ paridṛṣṭo dīrghasūkṣmaḥ.

बाह्य outer; external आभ्यन्तर internal स्तम्भवृत्तिः suppressed, paralysed, (stopped suddenly) modification देश (by) place काल time संख्याभिः (and) number परिदृष्टः measured; regulated दीर्घ prolonged सूक्ष्मः (and) subtle; attenuated.

50. (It is in) external, internal or suppressed modification; is regulated by place, time and number, (and becomes progressively) prolonged and subtle.

In the *Sūtra* given above the various factors involved in the practice of *Prāṇāyāma* have been dealt with in a very terse manner. The first factor is the position in which the breath is held. There can be three modes of performing *Kumbhaka* and the three kinds of *Prāṇāyāma* referred to in this *Sūtra* depend upon these. Either the breath is held outside after expiration, or held inside after inspiration or just stopped wherever it is at the moment. It is the position or manner in which the breath is held or stopped which determines the kind of *Prāṇāyāma*. The second factor is the place where *Prāṇāyāma* is performed. This will obviously have to be taken into account in determining the period for which *Prāṇāyāma* is performed, the food which is taken and other things. A *Sādhaka* who is practising *Prāṇāyāma* in the tropics will have to adopt a different regimen from the one which is suited for another practising high up in the *Himālayas*. The third factor is the time. Time here means not only the relative duration of *Pūraka*, *Recaka* and *Kumbhaka* but also the time of the year in which *Prāṇāyāma* is being practised. Diet etc. has to be changed according to the season. Number, obviously, refers to the number of rounds at each sitting and the number of sittings in one day. The *Sādhaka* generally starts with a small number of rounds at each sitting and gradually and cautiously increases the number according to the instructions of his teacher.

After pointing out the factors which are involved in regulating the practice of *Prāṇāyāma* the author gives two words which indicate the nature of the objective towards which the efforts of the *Sādhaka* should be directed. In the first place, the period of *Kumbhaka* has to be very gradually and cautiously prolonged. The fourth kind of *Prāṇāyāma* referred to in the next *Sūtra* cannot be practised until the *Sādhaka* has acquired the capacity to practise *Kumbhaka* for fairly long periods of time. Not only has he to prolong the period of *Kumbhaka* but he has also to work in the direction of gradually transferring the process from the outer to the inner invisible plane. This means that the *Prāṇāyāma* from being merely a control and manipulation of the visible process of breathing becomes a process of controlling and manipulating the *Prāṇic* currents flowing in the *Prāṇamaya Kośa*. This transference of activity from the outer to the inner plane can come only after *Kumbhaka* can be practised easily without any strain for fairly long periods, but it must come if *Prāṇāyāma* is to be used for its real purpose in *Yogic* discipline.

५१. बाह्याभ्यन्तरविषयाक्षेपी चतुर्थः ।

Bāhyābhyantara-viṣayākṣepī caturthaḥ.

बाह्य external अभ्यन्तर (and) internal विषय range; sphere; domain आक्षेपी going beyond चतुर्थः (is) the fourth (variety of *Prāṇāyāma*.)

51. That *Prāṇāyāma* which goes beyond the sphere of internal and external is the fourth (variety).

The fourth and the highest kind of *Prāṇāyāma* referred to in this *Sūtra* transcends the movements of the breath altogether. The external breath is kept suspended in any position, external or internal, and there is nothing to show that any kind of activity is going on. And yet the *Prāṇic* currents in the *Prāṇamaya Kośa* which are now under the complete control of the *Sādhaka* are being manipulated and directed with a view to bring about the desired changes in the vehicle.

For conducting operations of such delicacy and importance it is necessary that the *Sādhaka* should be able to see clearly the mechanism of the *Prāṇamaya Kośa* and direct the currents of *Prāṇa* deliberately and unerringly. Such direct vision which means clairvoyance of the lowest kind, develops naturally and automatically during the course of *Prāṇāyāma* practice.

The fourth kind of *Prāṇāyāma* referred to in the *Sūtra* under discussion is the real *Prāṇāyāma* for which all the previous practices are merely a preparation. What takes place during the course of these practices, how the *Prāṇic* currents are used to arouse *Kuṇḍalinī*, how the *Kuṇḍalinī* activates the *Cakras* in the *Suṣumnā* is not mentioned by Patañjali because all these things of a practical nature which are fraught with dangerous possibilities are taught by the *Guru* personally to the *Celā*. Patañjali has throughout dealt with general principles and left out instructions with regard to practical details.

५२. ततः क्षीयते प्रकाशावरणम् ।

Tataḥ kṣīyate prakāśāvaraṇam.

ततः then; from that क्षीयते dissolves; disappears प्रकाश (of) light आवरणम् covering.

52. From that is dissolved the covering of light.

In this *Sūtra* and the next are given two results of *Prāṇāyāma* practice which are of great importance to the *Yogi*. The first is the disappearance of the covering of light. Many commentators have gone completely off the track in the interpretation of the *Sūtra* under discussion, mistaking this light to be the light of the soul. They thus attribute to *Prāṇāyāma* practice accomplishment of results which appear after considerable success has been gained in the subsequent practices of *Dhāraṇā*, *Dhyāna* and *Samādhi*. This misinterpretation is all the more surprising in view of the *Sūtra* which follows. If *Prāṇāyāma* prepares the mind for the practice of *Dhāraṇā* which is the first step in mental control how can it bring about the removal of the covering of light of the soul which is the culmination of mental control?

The covering of light referred to in this *Sūtra* is obviously not used in reference to the light of the soul but to the light or luminosity associated with the subtler vehicles associated with and interpenetrating the physical vehicle. The distribution of *Prāṇa* in the *Prāṇamaya Kośa* and the development of the psychic centres in the ordinary individual is such that he is quite insensitive to these subtler planes. When, through the practice of *Prāṇāyāma*, the necessary changes in the distribution of *Prāṇa* have been made and the psychic centres have been activated, the mechanism of the subtler bodies comes into close and more intimate touch with the physical brain and it is possible to become aware of the subtler vehicles and the luminosity which is associated with them.

An additional advantage to the *Sādhaka* of this 'contact' with the subtler vehicles is that the mental images which he has to work with in *Dhāraṇā* and *Dhyāna* become very precise and almost tangible. The cloudy and blurred mental images which an ordinary person is able to form in his brain are replaced by clear-cut and sharp images in the subtler vehicles. These are manipulated and controlled with far greater ease.

५३. धारणासु च योग्यता मनसः ।

Dhāraṇāsu ca yogyatā manasaḥ.

धारणासु for (stages of) concentration च and योग्यता fitness मनसः of the mind.

53. And the fitness of the mind for concentration.

The second result of *Prāṇāyāma* practice is that it prepares the mind for the practice of *Dhāraṇā*, *Dhyāna* and *Samādhi*—*Antaraṅga*

Yoga. The capacity to form vivid and sharp mental images and to be able to see them clearly is necessary for practising *Dhāraṇā* effectively. As long as our mental images are blurred and confused it is not easy to concentrate on them or manipulate them, as all people who try to meditate know from practical experience. The mind does not seem to get a good hold on them and they tend to slip away easily. *Prāṇāyāma* by removing this difficulty facilitates concentration to a great extent. To say that *Prāṇāyāma* is absolutely necessary for *Dhāraṇā* will perhaps not be justifiable in view of the success attained by followers of other schools of *Yoga* also. But that it helps enormously in the practice of *Dhāraṇā* there can be no doubt. That is why Patañjali has made it an integral part of his *Yogic* technique.

५४. स्वविषयासंप्रयोगे चित्तस्वरूपानुकार इवेन्द्रियाणां प्रत्याहारः ।

Sva-viṣayāsaṃprayoge citta-svarūpānukāra ivendriyāṇāṃ pratyāhāraḥ.

स्व (with) their own; their respective विषय objects असंप्रयोगे not coming into contact चित्त (of) the individual mind's स्वरूप own form; nature अनुकारः the imitating or functioning according to इव as if; like इन्द्रियाणां by the senses प्रत्याहारः abstraction (fifth constituent of *Yoga*).

54. *Pratyāhāra* or abstraction is, as it were, the imitation by the senses of the mind by withdrawing themselves from their objects.

Pratyāhāra is the next *Aṅga* or component part of *Yoga* after *Prāṇāyāma.* There seems to exist a good deal of uncertainty in the mind of the average student with regard to the nature of this *Yogic* practice. Patañjali has disposed of the subject in two *Sūtras* and the commentaries are not very illuminative. In order to understand what *Pratyāhāra* really means let us recall how mental perception of objects in the outer world takes place. We perceive an object when different kinds of vibrations which emanate from it strike our sense-organs and the mind is then joined to the sense-organs thus activated. As a matter of fact, from the physiological and psychological points of view there are many stages intervening between the reception of the vibration by the sense-organs and the perception by the mind but let us, for the sake of simplicity, confine ourselves to the simple representation of the mechanism of sense-perception as generally understood. This may be represented diagrammatically as follows:

Bhūtas (elements)	*Indriyas* (sense-organs)	*Tanmātras* (sensations)	*Citta* (mind)	*Buddhi* (perception)	*Ātmā* (Spirit)
Prithvī (earth) →	nose →	smell →	MIND	←	☼
Jala (water) →	tongue →	taste →			
Tejas (light) →	eye →	sight →			
Vāyu (air) →	skin →	touch →			
Ākāśa (ether) →	ear →	hearing →			

Now, it is a matter of common experience that the corresponding vibrations may be striking against any particular sense-organ but if the mind is not joined, as it were, to that sense-organ the vibrations remain unperceived. The clock in our room keeps ticking constantly but we rarely hear the ticking. Although the vibrations of sound are striking the ear constantly the conscious mind is not joined to the organ of hearing as far as those vibrations are concerned. When we pass down a road vibrations from hundreds of objects strike our eye but we notice only a few, the rest not entering our consciousness at all because of this lack of contact between the mind and those vibrations. Innumerable vibrations from all kinds of objects are thus constantly impinging upon our sense-organs but most of these remain unnoticed. Still, a few do manage to catch our attention and these in their totality constitute the content of our awareness of the external world.

A very interesting fact about this process of sense-perception is that although the mind is automatically ignoring the vast majority of vibrations bombarding its sense-organs it cannot shut out all of them voluntarily if it wants to. A few vibrations always manage to catch the attention and the mind is generally helpless against the inroads of these unwanted intruders. In fact, the more it tries to shut them out the more numerous and insistent they become as anyone can find out for himself by making a few efforts in this direction.

But, for the practice of *Rāja Yoga* the outer world has to be shut out completely, whenever necessary, in order that the *Yogi* may have his mind alone to grapple with. Let us go into this question a little more in detail. If we examine the contents of our mind at any time when we are not making any particular mental effort we shall find that the mental images which are present and changing constantly may be divided into the following three categories: (1) Ever-changing impressions produced by the outer world through the vibrations impinging upon the sense-organs. (2) Memories of past experiences floating in the mind. (3) Mental images connected with anticipations of the future. (2) and (3) are wholly mental, not depending upon any objective reality outside the mind while (1) are the direct result of contact with the outer world. The object of *Pratyāhāra* is to eliminate (1) completely from the mind, thus leaving only (2) and (3) which are then mastered through *Dhāraṇā* and *Dhyāṇa*. *Pratyāhāra* interposes, as it were, a shutter between the sense-organs and the mind and isolates the latter completely from the external world.

In the light of what has been said above it should be easy to understand the meaning of the rather enigmatic *Sūtra* we are discussing. It will help us to appreciate the manner in which the idea has been expressed if we remember that according to *Yogic* psychology the senses are really a part of the lower mind. They are, as it were, the outposts of the mind in the external world and should follow the lead of the mind. When the mind wants to put itself in touch with the external world they should begin to function. When it decides to withdraw they should be able to withdraw with it, thus breaking all connection with the world outside. This relation between the mind and the senses has been likened very aptly to the relation existing between the bees in a hive and the queen bee. The bees follow the queen in a body as it flies from one place to another, and do not function independently of the queen.

Is this complete severance of connection with the world outside in the manner indicated possible? It is not only possible but absolutely necessary if the higher stages of the *Yogic* path are to be trodden. But in order that success may be attained the *Yogic* life has to be adopted as a whole. All the different steps or component parts of *Yogic* discipline are linked with one another, and success in tackling any particular problem depends to a great extent upon how far the other related problems, especially those going before, have been mastered. If *Yama* and *Niyama* have not been practised sufficiently and all emotional disturbances eliminated, if *Āsana* and *Prāṇāyāma* have not been mastered and the physical body brought under complete control, then surely, the practice of *Pratyāhāra* is bound to end in failure. But if the whole of the *Sādhaka's* life conforms to the *Yogic* ideal and all his energies are bent on achieving his ultimate goal then success must come sooner or later.

It should also be mentioned here that though *Pratyāhāra* appears to be a control of the senses by the mind, the essential technique is really the withdrawal of the mind into itself. It is a kind of abstraction so complete that the sense-organs cease to function. Any school boy who is intensely interested in a novel cuts himself off from the outer world. Any inventor like Edison who is absorbed in a problem can forget the external world completely. But in all such cases, although a high degree of abstraction is attained the abstraction is involuntary and there is something in the external world on which the mind is concentrated. In *Pratyāhāra* the abstraction is voluntary and the mind has no object of attraction in the external world. Its field of activity is entirely within itself and the external world is kept out by the sheer force of will, as in *Rāja Yoga*, or by the supreme attractive power of an object of love within, as in *Bhakti Yoga*.

५५. ततः परमा वश्यतेन्द्रियाणाम् ।

Tataḥ paramā vaśyatendriyāṇām.

ततः then; from that परमा the highest; the greatest वश्यता mastery इन्द्रियाणाम् over the senses.

55. Then follows the greatest mastery over the senses.

The successful practice of *Pratyāhāra* as we have seen in the previous *Sūtra* gives complete control over the *Indriyas* in the sense that we no longer remain their slaves but become their master, switching them off and on as we switch off and on the electric light in our room. What such a power will mean to an ordinary man can be easily imagined, but for a *Rāja Yogi* it is a *sine qua non.*

It is interesting to note how the first five *Aṅgas* of *Yoga* eliminate one after another different sources of disturbance to the mind and prepare it for the final struggle with its own *Vṛttis.* First to be eliminated by *Yama-Niyama* are the emotional disturbances due to moral defects in one's nature. Next to be eliminated by the practice of *Āsana* are the disturbances which arise in the physical body. Then come the disturbances caused by the irregular or insufficient flow of vital forces in the *Prāṇic* sheath. All these are removed completely by the practice of *Prāṇāyāma.* And lastly, through *Pratyāhāra* is removed the major source of disturbances coming through the sense-organs. Thus is accomplished *Bahiraṅga* or external *Yoga* and the *Sādhaka* becomes capable of treading the further stages of *Antaraṅga* or internal *Yoga.*

SECTION III

VIBHŪTI PĀDA

VIBHŪTI PĀDA

१. देशबन्धश्चित्तस्य धारणा ।

Deśa-bandhaś cittasya dhāraṇā.

देश place; spot बन्धः binding; confining; fixing चित्तस्य of the mind धारणा concentration.

1. Concentration is the confining of the mind within a limited mental area (object of concentration)

As has been pointed out already, the first five *Aṅgas* of *Yoga* eliminate, step by step, the external causes of mental distraction. *Yama* and *Niyama* eliminate the disturbances which are caused by uncontrolled emotions and desires. *Āsana* and *Prāṇāyāma* eliminate the disturbances arising from the physical body. *Pratyāhāra*, by detaching the sense-organs from the mind, cuts off the external world and the impressions which it produces on the mind. The mind is thus completely isolated from the external world and the *Sādhaka* is thus in a position to grapple with it without any interference from outside. It is only under these conditions that the successful practice of *Dhāraṇā*, *Dhyāna* and *Samādhi* is possible.

Although the different *Aṅgas* of *Yoga* appear to be independent of each other and it may be possible to a certain extent to practise *Āsana*, *Dhyāna*, etc. independently of other *Aṅgas*, still, we have to keep in mind that they have also a sequential relationship and the effective practice of one *Aṅga* requires at least a partial mastery of those which precede it. The main reason why the vast majority of aspirants for the *Yogic* life keep struggling with the mind year after year and then generally give up the effort as a hopeless task, lies in the lack of systematic preparation without which even the elementary practice of *Dhāraṇā* is very difficult, to say nothing of the further stages of *Dhyāna* and *Samādhi*. Theoretically, it is possible for the student to start right away with the mind and he may succeed in practising meditation to a certain extent but he cannot go very far in this manner and his progress is bound to come to a stop sooner or later. It is only when he has prepared himself in the manner indicated above that he can go on steadily right up to the end. In the rare cases where people have practised meditation successfully without any other kind of preparation it will be found that they had already developed the necessary qualifications, even though they did not go through all the practices in this life. It is the possession of the qualifications and not going through the prescribed practices which determines the fitness of the *Sādhaka* for taking up the practice of *Dhāraṇā*, *Dhyāna* and *Samādhi*. These qualifications for the *Yogic* life are the cumulative result of several lives of effort in this direction and one need not go through every practice in a particular life. Some people are born, for example, with a high degree of *Vairāgya* and show even in their childhood a remarkable capacity for controlling their vehicles. They have not to go through the long and tedious discipline which is essential for the ordinary man. Anyway, Patañjali has pointed out unambiguously the necessity of going through the first five *Aṅgas* of *Yoga* before taking up the practice of *Dhāraṇā*, as for example in II-53.

Before dealing with the question of *Dhāraṇā* it is necessary to point out that though the word concentration has to be used for translating *Dhārāṇā* there is a great deal of difference between what an ordinary man means by concentration of mind and what this phrase means in *Yogic* psychology. Without going into details it may be stated that the main difference, and a very fundamental difference, is that according to modern psychology the mind cannot be made to remain fixed on any object for any considerable time. It must remain moving even when concentration of the highest degree has been attained. Concentration according to this view is the controlled movement of the mind within a limited sphere and by keeping the mind confined in this manner all the remarkable results of concentrated mental effort can be obtained. But according to Eastern psychology upon which the Science of *Yoga* is based, though concentration begins with the controlled movement of the mind it can reach a state in which all movement or change stops. In this ultimate stage the mind becomes one with the essential nature of the object concentrated upon and can thus move no further.

Eastern psychology recognizes the uses of the ordinary type of concentration but it holds that there are two limitations in this kind of concentration. One is that the mind can never fully realize the essential nature of the object concentrated upon. However deep it may penetrate, it still touches only the fringe or superficial aspects of its nature and can never reach the core. The second limitation is that with this kind of concentration consciousness always remains confined within the prison-house of the intellect. It cannot be released from the limitations of the intellect to be able to function at the deeper levels through the subtler vehicles. For, to be able to jump from one plane to another the mind must be brought first to that condition in which it is without movement though ' shining ' with the object which holds the field of consciousness. This point has been elaborated elsewhere and we need not go further into it here.

Let us now come to the particular stage of concentration dealt with in this *Sūtra*. In *Dhāraṇā*, as this first stage is called, the mind is confined within a limited sphere defined by the object which is being concentrated upon. The phrase *Deśa-Bandha* means confinement within a territory which allows a limited freedom of movement. The mind is interned, as it were, within the limited mental territory and has to be brought back immediately if it strays out. The reason why a limited freedom of movement is possible when the mind is being concentrated upon a particular object will be seen if we remember that every object has innumerable aspects and the mind can consider these aspects only one by one. So that, while it takes up one aspect after another it is moving and yet really fixed on the object of concentration. Or it may be that the object may involve a process of reasoning consisting of many steps connected logically with each other and forming an integrated whole. Here also there can be movement without really leaving the object of concentration. It is only when the mind gets out of touch with the object and an unconnected and irrelevant object enters it that *Dhāraṇā* may be considered to be broken. The main work in *Dhāraṇā* therefore consists in keeping the mind continuously engaged in the consideration of the object and to bring it back immediately as soon as the connection is broken. The objective which the *Sādhaka* should place before himself is to reduce progressively the frequency of such interruptions and to eliminate them completely ultimately. But it is not only the elimination of interruptions which has to be aimed at but complete focussing of the mind on the object. Vague and blurred impressions should be replaced by sharply defined mental images by increasing the degree of alertness and power of attention. So, the condition of the mind during the period when it is engaged with the object is as important as the frequency of the interruptions which break the connection. But as the nature of this stage of concentration is generally understood we need not elaborate this point further.

२. तत्र प्रत्ययैकतानता ध्यानम् ।

Tatra pratyayaikatānatā dhyānam.

तत्र there; in that (place) प्रत्यय content of consciousness; एकतानता stretching or streaming unbrokenly as one ध्यानम् meditation; contemplation.

2. Uninterrupted flow (of the mind) towards the object (chosen for meditation) is contemplation.

It was pointed out in the previous *Sūtra* that the *Sādhaka* should aim at eliminating the intruding thoughts which are called distractions and should see that such interruptions are reduced in frequency in a progressive manner. When he succeeds in eliminating the distractions completely and can continue the concentration on the object without any interruptions for as long as he decides to do so he reaches the stage of *Dhyāna*. It will be seen, therefore, that it is the occasional appearance of distractions in the mind which constitutes the essential difference between *Dhāraṇā* and *Dhyāna*. Since this *Sūtra* is very important from the practical point of view let us first examine the significance of the various *Saṃskṛta* words used in defining *Dhyāna*.

Let us first take the word *Pratyaya* which is used frequently in the *Yoga-Sūtras*. This word covers a wide range of notions such as concept, idea, cause, etc. but in *Yogic* terminology it is generally used for the total content of the mind which occupies the field of consciousness at a particular time. As the mind is capable of holding a large variety of objects simultaneously a word has to be used to denote all these objects taken together irrespective of their nature. *Pratyaya* is a technical word for this total content of the mind. In view of what has been said above about *Dhāraṇā*, it will be seen that this *Pratyaya* with which the mind remains in continuous contact in *Dhyāna* is fixed and yet a variable thing. It is fixed in the sense that the area within which the mind moves is defined and remains the same. It is variable because within that limited area or sphere there is movement. A few illustrations will make this point clear. When a scientist focusses his microscope on a drop of dirty water the field of vision is defined and limited within a circle and he cannot see anything outside it. But within that circular patch of light there are constant movements of all kinds. Or, take a river which is flowing within well-defined banks. There is constant movement of the water and yet this movement is confined within the banks of the river. A person who looks at a river from an aeroplane sees a thing which is fixed and moving at the same time. These illustrations help us to understand the dual nature of the *Pratyaya* in *Dhyāna* and the possibility of keeping the mind moving within the limits defined by the object of meditation.

The *Saṃskṛta* word *Tatra* means ' in that place ' and obviously refers to the *Deśa* or place or mental territory within which the mind is confined. The mind has to remain united with the *Pratyaya* within the limits defined in *Dhāraṇā*. The mind of any person remains united with the *Pratyaya* while he is in waking consciousness. But not only is the *Pratyaya* changing all the time but the mental territory is also changing because the mind is flitting from one subject to another.

Ekatānatā which means ' extending continuously or unbrokenly ' refers to the absence of interruptions from distractions which are present in *Dhāraṇā*. In fact, as pointed out above, continuity of the *Pratyaya* is the only thing which distinguishes *Dhāraṇā* from *Dhyāna* from the technical point of view. This continuity may be compared to the continuity of the flow of water in a river or that of oil being poured from one vessel into another. Why is it essential to achieve this kind of continuity before *Samādhi* can be practised? Because every break in the continuity means distraction and distraction means lack of adequate concentration and grip over the mind. If the mind is diverted from the chosen object it means that some other object has taken its place, for there must be continuity in the movement of the mind. It is only in *Nirodha* that the continuity of the movement can be broken without any other object occupying the mind. Now, if a distraction breaks the continuity, apparently, there is not much harm done, for the mind can take up the thread immediately and continue with its work of diving deep into the subject. But actually, the appearance of the distraction is not as innocuous as it appears. It shows the absence of sufficient grip over the mind and a corresponding lack in the depth of concentration. In practising *Dhāraṇā* it is found that as the depth of abstraction increases and the grip over the mind becomes stronger, the frequency with which the distractions appear becomes smaller. So, continuity should be regarded as a gauge for measuring the necessary control over the mind and intensity of concentration. The attainment of *Dhyāna Avasthā* shows that the mind is getting ready for the last stage and the real practice of *Yoga*. Unless and until this condition is fulfilled the practice of *Samādhi* cannot be begun and the real secrets of *Yoga* will remain hidden from the *Sādhaka*.

३. तदेवार्थमात्रनिर्भासं स्वरूपशून्यमिव समाधिः।

Tad evārthamātra-nirbhāsaṃ svarūpa-
śūnyam iva samādhiḥ.

तदेव (तत्+एव) the same अर्थ the 'object'; the thing being meditated upon मात्र only निर्भासं 'shining' or appearing therein

स्वरूप true or essential form शून्यम् empty; void; cipher इव as if समाधिः (is) *Samādhi*; trance.

3. The same (contemplation) when there is consciousness only of the object of meditation and not of itself (the mind) is *Samādhi*.

Now we come to the last stage of the concentration of the mind. This marks the culmination of the previous preparation to make it fit to dive into the realm of realities which lie hidden behind the phenomenal world. The subject of *Samādhi* has been dealt with thoroughly in Section I. But in that Section its more general and deeper aspects were considered. In the present context it is therefore necessary to deal only with its introductory aspects especially with its relation to *Dhāraṇā* and *Dhyāna*. On account of the unusual manner in which the subject of *Samādhi* has been dealt with by Patañjali it will be necessary for the student to study carefully its various aspects several times before he can grasp its essential nature and technique. But the time and mental energy which he spends will be worth while for he will acquire in this manner an understanding of the essential technique of *Yoga*, the only technique which can unlock the gates of the world of Reality.

When the state of *Dhyāna* has been well established and the mind can hold the object of meditation without any distractions it is possible to know the object much more intimately than in ordinary thinking, but even then a direct knowledge of its very essence is not obtained and the reality hidden within the object seems to elude the *Yogi*. He is like a general who has reached the very gates of the fort which he has to conquer but the gates are closed and he is unable to enter the fort. What is standing between him and the reality of the object which he wants to know? III-3 gives an answer to this question. The mind itself is preventing the realization of the very essence of the object of meditation. All the distractions have been completely eliminated and the consciousness is fully focussed on the object of meditation. How does the mind interfere with the realization of the very essence of the object? By interposing consciousness of itself between the reality hidden behind the object and the consciousness of the *Yogi*. It is this self-consciousness or subjectivity, pure and simple, which serves as a veil to keep it separated from the object and to hide the reality he is seeking.

To understand how consciousness of the mind of itself can become a bar to further progress, let us recall how this self-consciousness interferes with intellectual work of the highest order. A great musician is able to create his best productions when he loses himself completely in his work. An inventor solves his greatest problems when he is not conscious of solving any problem. It is at such moments that these people get their inspirations and contact with what they are seeking, provided, of course, they have mastered the technique and their mind is fully concentrated. It is the disappearance of self-consciousness which somehow opens the door to a new world which they cannot enter normally.

Something similar though at a much higher level takes place when *Dhyāna* passes into *Samādhi* and the gate which leads into the world of realities opens. Patañjali calls this disappearance of the mind's awareness of itself as *Svarūpa śūnyam iva*. 'The mind's "own-form" or essential nature disappears, as it were.' Let us examine this phrase carefully because each word in it is significant. What is *Svarūpa*? Everything in manifestation has two forms. An external form expressing its superficial and non-essential nature which is called *Rūpa* and an internal form which constitutes the very essence or substance of its true nature which is called its *Svarūpa*. In the case of the mind in the state of *Dhyāna* the *Rūpa* is the *Pratyaya* or the object of meditation. It is through this that the mind finds expression. The *Svarūpa* is the residual consciousness of its own action or role in the process of *Dhyāna* and is essentially the subjective nature of the mind. This consciousness steadily becomes weaker as *Dhāraṇā* passes into *Dhyāna* and the concentration of the mind in *Dhyāna* increases. But still, it is present, even though in a weak form, in all stages of *Dhyāna*, and it is only when it disappears completely that *Dhyāna* passes into *Samādhi*.

The word *Śūnyam* means a void or cipher and here it must be interpreted as cipher, because it is a question of reducing the residual self-awareness to the vanishing point and not of emptying anything to the utmost limit. In fact, as the objects of meditation continue to fill the mind completely there can be no question of emptying the mind. *Svarūpa Śūnyam* therefore means reducing the self-awareness or the subjective role of the mind to the utmost limit. Lest the student may imagine that the *Svarūpa* really disappears when the *Samādhi* takes the place of *Dhyāna* the author adds the word *Iva* which means 'as if'. The *Svarūpa* only seems to disappear but does not in reality because when the *Samādhi* comes to an end it manifests again immediately.

The question as to how it is possible to know the innermost nature of an object of meditation by fusing the mind with it is a very interesting one and has been dealt with fully in considering I-41. It will suffice to point out here that the apparent disappearance of the self-awareness means really dissolution of the subject-object relationship and their fusion in consciousness. With the disappearance of the mental *Svarūpa* a faculty higher than the intellect comes into play, and the perception of the reality hidden behind the object takes place through the instrumentality of this faculty which perceives by becoming one with the object of perception. The perceiver, the object of perception and perception become fused in one state.

When the self-awareness has disappeared, what is left in the mind? Only the object of meditation can remain, for all kinds of distractions have to be eliminated before the state of *Dhyāna* can be firmly established. This is the meaning of the phrase *Artha-mātra-Nirbhāsaṃ*. The phrase *Tad eva* means 'the same' and is used here to emphasize the fact that *Samādhi* is merely an advanced phase of *Dhyāna* and not a new technique. The only difference between them as we have seen is the absence of the mental self-awareness which makes the object shine in a new light.

The difference between the three phases of the same process which culminates in *Samādhi* may be represented in the following way. If A is the object chosen for *Saṃyama* and B, C, D, E, etc. are distractions, then the content of the mind at regular intervals of successive moments in the three phases may be represented by the following series of *Pratyayas* present in the mind. The circle round the letters represents the mental self-awareness referred to above.

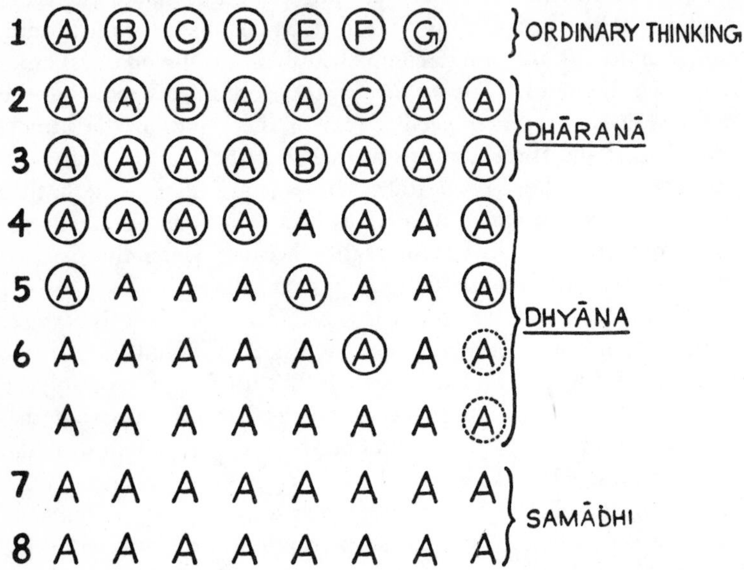

It will be seen that the frequency of distractions goes on decreasing in *Dhāraṇā* and frequency and degree of mental self-awareness goes on decreasing in *Dhyāna.* In *Samādhi* there is complete freedom both from distractions and self-awareness and the object alone remains in the field of consciousness. It is true that further changes are possible but these changes are connected with the object itself and do not affect the two conditions which determine the state of *Samādhi.* But these further developments have been discussed in connection with I-42-49.

It will be seen that the transformations which take place in *Dhāraṇā*, *Dhyāna* and *Samādhi* are purely mental phenomena and are related to consciousness. The mind has already been disconnected from the body and whatever takes place in the realm of the mind cannot be judged by the condition of the body. The physiological functions go on perfectly but there is no response of the body either to the world outside or inside. This lack of response to outer stimuli in the physical body in the state of *Samādhi* makes many people mistake ordinary trance for *Samādhi.* But mere trance cannot be a proof of the attainment of *Samādhi.* The body becomes unresponsive in sleep or under the influence of anaesthetics or drugs. It also becomes unresponsive when, in the case of psychics, the subtler vehicles withdraw from the physical body and consciousness begins to function in the subtler world next to the physical. In all such cases the body is inert but the lower mind is functioning partially or fully in the next subtler vehicle. It is still under the full domination of distractions as before. The mental processes leading up to *Samādhi* take place in the lower mental body and require the quiescence of the lower vehicles. Therefore, the fact of a person being in real *Samādhi* is determined solely by the condition of his mind and not at all by the inertness of the physical body.

It is necessary to draw attention to these obvious facts because those who are not well versed in the philosophy of *Yoga* and dabble in lower psychism generally confuse the inertness of the physical body with *Samādhi* and a person who can manage to remain unconscious for any length of time is regarded as a great *Yogi*! This condition of mere inertness is generally referred to as *Jaḍa-Samādhi* and has really no relation with true *Samādhi* although outwardly they appear very much alike. A person who comes out of true *Samādhi* brings with him the transcendent knowledge, wisdom, peace and strength of the inner life while a person who comes out of *Jaḍa-Samādhi* is no wiser than a person who comes out of sleep. Sometimes, when he is psychic he may be able to bring down into the physical brain clear or confused memory of some of his experiences on the next subtler plane but there is nothing remarkable or reliable about these experiences and certainly there is nothing in common with the transcendent knowledge which is gained in true *Samādhi*.

The extent of ignorance prevailing with regard to these things is sometimes amazing. Some time ago an article was published in a well-known *Hindi* journal dealing with the different stages of *Samādhi*. In this article were given a series of photographs of a *Yogi* supposed to be passing into different stages of *Samādhi* one after another. The series of photographs, as far as could be seen, merely showed an increasing dullness of the eyes but what was astounding was that they showed more and more *physical* light coming out of the physical body in the advanced stages of *Samādhi*!

As if the light which dawns in the consciousness of the *Yogi* in *Samādhi* can be photographed! But such is the power of ignorance to distort and vulgarize the highest truths of life and to consider everything in terms of the physical which is the only part of life which is tangible and visible to the common man.

४. त्रयमेकत्र संयमः ।

Trayam ekatra saṃyamaḥ.

त्रयम् the three एकत्र in one place; jointly संयमः (is) *Saṃyama*; a technical word meaning *Dhāraṇā, Dhyāna* and *Samādhi* taken together.

4. The three taken together constitute *Saṃyama*.

It should be clear from what has been said previously in dealing with *Dhāraṇā, Dhyāna* and *Samādhi* that these are really different phases of the same mental process, each succeeding stage differing from the preceding in the depth of concentration which has been attained and the more complete isolation of the object of contemplation from distractions. The complete process beginning with *Dhāraṇā* and ending in *Samādhi* is called *Saṃyama* in *Yogic* terminology and the practical mastery of its technique opens the door not only to knowledge of all kinds but also to powers and superphysical accomplishments known as *Siddhis*.

It is necessary to keep in mind two facts about *Saṃyama*. First, it is a continuous process and the passage from one stage to another is not marked by any abrupt change in consciousness. Secondly, the time taken in reaching the last stage depends entirely upon the progress made by the *Yogi*. The beginner may have to spend hours and days in reaching the final stage while the Adept can pass into it almost instantaneously and effortlessly. As *Samādhi* does not involve any movement in space but merely sinking, as it were, towards the centre of one's own consciousness, time is not an essential factor in the process. The time taken by the *Yogi* is due entirely to the lack of mastery of the technique.

५. तज्जयात् प्रज्ञालोकः ।

Taj-jayāt prajñālokaḥ.

तत्-जयात् by mastering it प्रज्ञा the higher consciousness आलोकः light.

5. By mastering it (*Saṃyama*) the light of the higher consciousness.

It has already been pointed out in dealing with *Saṃprajñāta Samādhi* (I-17) that *Prajñā* is the higher consciousness which appears in the state of *Samādhi*. But as the word *Samādhi* covers a wide range of states of consciousness, so *Prajnā* stands for all the states of consciousness in *Samādhi* beginning with the *Vitarka* stage and ending with the *Asmitā* stage. There are two critical stages in the subtilization of *Prajñā*. One of these is referred to in I-47 where the light of spirituality irradiates the mental consciousness. The other is indicated in III-36 when the consciousness of the *Puruṣa* begins to illuminate the *Yogi's* consciousness. The role of *Prajñā* comes to an end when *Viveka Khyāti* or the pure awareness of Reality takes its place as indicated in IV-29.

६. तस्य भूमिषु विनियोगः ।

Tasya bhūmiṣu viniyogaḥ.

तस्य its भूमिषु in stages विनियोगः application; employment.

6. Its (of *Saṃyama*) use by stages.

This *Sūtra* brings out another important fact about the application of *Saṃyama*. *Saṃyama*, as has been pointed out already, is the composite process of *Dhāraṇā*, *Dhyāna* and *Samādhi* when applied to any object. But though the process will be essentially the same in every case, it will be more or less complicated according to the nature of the object to which it is applied. All objects in the

Universe are not equally mysterious if we may say so. The mystery which is hidden behind them depends upon the depth of the reality in which they are rooted. Take, for example, the following objects: a piece of stone, a rose and a human being. All the three objects have their physical casing and although the physical particles constituting the physical form are progressively more organized as we pass from the first to the third, still, there is not much difference between them if we consider only their physical nature. But what a tremendous difference there exists between them when we try to go behind the outer forms in order to unravel the mystery which lies hidden within them! Any fool can see that there is some difference between them although all three of them are physically on the same level. A rose arouses even in the ordinary man thoughts and emotions which a stone can never do and the mystery which is hidden behind the human form is one of the eternal riddles of the Universe. Materialistic philosophy may use all the logic which it can command to prove that essentially there is no difference between the objects except that of functions and structures and people may thoughtlessly repeat these dogmas of a mechanistic universe but in actual life nobody takes these dogmas seriously and even the rank materialist has to recognize and take into account these differences in his life. The voice of intuition cannot be silenced by these intellectual dogmas.

What causes the differences between 'objects' such as those mentioned above? Why is a rose a more mysterious object than a piece of stone and a human being infinitely more mysterious than a rose? To understand these differences it is necessary to bear in mind that the outer form of any physical or mental object is merely a covering of an inner reality and what we mentally see of the object does not constitute the totality of the object. As in the case of a ship the part which is submerged below the surface of water is much larger than the part that is visible, in the same way, what we mentally see in an object is merely a small fraction of what is hidden from our view. The researches made in the domain of Science have brought to our knowledge by methods of experiment and reasoning a part of these hidden realities but what we have come to know in this manner is very little and of comparatively less significance as compared with the totality of what lies beyond the range of scientific investigations. These submerged aspects of all objects can be exhaustively investigated only by the methods of *Yoga*, and *Saṃyama* is the key which unlocks the doors of these hidden worlds.

All objects in the manifested Universe, as has been pointed out already, are an expression of an Ultimate Reality but the roots of different objects lie at different levels of spirit-matter combinations through which this Reality is manifested. We may symbolize this fact diagrammatically by the following figure in which the centre of the concentric circles stands for the Ultimate Reality and the successive circles represent the different planes of existence in their increasing order of density.

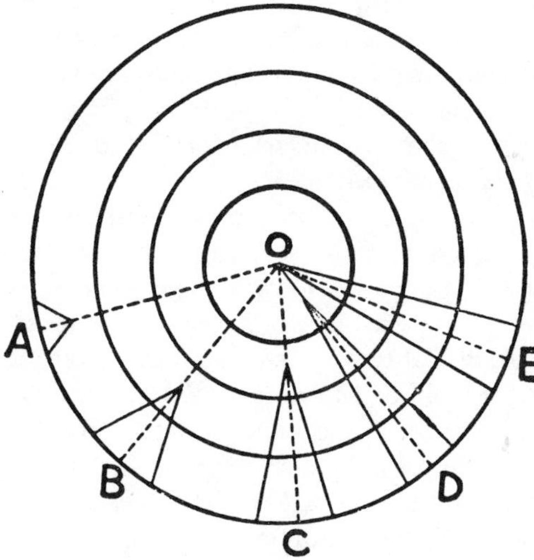

FIG. 8

The objects A, B, C, D represented by arcs of the outermost circle will be seen to have their roots in progressively subtler planes of existence, while the object E will be seen to be rooted in the Ultimate Reality Itself.

Taking the three objects mentioned above for comparison we can see easily that in the case of a piece of stone we have a mere conglomeration of physical matter with no design at its basis and so its roots cannot lie very deep. In the case of a rose also we have a conglomeration of different kinds of matter but this combination differs from that of a stone in two things. Firstly, it has the capacity for organic growth and decay inherent in it and secondly, its form corresponds to an archetype. Even to a superficial observer it should be obvious that a rose has got deeper roots in reality than a piece of stone. Coming to the human form we cannot help feeling that we are face to face with a profound mystery. We have here not only a more elaborate material structure but the form is the vehicle of complicated phenomena like thoughts and emotions and other aspects of consciousness. Whatever may be the nature and potentiality of human consciousness there cannot be the slightest doubt that the roots of a human being lie much deeper than those of a rose. How far they penetrate into the heart of the manifested Universe it is unnecessary to discuss here. According to the philosophy upon which the Science of *Yoga* is based they reach to the very Centre of Ultimate Reality. That is what the doctrine of the identical nature of *Jīvātmās* and *Paramātmā* really means.

The fact that there are enormous differences in the inner complexity of objects must be kept in mind if we are to understand why the technique of *Saṃyama* is a very complicated science and has to be mastered in stages. Some objects touch as it were the mere surface of reality while others go down very deep into it. Though *Saṃyama* is needed to unravel the underlying mystery in all the cases it cannot be the same in actual practice. That is why there is a world of difference between the beginner who has just mastered the technique of *Samādhi* and the Adept who can almost instantaneously pass out into the highest realms of existence without much effort. The whole science of mathematics is based upon the four operations of addition, subtraction, multiplication and division but the beginner who has mastered these operations has very far to go before he can become an expert mathematician.

In the language of the *Yoga-Sūtras* these different stages involved in the use of *Saṃyama* mean the attainment of the four successive stages of *Samprajñāta Samādhi* mentioned in I-17 and the stage of *Nirbīja Samādhi* mentioned in I-51. In the language of Occultism they mean the functioning of consciousness through increasingly subtler vehicles referred to in connection with I-17. But the fundamental basis of both is the same, namely, penetration into different depths of consciousness which finds expression through different grades of *Citta*. The *Yoga-Sūtras* deal with *Samādhi* from the functional point of view while Occultism deals with it from the structural point of view. That is why, outwardly, the two modes of treatment seem to differ. But the student who has grasped the nature of *Samādhi* will see that there is no essential difference between the two, because passing in *Samādhi* from one vehicle to another means coming into touch with the deeper levels and aspects of consciousness. The correspondences between these have been shown already in dealing with II-19.

७. त्रयमन्तरङ्गं पूर्वेभ्यः ।

Trayam antaraṅgaṃ pūrvebhyaḥ.

त्रयम् the three taken together अन्तरङ्गम् inner; internal पूर्वेभ्यः in relation to the preceding ones.

7. The three are internal in relation to the preceding ones.

The three mental processes of *Dhāraṇā*, *Dhyāna* and *Samādhi* constitute *Yoga* proper and the five preceding *Aṅgas* may be considered as merely preparatory. The whole process of *Saṃyama* takes place in the realm of the mind and no part of the visible man is involved in it. That is why it is called *Antaraṅgam.* This should not, however, be considered to mean that the first five *Aṅgas* which are external in relation to the last three are in any way not quite essential. In fact, without the preparatory work involved in the former it is impossible to undertake the more subtle and difficult task involved in the latter. At least, the essential conditions which it is the object of the first five *Aṅgas* to bring about must be produced though not necessarily by exactly the same means. They may be brought about by other *Yogic* practices or by *Īśvara-Praṇidhāna* as pointed out in I-23.

८. तदपि बहिरङ्गं निर्बीजस्य ।

Tad api bahir-aṅgaṃ nirbījasya.

तत् that अपि too बहिरङ्गम् external निर्बीजस्य to the seedless (*Samādhi*).

8. Even that (*Sabīja Samādhi*) is external to the Seedless (*Nirbīja Samādhi*).

The subject of *Nirbīja Samādhi* has already been dealt with in connection with I-51. Various other matters connected with *Nirbīja Samādhi* will also be discussed in Section IV. This *Sūtra* has been introduced here only to emphasize the distinction between *Sabīja* and *Nirbīja Samādhi* and to bring home to the student that *Nirbīja Samādhi* is a more advanced stage on the path of Self-realization than *Sabīja Samādhi*. *Sabīja Samādhi* is concerned with knowledge and powers exercised within the realm of *Prakṛti* on this side of the gate which leads to *Kaivalya*. *Nirbīja Samādhi*, on the other hand, aims at transcending the realm of *Prakṛti* and living in the state of Enlightenment implied in *Kaivalya*. The latter, therefore, is naturally internal in relation to the former. The *Puruṣa* has first to conquer all the realms of *Prakṛti* through *Sabīja Samādhi* and then, after conquering these realms, to gain complete Self-realization which makes him not only the Lord of these realms but also independent of them.

९. व्युत्थाननिरोधसंस्कारयोरभिभवप्रादुर्भावौ निरोधक्षणचित्तान्वयो निरोधपरिणामः ।

Vyutthāna-nirodha-saṃskārayor abhibha-va-prādurbhāvau nirodha-kṣaṇa-cittān-vayo nirodha-pariṇāmaḥ.

व्युत्थान outgoing; (that which is to disappear) निरोध incoming; (that which is opposing the outgoing impression) संस्कारयोः of the impressions अभिभव suppression; becoming latent प्रादुर्भावौ appearance निरोधक्षण (the unmodified state of the mind at) the moment of suppression चित्त mind अन्वय: permeation; pervasion निरोध suppression परिणाम: transformation.

9. *Nirodha Pariṇāma* is that transformation of the mind in which it becomes progressively permeated by that condition of *Nirodha* which intervenes momentarily between an impression which is disappearing and the impression which is taking its place.

After dealing with the three stages of meditation leading up to *Samādhi* Patañjali takes up the question of the three fundamental types of mental transformations which are involved in the practice of higher *Yoga*. These four *Sūtras* (III-9-12) bearing on this question are very important because they throw light on the essential nature of the mental processes which are involved in the practice of *Yoga* and further elucidate the technique of *Samādhi*.

The important point to note with regard to these three *Pariṇāmas* is that they are not states but modes of transformation, or to put it in other words, they do not represent static but dynamic conditions. In the progressive process of Self-realization through *Samādhi* the mind can pass from one stage to another through the use of three and only three kinds of transformations which are sequentially related to one another and really constitute three integral parts of a larger composite process which has to be repeated on each plane as consciousness withdraws, step by step, towards the Centre of Reality. The ordinary transformations of the mind take place according to the laws of association or reasoning or according to the stimuli applied by the external world through the sense-organs. The three kinds of transformations we are now considering are of a special kind and are used only in the practice of higher *Yoga* after the *Yogi* has acquired the capacity of passing into the *Samādhi* state at will.

The *Sūtra* under discussion defines *Nirodha Pariṇāma* or transformation which results in suppression of *Citta-Vṛttis*. In view of the fact that *Yoga* is described in I-2 as the suppression of *Citta-Vṛttis* it is easy to see how important it is to understand this *Sūtra* thoroughly. As soon as control of the mind is begun *Nirodha* comes into play. The word *Nirodha* in *Saṃskṛta* means both restraint and suppression and the earlier efforts at control of the mind beginning with *Dhāraṇā* involve *Nirodha* not so much in the sense of suppression as that of restraint. But a little careful thought will show that even in the preliminary practice of *Dhāraṇā*, *Nirodha*, in the sense of suppression, is involved to a certain extent. In trying to practise *Dhāraṇā* the will is trying all the time to suppress distractions and substituting in their place the one object on which meditation is to be performed. It will be obvious to anyone that in each of these efforts to replace a distraction by the chosen object there must be a momentary state in which neither the distraction nor the chosen object is present and the mind is really without any *Pratyaya*, just as when the direction of a moving object is suddenly reversed there must be a moment when the object is not moving but is at rest. It is because *Nirodha* in this limited sense enters the problem of controlling the mind from the very beginning that Patañjali has taken up *Nirodha Pariṇāma* first in his treatment of the subject but it should be noted that true *Nirodha* or complete suppression is the last in the cycle of transformations and comes after *Samādhi Pariṇāma* and *Ekāgratā Pariṇāma* in actual practice.

We have seen that *Nirodha* is that momentary unmodified state of the mind which intervenes when one impression which holds the field of consciousness is replaced by another impression. The impression which holds the field of consciousness is called *Vyutthāna Saṃskāra* and the impression which opposes or tries to replace the *Vyutthāna Saṃskāra* is called *Nirodha Saṃskāra* in this *Sūtra*. Between two successive impressions there must be a momentary state in which the mind has no impression at all or is present in an unmodified condition. The object of *Nirodha Pariṇāma* is to produce at will this momentary state and gradually extend it, so that the mind can exist for a considerable duration in this unmodified state. This extension of the *Niruddha* state by repeated efforts has been expressed by the phrase *Nirodha-Kṣaṇa-Cittānvaya* which means ' permeation of the mind by the momentary state of *Nirodha* or complete suppression of *Vṛttis*'. *Nirodha Pariṇāma* comprises the whole process beginning with the first effort at suppression of the 'seed' and ending with the firm establishment of the *Niruddha* state. The *Yogi* should be able to maintain the *Niruddha* state for a sufficiently long time to enable consciousness to pass through the 'cloud' or void and emerge into the next plane.

In passing from a condition in which the 'seed' of *Samādhi* holds the field of consciousness to a condition of complete *Nirodha* there is a struggle between two opposite tendencies, the tendency of the 'seed' to rise again in the field of consciousness and the tendency of the mind to remain in a condition of *Nirodha*. No other distraction can rise and occupy the field of consciousness because that tendency has already been eliminated in the previous two processes of *Samādhi Pariṇāma* and *Ekāgratā Pariṇāma*. *Samādhi Pariṇāma* has eliminated the tendency of distractions to appear in the field of consciousness and *Ekāgratā Pariṇāma* has established the tendency of the same impression—the 'seed'—to persist without interruption. That is why, when the force of will is applied to suppress the 'seed', it is only that particular seed which can appear again. This will also show why the *Samādhi* and *Ekāgratā* states must be attained before the will can be applied to produce the *Niruddha* state. If these techniques have not been mastered then after every effort of suppression a new *Pratyaya* or distraction may arise as happens in the case of the ordinary man who tries to practise *Nirodha*. The student will also be able to understand now the significance of the phrase *Abhyāsa Pūrvaḥ* in I-18, for *Asaṃprajñāta Samādhi* is nothing but the state of the mind in which the *Pratyaya* or 'seed' has been made to disappear by the practice of *Nirodha*. This condition of *Nirodha* is not a state of ordinary mental vacuum, but a state of *Samādhi* in which the *Yogi* is in complete control of the mind.

The first effort to suppress the 'seed' of *Saṃprajñāta Samādhi* produces a void only momentarily. The tendency of the 'seed' to emerge again into consciousness is so strong owing to the previous practice of *Ekāgratā* that it again takes possession of the mind and transforms it into its own image. The repetition of the effort at suppression, however, makes it slightly easier every time to bring about the *Niruddha* state and maintain the mind in that state a little longer. Continued practice of this kind gradually increases the tendency of the mind to remain in the *Niruddha* state and weakens the tendency of the 'seed' to reappear in the field of consciousness as pointed out in the next *Sūtra.*

A simple physical experiment will serve perhaps to illustrate the opposition of the two tendencies referred to above. OB is a rod attached to a stand OA and kept in the position OB by a spring at C.

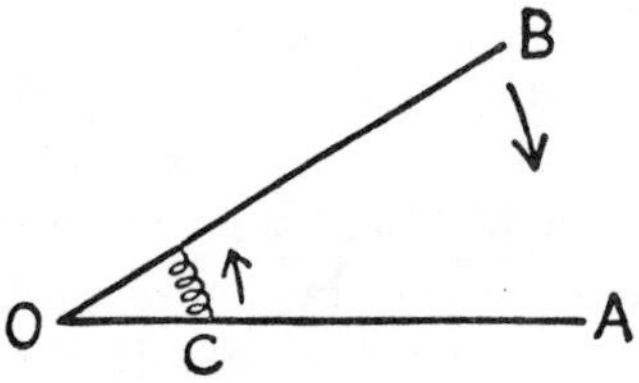

FIG. 9

If a child is asked to press the rod OB to the position OA he may be able to bring it to that position with difficulty and may be able to touch the stand OA only momentarily in the first attempt. Each successive attempt will, however, make it easier for him to bring the rod to the position OA and keep it in that position longer. And with sufficient practice the child may learn to keep the rod in the position OA as long as he likes. The tendency of the rod to spring upwards has been completely mastered by practice. In the same way the tendency of the 'seed' to spring back into the field of consciousness can be mastered by sufficient practice and the *Niruddha* state maintained for a sufficient length of time for the consciousness to pass through the *Laya* centre and emerge into the next higher plane.

१०. तस्य प्रशान्तवाहिता संस्कारात् ।

Tasya praśānta-vāhitā saṃskārāt.

तस्य its (of *Nīrodha Pariṇāma*) प्रशान्त peaceful; tranquil; undisturbed वाहिता flow संस्कारात् by (repeated) impression.

10. Its flow becomes tranquil by repeated impression.

The meaning of this *Sūtra* will be clear from what has been said in connection with the previous *Sūtra*. The tendency of the mind to remain in the *Niruddha* state also grows with practice and ultimately becomes so strong by the force of *Saṃskāras* that it can remain in that condition easily for any length of time. The significance of the phrase *Praśānta Vāhitā* should be noted. The flow of this *Niruddha* state becomes, after sufficient practice, easy and peaceful. There is no struggle which may be present in some degree in the earlier stages when the tendency has not been established firmly. Such a struggle would produce an unstable condition of the mind which is utterly unsuited for the purpose which has to be accomplished.

It may be pointed out here that the resistance encountered from the mind in bringing about the different transformations is due not so much to the mind itself as to the *Saṃskāras* of *Vāsanās* still hidden within it. If these have been removed to a sufficient degree the passage from one condition to another can take place without much resistance. In fact, if *Vairāgya* has been developed to a high degree the necessary changes may be brought about with comparative ease as shown by the life of great spiritual teachers of the world. That is why the *Yogi* has to rise on the two wings of *Vairāgya* and *Abhyāsa* as pointed out in I-12. Even in the last stage when *Dharma-Megha-Samādhi* is practised (IV-29) for the attainment of *Kaivalya* it is the practice of extreme *Vairāgya* which destroys the remaining *Saṃskāras* of the subtlest *Vāsanās* and liberates the consciousness of the *Yogi*.

११. सर्वार्थतैकाग्रतयोः क्षयोदयौ चित्तस्य समाधिपरिणामः ।

Sarvārthataikāgratayoḥ kṣayodayau cittasya samādhi-pariṇāmaḥ.

सर्वार्थता- 'all-objectness'; many-pointedness; a state of mental distraction -एकाग्रतयोः of one-pointedness; of concentratedness

क्षयोदयौ decay and rise चित्तस्य of the mind समाधि trance परिणामः transformation.

11. *Samādhi* transformation is the (gradual) setting of the distractions and simultaneous rising of one-pointedness.

The second kind of mental transformation which is involved in the different stages of *Samādhi* is *Samādhi Pariṇāma.* This transformation really begins with the practice of *Dhāraṇā* and continues until the *Ekāgratā* state is reached. As the definition of *Samādhi Pariṇāma* given by the author shows, its essential nature is the gradual reduction of the all-pointed condition of the mind to the one-pointed condition. First, the series of objects which in the case of the ordinary man occupy the mind, one after another, are replaced by one chosen object, the 'seed' of *Samādhi.* All the other objects except the object chosen for *Saṃyama* which are technically called 'distractions' are eliminated completely when *Dhyāna* is perfected. Then begins a new kind of movement or transformation of the mind in which consciousness begins to move in depth, as it were, and the object is denuded of its coverings or non-essential elements like name or form. The 'seed' is split open and its different layers exposed in order to get at the core which is its *Svarūpa.* When this process which is dealt with in I-43, has been completed and the object 'shines' in the mind in its real *Svarūpa* there is nothing further which can be done on that plane. The attainment of the *Nirvitarka* stage marks the completion of the *Samādhi Pariṇāma* as far as the *Vitarka* stage of *Saṃprajñāta Samādhi* is concerned. If the mind is kept concentrated on the object it can merely reproduce the irreducible *Svarūpa* of the object. Here the *Ekāgratā Pariṇāma* which is dealt with in the next *Sūtra* begins.

१२. ततः पुनः शान्तोदितौ तुल्यप्रत्ययौ चित्तस्यैकाग्रतापरिणामः

Tataḥ punaḥ śāntoditau tulya-pratyayau:
cittasyaikāgratā-pariṇāmaḥ.

ततः then पुनः again शान्त-उदितौ subsided and uprisen तुल्य- equal; exactly similar प्रत्ययौ cognitions; contents of the mind at two different moments चित्तस्य of the mind एकाग्रता one-pointedness परिणामः transformation.

12. Then, again, the condition of the mind in which the 'object' (in the mind) which subsides is always exactly similar to the 'object' which rises (in the next moment) is called *Ekāgratā Pariṇāma.*

The characteristic of the *Ekāgratā Pariṇāma*, which as we have seen is the consummation of the *Samādhi Pariṇāma*, is that exactly the same *Pratyaya* rises in the field of consciousness again and again and produces the impression as if a single fixed unchanging *Pratyaya* is occupying the field. The succession of exactly similar images in an apparently stationary *Pratyaya* is due to the intermittent nature of the manifested Universe which has been briefly explained in connection with IV-33. The whole Universe appears and disappears alternately but the interval called a *Kṣaṇa* is so small that it appears to be a continuous phenomenon. We see a continuous glow in an electric bulb with an alternating current but we know that the glow is discontinuous and periods of illumination follow periods of darkness alternately at very short intervals. It is not only in *Samādhi* that this discontinuity enters in the perception of the *Pratyaya.* It is present in all perceptions and thinking right from the plane of the lower mind up to the *Ātmic* plane. Wherever there is manifestation there must be discontinuity or succession which is called *Kramaḥ* in III-15 and IV-33.

The projection of a cinematographic picture on a screen may serve to illustrate, to some extent, the difference between the three *Pariṇāmas.* The moving picture on the screen is produced, as is explained in connection with IV-33, by a succession of dissimilar images falling on the screen at intervals of less than 1/10th second. This produces an illusion of continuity while there is actual discontinuity in the projection. If all the pictures on the film roll are made exactly similar there will be one stationary and unchanging image produced on the screen. But we know that the appearance of such a stationary and unchanging image is an illusion. What we see as an unchanging image is composed of a number of similar (*Tulya*) images following each other so rapidly as to be indistinguishable. If we slow down the speed of projection sufficiently the illusion will disappear and we shall be able to see similar images following each other at regular intervals. In the same way the *Pratyaya* of *Ekāgratā Pariṇāma* remains apparently the same but in reality it is composed of a series of similar (*Tulya*) *Pratyayas* following each other at inconceivably high speed. It is because the phenomenon is dynamic and not static that it is called a *Pariṇāma* (transformation) and not *Avasthā* (state).

Now, if we suppose that even this picture which produces an unchanging image on the screen is removed and each portion of the film corresponding to a single picture is quite transparent it is obvious that a uniform illumination will be seen on the screen. Here the analogy breaks down. The dropping or suppression of the *Pratyaya* of *Ekāgratā Pariṇāma* by means of *Nirodha* does not produce the illumination of Reality but the consciousness of the next subtler plane and the whole cycle of the three *Pariṇāmas* has to be repeated again on this plane to enable the consciousness to pass again into the next subtler plane. It is only when the *Pratyaya* of the last plane (*Ātmic*) is dropped or suppressed that the illumination of Reality or consciousness of the *Puruṣa* dawns.

The reason for the emergence of a *Pratyaya* of the next subtler plane when the 'seed' present in *Ekāgratā Pariṇāma* is suppressed is to be sought in the nature of the complex mechanism through which consciousness functions on the different planes and the nature of the *Saṃskāras* which bind consciousness to its vehicles. Theoretically, the *Nirodha* which follows the *Ekāgratā* state should lead to direct contact with Reality but this does not happen. As this question has been dealt with at another place (I-18) it is not necessary to enter into it here.

१३. एतेन भूतेन्द्रियेषु धर्मलक्षणावस्थापरिणामा व्याख्याताः ।

Etena bhūtendriyeṣu dharma-lakṣaṇā-
vasthā-pariṇāmā vyākhyātāḥ.

एतेन by this भूत (in) the elements इन्द्रियेषु in the sense-organs धर्म property लक्षण character अवस्था condition परिणामाः transformations; changes व्याख्याताः are explained.

13. By this (by what has been said in the last four *Sūtras*) the property, character, and condition-transformations in the elements and the sense-organs are also explained.

Since the mind gets its raw material for thinking from the *Bhūtas* through the instrumentality of the *Indriyas* it follows that, corresponding to the three *Pariṇāmas* dealt with previously in relation to *Citta*, there must be analogous *Pariṇāmas* in the field of *Bhūtas* and *Indriyas* also. These *Pariṇāmas* are referred to in this *Sūtra*, firstly, to emphasize their all-pervading character in every field of *Prakṛti* and, secondly, to facilitate the understanding of the *modus operandi* of many *Siddhis* which are dealt with in the remaining portion of this Section. Transformations of every kind in Nature are based according to *Yogic* philosophy on the changes in *Guṇas* and must therefore be governed by laws which are fundamentally the same. It is easy to understand, therefore, that the laws governing the three types of transformations which are utilized in the control and manipulation of *Citta* in *Yogic* practice must also hold true in the field of *Bhūtas* and *Indriyas*. But, owing to the difference in the medium, their mode of working, though analogous, will not be the same. Just as mastery over the technique of the three kinds of transformations in the field of *Citta* enables the *Yogi* to control and manipulate the working of *Citta*, in the same way, mastery over this technique in the field of *Bhūtas* and *Indriyas* enables him to control and manipulate natural phenomena. He can then exercise extraordinary powers which are called *Siddhis*.

Patañjali has merely referred to the applicability of the three laws of transformation to the field of *Bhūtas* and *Indriyas* without elucidating the idea further. The student is expected to work out the analogous relationships himself. Let us see how this can be done taking into consideration what has been said in relation to the functioning of *Citta*.

Let us take the field of *Bhūtas* or elements first. As has been explained elsewhere (II-19) it is by the action of *Bhūtas* on the *Indriyas* that sensuous perception takes place. What is the action of *Bhūtas* due to in the last analysis? Obviously, to the physical and chemical properties of different kinds of matter. It is these properties which make us see colours. hear sounds and produce the innumerable sensations which form the raw material of our mental life. It is these properties which are inherent in matter and appear under different conditions which are the specific instruments of *Bhūtas* and by their action on the *Indriyas* produce all kinds of sensuous perceptions. These properties in their totality are called *Dharma* in the present context.

According to the *Yogic* conception of matter all kinds of chemical and physical properties are not separate properties of different elements and compounds which Science has discovered. They inhere in one parent substance. The different elements and compounds merely serve as vehicles for making manifest the properties which are latent in the parent substance. This basic medium or repository of all properties is called *Dharmī* in the next *Sūtra*.

What is the significance of the three *Pariṇāmas* in relation to the *Bhūtas*? Corresponding to *Nirodha Pariṇāma* of *Citta* there will be reduction to the state of *Dharmī*, the basic medium in which all the properties have become latent and the *Dharmī* is present in a perfectly quiescent state. Corresponding to the *Samādhi Pariṇāma* of *Citta* there will be a concentration towards a particular set of properties instead of the properties changing continuously in a haphazard manner according to the prevailing natural conditions. Corresponding to *Ekāgratā Pariṇāma* of *Citta* there will be a stationary state in which one particular set of properties holds the field for the time being or the *Dharmī* remains in exactly the same state for a certain period.

The continuous changes in matter which are brought about by natural forces correspond to the condition of the ordinary mind which passes from one object to another in a haphazard manner according to the laws of mental association. Changes in matter which are brought about by deliberately regulating the conditions in a particular way are analogous to *Samādhi Pariṇāma*. This may be done either by the regulation of the external conditions, as is done by a scientist, or by going to the source of all properties and manipulating them from there, as is done by a *Yogi*. In the latter kind of technique lies the secret of many *Siddhis* such as *Bhūta Jaya* dealt with in III-45.

Since the sense-organs merely convert the properties which are present in an active form in the *Dharmī* into the corresponding sensations, the *Pariṇāmas* in the field of *Indriyas* are merely the counterparts of the *Pariṇāmas* in the field of *Bhūtas* and the analogous relationships can be worked out easily. We have merely to substitute *Lakṣaṇa* or characteristics in place of *Dharma* or properties. In this field also the *Yogi* who can perform *Saṃyama* can trace back the sensations to their ultimate source and acquire complete control over the sense-organs as shown in III-48.

It is easy to understand what is *Dharma Pariṇāma* and *Lakṣaṇa Pariṇāma* because these fall within the range of our common experience. What is *Avasthā Pariṇāma*? *Avasthā* means state and *Avasthā Pariṇāma* is therefore change of state. To understand the significance of this kind of transformation we should turn to III-45 and III-48. The *Bhūtas* and *Indriyas* exist in five states, each of the successive state mentioned being subtler than the preceding one. In fact, the grossest form of the *Bhūtas* or *Indriyas* is derived by the progressive condensation of the subtlest form through the intermediate three stages and can therefore be again reduced to the subtlest form by reversing the process. These changes from one state to another are referred to in the present *Sūtra* as *Avasthā Pariṇāma* and are analogous to the three kinds of *Pariṇāmas* which can be brought about by the *Yogi* in relation to properties and characteristics. This kind of transformation is beyond the range of common experience and can be utilized only through the practice of *Saṃyama*.

१४. शान्तोदिताव्यपदेश्यधर्मानुपाती धर्मी ।

Śāntoditāvyapadeśya-dharmānupātī
dharmī.

शान्त the subsided; the latent उदित the uprisen, the manifest अव्यपदेश्य the unmanifest; as yet in the future धर्म the properties अनुपाती correlated; common to धर्मी the substratum in which the properties inhere.

14. The substratum is that in which the properties—latent, active or unmanifest—inhere.

As has been pointed out already in the last *Sūtra* all properties of different elements whether manifest or unmanifest, are considered to inhere in, and to be derived from one substratum which is called *Dharmī*. This substratum which is the root of all properties is none other than *Prakṛti*. When a particular property disappears we may say that it has become latent in *Prakṛti*. When it becomes manifest we may say that it has taken an active form in *Prakṛti*. So the appearance and disappearance of all kinds of properties in Nature through the medium of different elements and compounds is merely a question of their being manifest or unmanifest. All of them are present eternally in *Prakṛti* and can be made active or latent by bringing about the necessary conditions.

The view that all natural phenomena are due to the continual appearance and disappearance of all kinds of properties in a substratum which is their repository may appear fantastic to people familiar with modern scientific ideas but deeper thought will show the fascinating nature of this idea and convince the student that it is not as absurd as it appears on first sight. In fact, those who are in touch with the latest developments in Science and are familiar with the trends of modern scientific thought will see in these developments a closer approach to the *Yogic* doctrine than to materialism. The fact that all elements are composed of a few fundamental types of particles like the protons and electrons, that mass and energy are interconvertible and other discoveries of this nature have really shaken the foundations of orthodox materialism and shown that the doctrines on which the *Yogic* philosophy is based are not after all as fantastic as they appear at first sight. The theory that the properties of all elements depend upon the number and arrangement of the electrons in those elements is only one or two steps removed from the doctrine that all properties of matter are derived from, and exist in a potential form in a substratum.

१५. क्रमान्यत्वं परिणामान्यत्वे हेतुः ।

Kramānyatvaṃ pariṇāmānyatve hetuḥ.

क्रम succession; underlying process; natural law अन्यत्वं difference; variety; परिणाम transformation; change अन्यत्वे in variation or difference हेतुः cause.

15. The cause of the difference in transformation is the difference in the underlying process.

The progress of modern Science has shown conclusively that behind various phenomena which we observe in different spheres of life there is a hidden framework of laws of Nature which bring about and regulate these phenomena with mathematical precision. Formerly, man was mystified by natural phenomena and as he did not know that they were based on natural laws he felt helpless before them. But the advent of Science, and the discovery of natural laws to which it has led, has given him power and confidence. He knows that if he can find the underlying laws in any sphere of natural phenomena he can control and manipulate them with utter certainty. He also knows that behind the external changes which he observes there are inner processes which bring about and account for the external changes, and much of the scientific work which is being done these days aims at tracing these inner processes and through their control and manipulation bringing about any desired result in the physical world.

It is this idea of a hidden process or natural sequence underlying the multifarious phenomena of Nature which is embodied in the *Sūtra* under discussion. The *Saṃskṛta* word *Krama* almost exactly expresses the idea behind a law of Nature. A law of Nature is nothing but a particular invariable order and manner in which things happen under a particular set of circumstances. We do not know really why things happen in certain ways under certain circumstances. We only know how they happen and an exact formulation of this mode of action is a law of Nature. This is also the essential idea behind the word *Krama* operating in the field of natural phenomena. The previous *Sūtra* points out that all phenomena whether brought about by the action of natural forces or by the will of the *Yogi* are due to the appearance and disappearance of the corresponding properties in *Prakṛti*. This *Sūtra* emphasizes that these changes do not take place in a haphazard manner but according to definite and exact natural laws which determine with mathematical precision the manner and order of the changes.

The need of bringing home to the student this important fact will be seen if we remember that all the following *Sūtras* of this Section deal with different kinds of *Siddhis* which can be acquired by the practice of *Saṃyama*. Some of these powers or attainments are of such an extraordinary nature that the student might well get away with the idea that they are acquired by some miraculous means. This would not only give an incorrect idea with regard to the nature of these attainments but also undermine the confidence of the *Yogi* in his ability to acquire them by *Yogic* processes. For there is always an element of uncertainty associated with the idea of miracles. A miracle may or may not happen. But a scientific process *must* produce the desired result if the right conditions are provided. It is the scientific nature of *Yogic* technique which provides the guarantee for success through them.

It is especially necessary to emphasize this fact because of the strange attitude of the present-day scientists towards all phenomena which are not of a purely physical character and cannot be dealt with in a scientific laboratory through physical instruments. They not only distrust all things which cannot be investigated through physical instruments; they also consider them outside the realm of law. To them only physical phenomena are governed by natural laws. All other phenomena connected with the mental, psychic and spiritual experiences of mankind belong implicitly to a world of chaos in which there are no definite and exact laws and th refore no possibility of investigating them in a scientific manner.

The *Yogic* philosophy takes a more sensible and scientific view. It considers the whole of the manifested Universe as a cosmos. It declares emphatically that all phenomena within this Universe—superphysical as well as physical—are subject to natural laws which work with mathematical precision. It provides the means by which the superphysical phenomena can be investigated and the underlying laws discovered. The student is thus not only free to decide which is the more rational view of the Universe but also to test by his own experiences and experiments which is the correct view.

१६. परिणामत्रयसंयमादतीतानागतज्ञानम् ।

Pariṇāma-traya-saṃyamād atītānāgata-jñānam.

परिणाम transformations त्रय the three संयमात् by performing *Saṃyama* on अतीत past अनागत future ज्ञानम् knowledge.

16. By performing *Saṃyama* on the three kinds of transformations (*Nirodha*, *Samādhi* and *Ekāgratā*) knowledge of the past and future.

Beginning with III-16 the remaining *Sūtras* of this Section deal with the *Siddhis* or attainments which can be acquired by the practice of *Saṃyama*. Before dealing with the individual *Sūtras* it is necessary to point out a few facts, by way of introduction, on this difficult but interesting subject. The word *Siddhis* is used generally for the extraordinary powers acquired through the practice of *Yoga* but its real meaning is best expressed by the words 'attainments' or 'accomplishments' connected with the superphysical worlds. It is chiefly in this latter sense that the word *Siddhis* should be taken in the present context because many of the *Siddhis* dealt with in the latter portion of this Section are concerned with the attainment of the highest states of consciousness and not with the development of occult powers as they are usually called. In these introductory remarks it is possible only to touch upon the more general and important aspects of the subject which will enable the student to see *Siddhis* in their correct perspective in the life of the *Yogi*.

The first point that may be noted with regard to occult powers as distinguished from the more important attainments in higher *Yoga* is the comparative unimportance of the former. These have a peculiar fascination for the neophyte who has merely acquired a superficial interest in the subject, but the more thoroughly he understands the philosophy of *Yoga* the more is his interest transferred to the final objective. When an ordinary student gets interested in *Yoga* he is still under the domination of ordinary desires, the desire for power and fame being one of them. He may not be conscious of this desire but deep down in his sub-conscious mind it lurks ready to come up when favourable conditions present themselves. Now, in the practice of *Yoga* his lower self sees an opening for acquiring extraordinary and spectacular powers of all kinds and in this lies in many cases the secret of the fascination which *Yoga* exercises on many people. But, if the student makes a deeper study of the subject he realizes that the *Yogic* philosophy is based on the philosophy of *Kleśas* and the occult powers which interested him so much are also part of that illusory side of life which it is the object of *Yoga* to transcend. The exercise of occult powers does not free him from the basic illusions of life and therefore cannot bring him Enlightenment and peace. Rather it tends to distract the mind more powerfully from his true goal and may bring about his downfall in the most unforeseen manner. It is only when he has completely conquered his lower nature and acquired true *Vairāgya* that he can safely exercise these powers for the helping of others, if necessary. Till then his interest in them should be merely scientific, as adding to the wonder and mystery of life which surrounds him and helping him to unravel that mystery. So when he finds these powers appearing spontaneously or as a result of the practice of *Saṃyama* he confines their use strictly to scientific purposes and maintains an attitude of utter indifference towards them.

The fact that real *Yogis* do not take the slightest pleasure or pride in the exercise of occult powers which they possess and refuse to yield to the common and vulgar desire of people to see 'miracles' probably accounts for the fact that they remain unknown to the outer world and the realities of the *Yogic* life have never been established to the complete satisfaction of the modern psychologist. The ordinary man who rushes out into publicity to proclaim any unusual ability or power that he may acquire cannot understand how any person can possess some of the most extraordinary *Yogic* powers and yet not even let other people know that he is in any way different from other people. He, therefore, naturally concludes that because such powers have never been exhibited in public under test conditions, they either do not exist or those who can exercise them are no longer living in the world. But a careful study of history and other relevant literature will prove conclusively that such powers have been exercised by people in practically all ages. And a persistent search among people who are in this line may also convince the student that there are people living in the present who can exercise these powers even though they may be difficult to find and may refuse to show these powers to any except those who are their tried and trusted disciples. Of course, there are present everywhere charlatans who pose as *Yogis* and dupe gullible people to serve their selfish and nefarious ends. There are also people who have acquired some of the lower *Siddhis* and who go about making an exhibition of these for the satisfaction of their petty vanities or for earning money. Though these people pose as great *Yogis* their vanity and worldly attitude betrays them and reveals their true status in *Yogic* life. The practice of higher *Yoga* and the unfoldment of spiritual life are the only sure means of coming into touch with true *Yogis* who are masters of this Science of sciences and who can undoubtedly exercise all the *Siddhis* mentioned in the *Yoga-Sūtras*.

The second important point to be borne in mind with regard to *Siddhis* is that their *modus operandi* can be explained only on the basis of *Yogic* psychology and those who try to fit into the extremely superficial and rather materialist framework of modern psychology the grand and all-inclusive facts of *Yogic* Science try to attempt an impossible task. Modern Science in the first flush of achievement, and owing to the capacity to produce spectacular results in the field of physical phenomena, may presume to pronounce judgments on the fundamental problems of life but as it knows practically nothing about these facts of the inner life its verdicts and opinions about them have no value except in the eyes of those who are, for the time being, hypnotized by the materialistic philosophy and are satisfied with a purely materialistic interpretation of the Universe.

This is not the place to deal at any length with the psychology upon which the whole structure of *Yogic* Science is based. The student will have to piece together the elements of this psychology from the relevant *Sūtras* scattered throughout the book and fill up the gaps by a careful and comprehensive study of other Eastern philosophical systems. He will then see that the philosophy and psychology upon which *Yogic* Science is based is the only one which is comprehensive enough to provide a sufficiently broad base for this Science. He will also realize that modern psychology which confines its investigations to the expressions of mind and consciousness through the imperfect and limited physical vehicle and is afraid of losing contact with the physical world in its investigations, is utterly inadequate for this purpose. Those who refuse to leave the shores of the physical world must content themselves with the limited knowledge and resources which they have got and should not sit in judgment on the experiences of those who have ventured on the high seas and found limitless lands of unimaginable splendour.

The best way of getting an insight into the *modus operandi* of *Siddhis* is to consider knowledge and power as two aspects of the same reality so that anyone who has the knowledge with regard to the inner working of any set of phenomena has also the power to manipulate those phenomena. There is nothing irrational in this assumption because the control and manipulation of physical forces by modern science follows the discovery of the physical laws underlying those forces. But Science has knowledge of only physical forces and can therefore control only physical phenomena. The *Yogi* acquires knowledge of the far subtler and powerful forces of mind and consciousness and can, therefore, exercise powers connected with those inner forces. And since mental forces lie also at the basis of physical forces he can manipulate even physical phenomena without using any physical aids.

It has been pointed out already in the previous *Sūtra* that according to the *Yogic* philosophy the whole of the manifested Universe, seen and unseen, is governed by natural laws and therefore there is no place for 'miracles' in this philosophy. When things are made to take place in a way which appears miraculous to the ordinary observer this is done by using forces which are still under the domain of natural law, though yet unknown to modern Science. There is, and can be, no violation of natural law, but it is possible to do things which seem to violate physical laws by employing laws of the superphysical realms. No one imagines that the law of gravitation is violated when a rocket soars into the sky. Why should it be necessary to assume that a miracle has happened when a man rises in the air by the practice of *Prāṇāyāma* or disappears from our sight as indicated in III-21?

To deny the existence of these powers because modern Science cannot accept or explain them is to attribute to the scientist omniscience which he himself does not claim. To assert that powers attributed to *Yoga* are not possible is not justified even from the scientific point of view. Things which were considered impossible before are passing into the realms of possibility as a result of new facts and laws which we are discovering. Scientists would do well to remember that they have not made the facts and laws, the discovery of which has enabled them to do so many marvellous things. They have merely discovered those facts. How can they say what other facts and laws are hidden within the bosom of Nature? The scientist may or may not show the true scientific spirit and humility which is a part of that spirit. But the true *Yogi* who discovers the infinitely more fascinating facts and powers of the inner worlds always attributes them to the Divine Life enshrined within him and in the world around him and when he uses those powers he uses them as an agent of that Life. And the day he forgets this important fact and loses this humble attitude his downfall is at hand.

Before dealing specifically with the *Sūtras* in which Patañjali has given some information with regard to *Siddhis* it is necessary to point out certain general facts regarding his manner of treating the subject.

The first thing we may note in this connection is that Patañjali has not dealt with the subject of *Siddhis* in an exhaustive manner. He has merely taken up a few well-known *Siddhis* and hinted at the principles underlying their exercise by way of illustration. Neither are the *Siddhis* named or classified though the student of *Yogic* literature will be able generally to identify the *Siddhi* dealt with in a particular *Sūtra* and correlate it with those mentioned in other schools of *Yoga*. It will also be seen that some of the *Sūtras* given in the last portion of Section III can hardly be said to deal with *Siddhis* in the sense of occult powers. They deal rather with stages of Self-realization leading up to the last stage of complete Liberation or *Kaivalya*. So close is the connection between the stages of Self-realization and the powers which inhere in those stages that it becomes almost impossible to differentiate between the two, though *Saṃyama* may have to be resorted to for the sake of learning the technique of certain specific processes.

The second important point we should impress upon our mind is that it is not the intention of Patañjali to give in these *Sūtras* a clear-cut technique for the development of the *Siddhis*. He merely hints in each *Sūtra* at the principle or *modus operandi* of the mental process whereby the particular result can be attained. This can be utilized only by the advanced *Yogi* who has already learnt the technique of *Saṃyama* to develop the particular *Siddhi*. Not only is the ordinary student unable to make any practical use of the hint given, but he is hardly in a position to understand its real significance. It is not enough merely to understand *Saṃyama* as an intellectual concept. The successive mental processes underlying it should be a matter of actual direct experience, as real as, for example, going from one room into another in one's own house. Let no one, therefore, be under the illusion that by carefully studying the various *Sūtras* and practising what is vaguely hinted at in them it is possible to develop the *Siddhis*. There is a price to pay and it is a very high price—a complete reorientation of one's life and its dedication to the *Yogic* ideal, an adoption of the *Yogic* discipline in its entirety and a fixed and unalterable determination to continue to strive, life after life, until the goal is reached. And in this ideal and the life which the *Yogi* adopts the *Siddhis*, in the sense of occult powers, have really a very subordinate position and are generally not striven after directly. The main emphasis is on finding the Ultimate Truth through Self-realization and the *Siddhis* are used merely as a means for gaining that end.

It will be seen from what has been said above that the subject of *Siddhis* is not taboo among *Yogis* and there is no need to adopt an attitude of morbid fear towards them as is sometimes advocated in certain schools of spiritual culture. There is no harm in studying the subject in an academic spirit with a view to acquire a better knowledge and comprehension of the Science of *Yoga*. The danger begins when a hankering for developing these powers takes possession of the mind of the neophyte and the possibility opens of his being side-tracked from the true Path of *Yoga*.

Even as regards this intellectual study the student should keep in mind his limitations and not expect too much from a careful and thorough study of the *Sūtras* bearing on *Siddhis*. As has been pointed out repeatedly the mental processes which are involved in the development of *Siddhis* are not only internal and subjective but beyond the range of the ordinary mind with which we are familiar. Even *Yogic* psychology cannot, therefore, explain everything. It can take the student only up to the border of the region with which he is familiar but cannot make him see through the veils which his lower mind has placed round his consciousness. All that can be hoped for, therefore, from the study of these *Sūtras* is an intelligent grasp of the general principles underlying the different mental processes involved in developing various *Siddhis*. And in some cases even this may not be possible.

The difficulty of understanding some of the *Sūtras* is further increased by the fact that the exact significance of the words used in them has been obscured through the passage of time or through the efforts of all kinds of commentators to interpret them in a rather fantastic manner. Add to this the fact that Patañjali has in some cases used blinds or deliberately vague expressions to prevent over-ambitious or foolish aspirants from injuring themselves by rushing into all kinds of dangerous practices and one can then see the difficulty in the way of acquiring a clear and satisfying grasp of the meaning of these *Sūtras* dealing with the *Siddhis*. But even with all these limitations the student will find the subject a fascinating one and well worth the trouble which he takes in studying it.

With this brief introduction regarding the treatment of *Siddhis* by Patañjali let us now turn to consider the different *Sūtras* in which he has dealt with the individual *Siddhis*. The first of these *Sūtras* which is under discussion deals with knowledge regarding the past and future. This *Sūtra* is sometimes interpreted as meaning that knowledge of the past and future (of anything) which arises by performing *Saṃyama* on the three kinds of transformations mentioned in III-13. With this kind of interpretation it becomes necessary to assume that the future of everything is fixed and so predetermination rules the manifested Universe. If we substitute for 'knowledge of the past and future' 'knowledge of the nature of past and future' the meaning becomes quite clear. How do we recognize the passage of time in which the future is constantly becoming the past? By the transformations of properties, characteristics and states which are taking place in things around us. If these transformations came suddenly to a stop time would cease to flow. So by performing *Saṃyama* on the nature of these three transformations the *Yogi* realizes the true nature of time.

It may be asked why the present has been left out of this classification of time into the past and future. The present as we all know has no reality. It is a mere concept for the ever-moving dividing line between the past and the future. In the incessant flow of time, as perceived by the change in properties, we can take a cross-section at any moment and that is the present, theoretically. Actually, the present has become the past before we realize its presence and, therefore, ever eludes us. But, though it has no reality of its own it is a thing of tremendous significance because beneath this dividing line between the past and future is hidden the Eternal Now, the Reality which is beyond Time.

Saṃyama on the three kinds of transformations makes the *Yogi* realize the nature of the ever-flowing current of time in the form of the past and the future. It does not enable him to transcend time and gain a glimpse of the Eternal which is hidden behind time. This is brought about by a different process given in III-53.

१७. शब्दार्थप्रत्ययानामितरेतराध्यासात् संकरस्तत्प्रविभागसंयमात् सर्वभूतरुतज्ञानम् ।

Śabdārtha-pratyayānāṃ itaretarādhyāsāt
saṃkaras tat-pravibhāga-saṃyamāt
sarva-bhūta-ruta-jñānam.

शब्द word; sound अर्थ object; purpose प्रत्ययानाम् (of) idea; content of the mind इतरेतराध्यासात् because of superimposition on each other संकर: mixture; confusion तत् (of) them प्रविभाग separation; differentiation; resolution संयमात् by performing *Saṃyama* on सर्व all भूत living beings, रुत sounds ज्ञानम् knowledge; comprehension.

17. The sound, the meaning (behind it) and the idea (which is present in the mind at the time) are present together in a confused state. By performing *Saṃyama* (on the sound) they are resolved and there arises comprehension of the meaning of sounds uttered by any living being.

If we are to understand how the *Yogi* can comprehend the meaning of the sounds uttered by any living being we have to consider the composite mental process which produces the sounds. Take, for example, a nightingale calling to its mate. We hear only the external sound but that sound is the final expression of a complex process in which two other elements are involved. One is the image of its mate present in the mind of the nightingale and the other is the desire or purpose (*Artha*), namely, to see the mate. Without both these elements the sounds could not be produced. If anyone could enter the mind of the nightingale he would become aware of both these factors and gain immediately a comprehension of the meaning of the external sounds. Now, it has been shown already in explaining I-42 that when several factors of this nature are present together in a complex mental process they can be resolved and separated from each other by performing *Saṃyama* on the factor which is outermost. The three factors together constitute a 'seed' which can be split open and the meaning separated out as explained already. This will immediately enable the *Yogi* to comprehend the meaning of the sound uttered by the nightingale. Since the sounds uttered by all living beings are produced by the same kind of mental process referred to above, the *Yogi* can always come to know their meaning through *Saṃyama*.

It is not necessary for the *Yogi* to sit down in meditation to know the meaning of such sounds. Once the technique of *Saṃyama* is mastered and he has learnt to resolve the complex process which results in the external sounds he can go through the process almost instantaneously and thus know the meaning on hearing the sounds.

१८. संस्कारसाक्षात्करणात् पूर्वजातिज्ञानम् ।

Saṃskāra-sākṣātkaraṇāt pūrva-jātijñānam.

संस्कार impressions साक्षात्-करणात् by observation; by direct perception पूर्व earlier; previous जाति (of) birth ज्ञानम् knowledge.

18. By direct perceptions of the impressions a knowledge of the previous birth.

It is a part of the doctrine of reincarnation that all the experiences which we pass through in life produce impressions upon our vehicles and can thus be recovered from them by the application of proper methods. Experiments in hypnotism have shown conclusively that experiences which a person has passed through in physical life are indelibly impressed upon his brain even though he may not be able to remember them. This is proved by the fact that they can be recovered by putting him under hypnosis. In fact, by pushing hypnosis to deeper levels even impressions of previous lives can be revived. For example, a person who did not know even the rudiments of a language was found under hypnosis to talk fluently in that language and to show the characteristics of an entirely new personality. This shows that impressions connected with all the lives we have passed through are present somewhere within us and by diving sufficiently deep into our own consciousness it should be possible to revive the experiences which have produced those impressions, just as by playing a gramophone record it is possible to recover the sounds which produced the impressions on the record.

These impressions of previous lives can be present only in some vehicle which has passed through all those lives and has not been newly formed with each incarnation like the physical body. This vehicle is called *Kāraṇa Śarīra* or causal body and is referred to as *Karmāśaya* in II-12 because in it lie hidden all the 'seeds' of *Karma* which will fructify in the present and future lives. All *Yogis* of a high order who can withdraw their consciousness into their causal vehicles and can thus come in direct contact with these impressions are thus able to obtain knowledge of previous lives of others and their own. The technique of this can be acquired through *Saṃyama.*

१९. प्रत्ययस्य परचित्तज्ञानम् ।

Pratyayasya para-citta-jñānam.

प्रत्ययस्य of the content of the mind पर another's चित्त (of) mind ज्ञानम् knowledge.

19. (By direct perception through *Saṃyama*) of the image occupying the mind, knowledge of the mind of others.

The meaning of the word *Pratyaya* has been explained fully elsewhere. It is the content of the mind functioning through a particular vehicle. As the consciousness of an ordinary individual in the waking state is functioning through his mental body the *Pratyaya* in his case will be the mental image occupying his mind. Anyone who can see this mental image can gain knowledge of that mind. This can be done by performing *Saṃyama* and establishing clairvoyant contact between the two vehicles. As this *Sūtra* follows immediately after III-18 the words *Sākṣātkaraṇāt* may be considered to be understood after *Pratyayasya.*

२०. न च तत् सालम्बनं तस्याविषयीभूतत्वात् ।

Na ca tat sālambanaṃ tasyāviṣayī-bhū-tatvāt.

न not च and तत् that सालम्बनं which support (आलम्बन is that from which a thing hangs or by which it is supported) तस्य its अविषयीभूतत्वात् because of (its) not being the object (of *Saṃyama*).

20. But not also of other mental factors which support the mental image for that is not the object (of *Saṃyama*).

It is obvious that by perceiving the mental image in the other mind the *Yogi* cannot automatically gain knowledge of the motive or purpose which is present behind the mental image. For this he will have to go deeper into the other mind. An example will make this clear. Suppose the *Yogi* sees the image of the sun in the other mind. This image may be produced by thinking of the sun by an astronomer who is interested in the sun as an astronomical object. It may be produced by an artist who is admiring the beauty of the sun. It may be produced by a sun-worshipper who is worshipping the sun as an expression of Divine Life. The image in all these cases will be the same but the mental background will be entirely different. The *Sūtra* points out that by merely perceiving the mental image the *Yogi* will not be able to obtain knowledge of the other factors which are present in the background and which are responsible for the production of the image. This merely serves to emphasize that the world of names and forms is different from, and is easier to reach than the world of motives, etc. which produces movements in the lower mind.

२१. कायरूपसंयमात् तद्ग्राह्यशक्तिस्तम्भे चक्षुःप्रकाशासंप्रयोगेऽन्तर्धानम् ।

Kāya-rūpa-saṃyamāt tad-grāhya-śakti-stambhe cakṣuḥ-prakāśāsaṃprayoge 'ntardhānam.

काय the body रूप form; visibility संयमात् by performing *Saṃyama* on तत् from it; thence ग्राह्य receptive; apprehensible शक्ति

(of) power; capacity स्तम्भे on suspension चक्षुः (of) the eye प्रकाश with the light असंप्रयोगे on there being no contact अन्तर्धानम् disappearance; invisibility.

21. By performing *Saṃyama* on *Rūpa* (one of the five *Tanmātras*), on suspension of the receptive power, the contact between the eye (of the observer) and light (from the body) is broken and the body becomes invisible.

The power of making oneself invisible is one of the well-known *Siddhis* which can be acquired by *Yoga*. How can the *modus operandi* of this *Siddhi* be explained? According to modern Science a body becomes visible when the light reflected from it strikes the eye of the perceiver. If this contact between the eye and the light can be prevented the body will become invisible. This can be done by performing *Saṃyama* on *Rūpa Tanmātra*. The interrelations between the *Tattvas*, *Tanmātras* and the organs of sensation and their correspondences are well known and form an integral part of the psychology upon which the Science of *Yoga* is based. All the visual phenomena are dependent upon the interplay of the *Tanmātra* which is called *Rūpa*, the *Tattva* which is called *Tejas*, and the organ of sensation which is called *Cakṣuḥ* (eye). By performing *Saṃyama* on the *Rūpa Tanmātra*, the *Yogi* gains knowledge of the forces which connect the *Tattva*, the *Tanmātra* and the organ of sensation and can manipulate these forces as he likes. He can, therefore, prevent the light from his body reaching or affecting the eyes of the perceiver and thus make himself invisible.

२२. एतेन शब्दाद्यन्तर्धानमुक्तम् ।

Etena śabdādy antardhānam uktam.

एतेन by this; by the above शब्द sound आदि and others; etc. अन्तर्धानम् disappearance उक्तम् has been said or described.

22. From the above can be understood the disappearance of sound, etc.

The principle referred to in the previous *Sūtra* in relation to visual phenomena is also applicable to the other four organs of sensation. Thus by performing *Saṃyama* on the *Śabda Tanmātra* and gaining knowledge of the forces acting between the *Tattva* which is called *Ākāśa*, the *Tanmātra* which is called *Śabda* and the organ of sensation which is called *Śrotra* (the ear) the *Yogi* can control phenomena connected with sound. If the vibrations which affect any sense-organ and produce the corresponding sensations can be cut off the source of those vibrations naturally becomes imperceptible as far as that sense-organ is concerned. This *Sūtra* is omitted in some of the texts, obviously because what is pointed out in it can be inferred from the previous *Sūtra*.

२३. सोपक्रमं निरुपक्रमं च कर्म तत्संयमादपरान्तज्ञानमरिष्टेभ्यो वा ।

Sopakramaṃ nirupakramaṃ ca karma
tat-saṃyamād aparānta-jñānam
ariṣṭebhyo vā.

सोपक्रमं energetically operative; active निरुपक्रमं slowly working; without intensive activity; dormant च and कर्म (sum of person's) actions (viewed as determining his future) तत् them संयमात् by performing *Saṃyama* on अपरान्त of death; of the final end ज्ञानम् knowledge अरिष्टेभ्यः from omens or portents वा or.

23. *Karma* is of two kinds: active and dormant; by performing *Saṃyama* on them (is gained) knowledge of the time of death; also by (performing *Saṃyama* on) portents.

Those who are familiar with the doctrine of *Karma* will recall that *Karma* is of three kinds: *Prārabdha*, *Saṃcita* and *Kriyamāṇa*.

Saṃcita Karma is the total stock of accumulated *Karma*, generated by an individual during the present and previous lives, which has still to be worked out. *Prārabdha* is that portion of this total stock which has to be worked out in the present incarnation. This portion is selected out of the total stock at the beginning of each incarnation according to the opportunities provided by the circumstances of the incarnation for the working out of particular types of *Karma*. *Kriyamāṇa* is the *Karma* which is generated from day to day. Some of this is exhausted immediately while the remainder goes to swell the accumulated stock.

It will be clear from what has been said above that *Prārabdha Karma* is distinguishable from *Saṃcita Karma* by its potentiality for finding expression in the present life and it should be possible for anyone who can obtain a bird's-eye view of the whole landscape of *Saṃskāras* to separate this active *Prārabdha Karma* from the dormant *Saṃcita Karma*. If this can be done then the determination of the time of death should be quite easy. It will be the moment when all the *Karmas* included in *Prārabdha* are due to be exhausted. This is what *Saṃyama* on the *Saṃcita* and *Prārabdha Karma* brings about. But this *Siddhi* implies the power to raise the consciousness to the plane of the *Kāraṇa Śarīra*. It is this body which is the repository of all *Kārmic Saṃskāras* and it is only when the *Yogi* can function consciously in this body that he can investigate successfully the *Kārmic* potentialities of his own life or those of others.

Another method by which the *Yogi* can determine the time of death is by observing a certain omen and performing *Saṃyama* on that. The coming of the scientific age has relegated all such things as omens or portents to the realm of superstitions, and there is no doubt that prior to the advance of Science the subject of portents had become surrounded by the grossest superstitions and fancies of the ignorant masses. But, it must be understood that there is nothing inherently absurd in obtaining an indication of future events which are imminent by means of certain signs or symptoms that may be available, because coming events do sometimes cast their shadows before they actually take place.

When a doctor is called in to see a patient in the last stages of a critical illness he can, by simply placing his hand on the pulse of the patient, sometimes say with certainty that the patient is about to pass away. The pulse gives an indication of his general condition and on the basis of that he can, almost with certainty, foretell the death of the patient. His prediction is not the result of guess work but of drawing an inference from certain observations he has made. Every man cannot foretell such an event. It requires medical knowledge and experience. A real portent is such a significant sign which gives an indication of the coming event. In itself it may be trivial and have no rational connection with the thing predicted but to the man who can peer into the inner side of natural phenomena it may provide a definite indication of what is to come in the future. But it is obvious that only those whose inner eyes have been opened and who are able to trace effects to their causes by means of *Saṃyama* can recognize such an omen and interpret it correctly.

२४. मैत्र्यादिषु बलानि ।

Maitry-ādiṣu balāni.

मैत्री-आदिषु on friendliness, etc. बलानि strengths or powers.

24. (By performing *Saṃyama*) on friendliness etc. (comes) strength (of the quality).

It is a well-known law of psychology that if we think of any quality persistently that quality tends to become more and more a part of our character. This effect is heightened by meditation in which the concentration of mind is far more intense than in ordinary thinking. The effect is increased tremendously in *Samādhi* for the following reason. When the *Yogi* performs *Saṃyama* on any quality his mind becomes one with that quality for the time being as has been explained in I-41. The positive qualities like courage, compassion etc. are not vague nebulous things as they appear to the lower mind but real, living, dynamic principles of unlimited power which cannot manifest fully in the lower worlds for lack of adequate instruments. A principle or quality merely sheds its radiance feebly, as it were, while we merely think of the quality, the radiance becoming more and more bright as the thinking becomes deeper and more persistent and the mind gets more and more attuned to the quality. But when *Saṃyama* is performed on the particular quality and it fuses with the mind it can manifest through it to an unlimited extent. Even when this condition of being *en rapport* with the quality ends on the cessation of *Saṃyama* the effect of this direct contact is to make a permanent impression on the mind and to increase enormously its power to manifest that quality under normal conditions. And with repeated *Saṃyama* the mind gets so attuned to the quality that its perfect expression in normal life becomes easy and natural.

That is how the advanced *Yogi* can make himself the very embodiment of the powers of love, sympathy, courage, patience, etc. and can express them to an extent which seems wonderful to the neophyte who is still struggling to acquire those qualities. *Saṃyama*, therefore, provides the *Yogi* with the most efficient technique of character-building.

२५. बलेषु हस्तिबलादीनि ।

Baleṣu hasti-balādīni.

बलेषु by *Saṃyama* on strengths; powers (pl.) हस्ति-बलादीनि strength of elephant, etc.

25. (By performing *Saṃyama*) on the strengths (of animals) the strength of an elephant, etc.

What has been said above with regard to qualities which may be called human traits of character applies equally to powers which are special characteristics of animals. Thus, if the *Yogi* performs *Saṃyama* on strength which is possessed in different degrees by different animals he can acquire strength, even that of an elephant. Of course, the elephant does not indicate the limit of the strength which can be acquired, this animal being mentioned merely because it is supposed to be the strongest animal known to us. What that limit is it is difficult to say.

What we should note, however, is that all these qualities or powers like strength, speed, etc. which involve generally physical forces are not mere abstractions but living principles or *Tattvas* having their source in the consciousness of the Logos. The *Yogi* who gains direct contact with these principles is therefore in touch with a source whose potentialities are unlimited as far as we are concerned.

२६. प्रवृत्त्यालोकन्यासात् सूक्ष्मव्यवहितविप्रकृष्टज्ञानम् ।

Pravṛtty-āloka-nyāsāt sūkṣma-vyavahita-viprakṛṣṭa-jñānam.

प्रवृत्ति higher sensuous activity; superphysical faculty आलोक light न्यासात् by directing or projecting सूक्ष्म (of) the small; fine; subtle व्यवहित the hidden; the obscure विप्रकृष्ट the distant ज्ञानम् knowledge.

26. Knowledge of the small, the hidden or the distant by directing the light of superphysical faculty.

That interpenetrating the physical plane there are several super-physical planes of progressively increasing subtlety is a well-known doctrine of Occult philosophy. Patañjali has not definitely mentioned and classified the different planes but their existence is implicit in his doctrines of different levels of consciousness (1-17) and the stages of the *Guṇas* (II-19). His reference to higher sensuous activity or superphysical faculties in the *Sūtra* also shows that he took for granted the existence of the superphysical worlds, and the exercise of faculties pertaining to them. Another reason, perhaps, why the different planes of existence are not mentioned by him specifically is that such a division of the material side of the Universe is not necessary for the purpose of *Yoga*. *Yoga* as a practical Science is concerned mainly with the raising of human consciousness into progressively higher levels of existence and since all the planes really form one heterogeneous mass of particles of matter, they may, for the sake of convenience, be taken as one.

Subtlety, obscurity and remoteness to which reference is made in this *Sūtra* are all due to the limitations of the sense-organs. These limitations are sought to be overcome by Science by enlarging the scope of the sense-organs through the use of highly refined physical instruments. Thus enormous help is given to the eyes in seeing what is distant by the use of a telescope, in seeing what is small by the use of a microscope and in seeing what is hidden by the use of an X-ray apparatus. But these instrumental aids afforded to our physical sense-organs, though wonderful in some ways, suffer from enormous limitations of various kinds. In the first place, their sphere of observation, however enlarged it may be, is confined within the physical world. All the superphysical worlds by their very nature will always remain hidden from the most sensitive physical instruments that may be devised. And since the physical world is merely the outermost shell of the manifested Universe our knowledge of this Universe is bound to remain fragmentary and extremely partial. In the second place, it is never possible to reach the final truth with regard to fundamental scientific questions in this way. Wonderful though our knowledge is with regard to matter and energy we should not forget that much of this knowledge is inferential and therefore subject to doubt and error. The rapid supersession of different theories, one after another, which has marked the advance of Science in the fields of chemistry and physics has created so much confusion and uncertainty with regard to the fundamental questions concerning the nature of the manifested Universe that the scientist does not seem to be sure about anything now except the empirical facts which he has obtained and utilized in such a marvellous manner. This is inevitable as long as we continue to investigate, exclusively by physical instruments and mathematical analysis, a Universe whose foundations lie in the realms of mind and consciousness.

Now, the *Yogic* method is entirely different. It discards completely all external aids and relies on the unfoldment of inner organs of perception. These organs are present in a more or less perfect state of development in all evolved human beings and require only to be put to use by proper training through *Yogic* methods. The unfoldment of these organs, corresponding to all levels of consciousness and subtlety of matter, step by step, opens up naturally all the subtle realms of matter to the *Yogi* right up to the last stage where matter disappears into consciousness. And incidentally, it provides him with the means of investigating the phenomena even of the physical world and manipulating its forces far more simply and effectively than a scientist can do, as the nature of many *Siddhis* clearly shows. It is true that the *Yogic* method is individual, incapable of public demonstration and requires prolonged and rigorous self-discipline. But those who can see the illusions of life and are determined to know the Truth are bound to prefer it when they realize that the scientific method can give them only the superficial knowledge of the physical plane, and does not hold out any hope of freeing them from the limitations of life.

The powers referred to in the *Sūtra* are decidedly of a lower order than the more important and real *Siddhis* because there are a few people scattered throughout the world who can undoubtedly exercise such powers in a limited way. Psychic powers like clairvoyance or clairaudience are so common now that their possibility is no longer denied by the majority of thoughtful people even though they may not have found recognition in strictly scientific circles. But when they are exhibited by people in the ordinary way either from pecuniary considerations or to satisfy the curiosity of people they will be found to be developed not by strictly *Yogic* methods but by other methods to which Patañjali has made reference in IV-1.

२७. भुवनज्ञानं सूर्ये संयमात् ।

Bhuvana-jñānaṃ sūrye saṃyamāt.

भुवन (of) the Solar system ज्ञानं knowledge सूर्ये on the Sun संयमात् by performing *Saṃyama* on.

27. Knowledge of the Solar system by performing *Saṃyama* on the Sun.

This *Sūtra* and the next two deal with the method of acquiring knowledge regarding the heavenly bodies. There are three basic questions involved in this knowledge. The first is the structure of a Solar system which is the fundamental unit in the whole Cosmos. The second is the arrangement of the stars in different kinds of groups such as galaxies, etc. The third is the law which underlies their movements. Knowledge with regard to these primary questions is obtained by performing *Saṃyama* on three different objects in the sky as indicated in these *Sūtras*. To understand how this is possible the student should recall what has been said in connection with I-42 concerning the different principles underlying *Saṃyama* for different purposes.

The *Sūtra* under discussion deals with the method of acquiring knowledge concerning the structure of a Solar system. This knowledge includes not only the physical aspect which has been studied so thoroughly by modern astronomers but also the superphysical aspects which are hidden from our view but are far more interesting and significant. A general knowledge regarding our Sun as obtained by scientific methods will convince anyone that the Sun is in some mysterious manner the very heart and soul of the Solar system. Occult investigations based on *Yogic* methods have shown that this appearance of all life in the Solar system being centred in the Sun has a deeper significance and is due to the fact that the Solar system is a vehicle for the expression of the life and consciousness of a Mighty Being whom we call an *Īśvara* or a Solar Logos. This life and consciousness expresses itself at different levels through the different planes of the Solar system which interpenetrate one another and form one integrated whole.

Since the different planes of the Solar system are organically related to one another and the physical Sun is the centre of this complex organism, it is easy to see how *Saṃyama* on the Sun will unfold in the mind of the *Yogi* the whole pattern of the Solar system and give him a comprehensive knowledge not only with regard to the structure of our Solar system but all Solar systems which constitute the Cosmos. For these Solar systems though separated from one another by tremendous distances are not really independent of one another. They are rooted in the One Ultimate Reality, derive their life from one 'Common Source' and are modelled on one pattern.

२८. चन्द्रे ताराव्यूहज्ञानम् ।

Candre tārā-vyūha-jñānam.

चन्द्रे (by performing *Saṃyama* on) the moon तारा (of) star व्यूह organization; interlinking arrangement ज्ञानम् knowledge.

28. (By performing *Saṃyama*) on the moon knowledge concerning the arrangement of stars.

This *Sūtra* provides an illustration of the principle that by performing *Saṃyama* on an external phenomenon it is possible to obtain knowledge of the basic law or principle upon which that phenomenon is based. A study of the sky by astronomical methods has not only enlarged our horizon and given us knowledge of stars, galaxies, and universes beyond human ken but it has also enabled us to gain a glimpse into the relations which exist between these different groups of stars. With every increase in the power of magnification of telescopes new galaxies and universes come within the range of observation and prove the infinite nature of the Cosmos. All these heavenly bodies which appear to be scattered in the sky in a haphazard manner have been found by astronomers to be grouped in different ways, these groups being related to one another in a definite manner. Thus the satellites are grouped and move round a planet, the planets are grouped and move round a central sun, the suns which we see as stars form part of a much larger group called a galaxy and the galaxies are grouped together in a universe. The distances and times involved in these groupings and movements of stars are so stupendous as compared with the periods during which the observations have been made that no clear and over-all picture of the whole Cosmos can be obtained by purely physical methods, though anyone who has studied the subject with an open mind cannot fail to see that there is a Grand Design at the basis of the astronomical phenomena.

How can the *Yogi* obtain knowledge of this design? By performing *Saṃyama* on an astronomical phenomenon which is typical of the different groupings and movements. The movement of the moon round the earth is such a phenomenon on the smallest scale. It embodies the essential characteristics of all the groupings and movements and it is easy to see how *Saṃyama* on it will unfold in the mind of the *Yogi* the essential nature of the Cosmic Design.

२९. ध्रुवे तद्गतिज्ञानम् ।

Dhruve tad-gati-jñānam.

ध्रुवे (by performing *Saṃyama*) on the pole-star तत्-गतिः (of) their movement ज्ञानम् knowledge.

29. (By performing *Saṃyama*) on the pole-star knowledge of their movements.

What has been said above with regard to the general law which regulates the spatial relationships of the heavenly bodies applies equally to the law which regulates their relative movements. It is well known that motion is a purely relative thing and it is not possible to define or determine absolute motion. We can measure motion only in relation to another object which is fixed. This is the law upon which all other laws of motion are based. Now, there is only one star in the sky whose position is relatively fixed and which is, therefore, considered as a symbol of fixity. This is called *Dhruva* or pole-star. This star may, therefore, be taken to be a symbol of the fundamental law of motion referred to above. By *Saṃyama* on *Dhruva* is, therefore, meant not *Saṃyama* on the physical star which bears that name but on the law of motion of which it is a symbol.

How *Saṃyama* on this fundamental law will enable the *Yogi* to acquire knowledge of all the laws of motion governing the movements of the heavenly bodies will be clear if we remember that the different laws of motion are inter-related and by performing *Saṃyama* on the basic law it is possible to acquire knowledge of all. Those who are familiar with the philosophy of modern Science will recall how Science is always aiming to discover a simple and fundamental law which underlies a number of diverse laws working in a particular sphere. Such a search is based on the intuitive perception of the fundamental unity underlying manifestation. All laws of Nature operating in different spheres and apparently quite unrelated are really derived from the progressive differentiation of a single comprehensive Law which expresses the working of Nature in its entirety. That is why it is possible to integrate minor laws into more comprehensive laws progressively and by performing *Saṃyama* on one aspect of a law to acquire knowledge of all the other aspects.

३०. नाभिचक्रे कायव्यूहज्ञानम् ।

Nābhi-cakre kāya-vyūha-jñānam.

नाभिचक्रे (by performing *Saṃyama*) on the navel-disc (centre) काय the body व्यूह arrangement; organization ज्ञानम् knowledge.

30. (By performing *Saṃyama*) on the navel centre knowledge of the organization of the body.

The physical body is a wonderful living organism which serves in a remarkable manner as an instrument of consciousness on the physical plane. It is true that a part of the physical body and the most important part, is invisible and outside the purview of modern scientific methods. The whole system of *Prāṇic* distribution, for example, which works through the *Prāṇamaya Kośa* and supplies vitality to the *Annamaya Kośa* is unknown to Science. But even what can be investigated by scientific methods shows that the various activities of the body have been organized in the most scientific manner and seem to be guided by the highest intelligence.

A detailed study of this organization of the body shows also that it is organized on a set pattern and, therefore, all human bodies are structurally and functionally alike in essentials. The circulatory system, the nervous system, the lymphatic system, the glandular system and other systems work in the same way in all human bodies though they have also remarkable powers of adaptability. The reason for this similar behaviour of all human bodies is, of course, the presence of an archetype in the Universal Mind to which all bodies conform. That is why, in the case of billions and billions of human beings who are born under the most varied conditions, the same pattern in the outer form of the body and in its inner working is repeated with remarkable fidelity.

Anyone who can mentally contact this archetype of the human body will obtain full knowledge of the machinery of the physical body. This can be done by performing *Saṃyama* on the navel *Cakra* because this *Cakra* controls the sympathetic nervous system working in the body. But, of course, it is the archetype of the body which is the object of knowledge in performing *Saṃyama* and the navel *Cakra* is merely the gateway leading to that archetype. The navel centre is not the solar plexus but the centre of *Cakra* in the *Prāṇamaya Kośa* which is connected with the solar plexus.

३१. कण्ठकूपे क्षुत्पिपासानिवृत्तिः ।

Kaṇṭha-kūpe kṣut-pipāsā-nivṛttiḥ.

कण्ठकूपे (by performing *Saṃyama*) on the gullet (' throat-well '); क्षुत् (of) hunger पिपासा thirst निवृत्तिः cessation.

31. (By performing *Saṃyama*) on the gullet the cessation of hunger and thirst.

It is well known that sensations of hunger and thirst and similar other phenomena depend upon the secretions of glands situated in various parts of the body. A knowledge of the working of these glands and the capacity to regulate their secretions will, naturally, give power to the *Yogi* to control the sensations. There are several glands situated in and around the throat, and *Saṃyama* on the navel *Cakra* having revealed the presence of the gland which controls hunger and thirst, will enable the *Yogi* to make these sensations voluntary.

It may, however, be mentioned that it is really *Prāṇa* which controls secretions of glands and since *Prāṇa* is amenable to thought, once knowledge of the working of glands is acquired the *Yogi* can control all the phy iological actions in the body, even the movements of the heart and lungs. What a doctor tries to bring about by the action of drugs the *Yogi* can bring about by the control and regulation of *Prāṇic* currents in the body. The glands involved in these physiological actions have not been specified by Patañjali, obviously, to prevent foolish people from dabbling in these matters and injuring themselves.

३२. कूर्मनाड्यां स्थैर्यम् ।

Kūrma-nāḍyāṃ sthairyam.

कूर्मनाड्यां (by performing *Saṃyama*) on the *Kūrma-nāḍī*, i.e. the nerve which is the vehicle of the *Prāṇa* called *Kūrma* स्थैर्यम् steadiness; immovability.

32. (By performing *Saṃyama*) on the *Kūrma-nāḍī* steadiness.

Prāṇa is of many kinds, each kind having special functions in the body and a special *Nāḍī* as its vehicle. *Kūrma* is one of the well-known varieties of *Prāṇa* and the particular nerve which serves as its vehicle is called *Kārma-nāḍī*. This variety of *Prāṇa* has obviously something to do with the motions of the body for by controlling it the *Yogi* acquires the power to make his body motionless. This control can be acquired, as usual, by performing *Saṃyama* on the *Nāḍī* which is its vehicle.

All the physiological devices working in the physical body are meant to carry on their normal activities in an involuntary manner. But since each device is really the vehicle of a principle or *Tattva* it is possible by gaining voluntary control over its function to express that principle to any extent desired. It is this kind of voluntary control over the function of the *Kūrma-nāḍi* which enables the *Yogi* to perform feats of strength which appear miraculous to an ordinary person. But, of course, no real *Yogi* will make a demonstration of this kind.

३३. मूर्धज्योतिषि सिद्धदर्शनम् ।

Mūrdha-jyotiṣi siddha-darśanam.

मूर्धज्योतिषि (by performing *Saṃyama*) on the light under the crown of the head सिद्ध- (of) perfected Beings; Adepts दर्शनम् vision of.

33. (By performing *Saṃyama* on) the light under the crown of the head vision of perfected Beings.

Since the *Yogic* philosophy is based upon the immortality of the human soul and its perfection through evolution, the existence of those who have perfected themselves and are living in a state of the highest Enlightenment is taken for granted. Such Beings are called *Siddhas*.

These perfected Beings are above the necessity of reincarnation because they have already learnt all the lessons which embodied life has to teach and have completed the cycle of human evolution. They live on the spiritual planes of the Solar system and even when they retain bodies on the lower planes for helping humanity in its evolution their consciousness remains really centred in the higher planes. To come in contact with these Beings one has to rise to the plane on which their consciousness normally functions. Merely coming in physical contact with them in some way is not of much use because unless a person is attuned to their higher life he cannot derive real benefit from his contact with them.

How can one come into touch with these perfected Beings in the proper way? By performing *Saṃyama* on the light under the crown of the head. There is a small rudimentary organ in the brain which is called the pituitary body. Besides its other physiological functions known to medical science it has the important function of establishing contact with the spiritual planes on which the consciousness of the *Siddhas* functions. When it is made active by meditation it serves as a bridge between the higher and lower consciousness and enables the light of the higher worlds to penetrate into the brain. It is only then that the *Siddhas* really become accessible to the *Yogi* because he can rise to their plane and hold communion with them. But it is not by merely concentrating on this physical organ that this kind of communication can be established. It is by performing *Saṃyama* on the light for which the organ can serve as the physical vehicle.

३४. प्रातिभाद्वा सर्वम् ।

Prātibhād vā sarvam.

प्रातिभात् from intuitive (knowledge) वा or सर्वम् everything; all.

34. (Knowledge of) everything from intuition.

It is well known that all the *Siddhis* can be acquired by methods other than those outlined in the *Yoga-Sūtras* so far. For example, a *Bhakta* who follows the path of love comes in possession of many *Siddhis* though he has done nothing to develop them deliberately. This shows that there is a state of spiritual consciousness in which all these powers are inherent and, therefore, anyone who attains to this state by whatever method acquires the *Siddhis* automatically. The *Bhakta* attains to this state by union with the Beloved through love, *Jñāni* through discrimination. Patañjali has given in the next two *Sūtras* the method of developing this state of consciousness by the strictly *Yogic* method.

This state of consciousness in which *Siddhis* of all kinds are inherent also confers the power to perceive truth directly without the help of any instruments. The latter faculty which is called *Pratibhā* here has really no equivalent in English. The word which comes nearest to it in meaning is intuition. But this word intuition as used in Western psychology has a rather vague and general sense of apprehension of truth by the mind without reasoning. The emphasis is on the absence of reasoning and not on the transcendent nature of what is apprehended. It is true that some Western philosophers have used the word intuition in a more specific sense which comes nearer to that of *Pratibhā* but that is not the generally accepted meaning of the term.

The word *Pratibhā* as used in the *Yoga-Sūtras* stands for that transcendent spiritual faculty of perception which can dispense with the use of not only the sense-organs but also the mind. It can perceive everything directly mirrored, as it were, in consciousness itself and not through the instrumentality of the senses or the mind. Intuition, on the other hand, is at its best a vague and weak reflection of *Pratibhā* and may be called an echo or lower reverberation of *Pratibhā* in the realm of the mind. It lacks the directness and definiteness of perception implied in *Pratibhā.*

That there must be a faculty of non-instrumental perception is clear from the fact that *Īśvara* is conscious of everything everywhere without the use of the sense-organs or the mind. If omniscience is a fact then non-instrumental perception must also be a fact and *Pratibhā* is only the expression of this kind of perception through an individual in a limited manner. This is also the faculty which perfected Beings who have attained *Kaivalya* use in maintaining their contact with the lower worlds which they have transcended. Perception through the sense-organs should, therefore, be considered merely as a stage in the unfoldment of consciousness. After the higher consciousness has become unfolded the use of these organs becomes mostly unnecessary and is resorted to only for certain specific purposes. In evolutionary progress it is found frequently that a particular mechanism representing a lower stage is used only in unfolding a higher stage and disappears after it has achieved its purpose.

३५. हृदये चित्तसंवित्।

Hṛdaye citta-saṃvit.

हृदये (by performing *Saṃyama*) on the heart चित्तसंवित् awareness of the mind (consciousness which manifests in association with matter as mind).

35. (By performing *Saṃyama*) on the heart, awareness of the nature of the mind.

In this *Sūtra* and the next the method of unfolding intuitional consciousness is given. As the intuitional consciousness transcends mental consciousness the first step, naturally, is to acquire true knowledge concerning the nature of the mind and how it modifies pure consciousness, i.e. consciousness of the *Puruṣa*. This knowledge is gained by performing *Saṃyama* on the heart. What is meant by the heart?

On the form side the *Jīvātmā* is constituted of a set of concentric vehicles composed of matter of different degrees of subtlety just as the Solar Logos on the form side is constituted of a set of concentric planes irradiated by His consciousness. The former is called *Piṇḍāṇḍa*, the auric egg, while the latter is called a *Brahmāṇḍa*, the *Brāhmic* egg, the two being related to each other as microcosm and macrocosm and having a common centre. Just as the sun both in its physical and super-physical aspects forms the heart of the Solar system from which radiate all the energies which are needed in the Solar system, in the same way, the common centre of all the vehicles of the *Jīvātmā* which energizes them is referred to in occult and mystic literature as the heart. It is probably so called firstly, because of its proximity to the physical heart and secondly, because of its analogous function. The gateway to the mystic heart is the *Cakra* known as *Anāhata* and it is *Saṃyama* on this really which enables the *Yogi* to know the nature of the mind principle which functions through the different vehicles at different levels.

As *Citta* is merely the product of the interaction of consciousness and matter (I-2) it should be easy to see why the common centre of all the vehicles through which consciousness functions should also be the seat of *Citta*. The senses are merely the outposts of *Citta* and should be considered as part of *Citta*.

३६. सत्त्वपुरुषयोरत्यन्तासंकीर्णयोः प्रत्ययाविशेषो भोगः परार्थात् स्वार्थसंयमात् पुरुषज्ञानम् ।

Sattva-puruṣayor atyantāsaṃkīrṇayoḥ pratyayāviśeṣo bhogaḥ parārthāt svārtha-saṃyamāt puruṣa-jñānam.

सत्त्वपुरुषयोः of Sattva (one of the three *Guṇas*) representing refined *Buddhi* and *Puruṣa* अत्यन्त extremely असंकीर्णयोः (of) the immiscible; distinctive प्रत्यय (of) awareness अविशेषः non-distinction भोगः (is) experience परार्थात् apart from another's (interest) स्वार्थ Self-interest संयमात् by performing *Saṃyama* on पुरुष (of) *Puruṣa* ज्ञानम् knowledge.

36. Experience is the result of inability to distinguish between the *Puruṣa* and the *Sattva* though they are absolutely distinct. Knowledge of the *Puruṣa* results from *Saṃyama* on the Self-interest (of the *Puruṣa*) apart from another's interest (of *Prakṛti*).

This is one of those *Sūtras* which many students find it difficult to understand. This is due to the fact that it involves some fundamental doctrines of *Sāṃkhya* philosophy about which our ideas are not quite clear. If we clarify these ideas first the meaning of the *Sūtra* will become much clearer. Although the *Yoga-sūtras* are considered generally to be based entirely on *Sāṃkhya* they are best understood on the basis of both *Sāṃkhya* and *Vedāntic* doctrines and there is really no justification for the arbitrary exclusion of *Vedāntic* doctrines in discussing the problems of higher *Yoga*.

The first idea which we should try to grasp is that the *Puruṣa* is a Centre in the Ultimate Reality (*Brahman*) and transcends manifestation and its limitations. His descent into manifestation through association with *Prakṛti* does not alter his transcendental nature although it modifies *Prakṛti* through which his triple nature denoted by *Sat-Cit-Ānanda* expresses itself. This triple nature is reflected in the three *Guṇas*, the correspondences between the aspects of consciousness and *Guṇas* being represented by the following diagram:

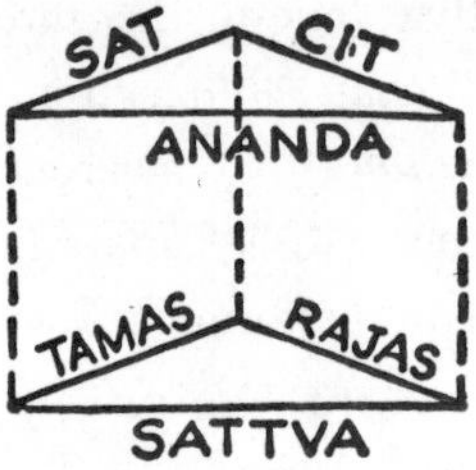

FIG. 10

It will be seen from the above diagram that the principle of cognition or awareness which is included in *Ânanda* of the *Vedāntic* terminology corresponds to the *Sattva Guṇa.* It is because the object of *Yoga* is Self-realization or obtaining awareness of one's true nature (I-3) that *Sattva Guṇa* plays such an important part in the exposition of its doctrines.

When the consciousness of the *Puruṣa* manifests in the realm of *Prakṛti* it appears as awareness of the Not-Self and this awareness which expresses itself through the action of *Sattva Guṇa* is called *Buddhi.* Some confusion is always caused by the use of the same word—consciousness—both for the transcendent consciousness of the *Puruṣa* which is *above* the realm of *Prakṛti* and its reflection as awareness *within* the realm of *Prakṛti.* When we use the word consciousness in its ordinary sense we always mean the latter, but there is really no word in English corresponding to the transcendent consciousness of the *Puruṣa* of which the consciousness of modern psychology is a partial and limited manifestation. The word used in *Saṃskṛta* for pure transcendent consciousness of *Puruṣa* is *Citi-Śakti* (IV-34) or more generally *Caitanyam* while the conditioned consciousness is called generally *Saṃvit* (III-35).

When the pure consciousness of the *Puruṣa* is associated with *Prakṛti* it becomes increasingly conditioned as it descends, plane by plane, these different degrees of conditioning being represented by the four stages of the *Guṇas* (II-19). It should, however, be borne in mind that *Sāṃkyha* is based upon the absolute transcendence of the *Puruṣa.* According to it the *Puruṣa* does not descend into *Prakṛti* but is merely associated with *Prakṛti* in an undefined manner. The mere propinquity of *Puruṣa* brings about changes in

Prakṛti, one of these changes being the development of conditioned consciousness. It is because the *Puruṣa* is always quite separate and distinct from *Prakṛti* that all phenomena of consciousness or awareness are considered purely *Prākṛtic*, based on *Sattva Guṇa*. For all practical purposes the word *Sattva* as used in the present context may be taken as the principle of awareness expressing through the faculty of *Buddhi*. The *Puruṣa* remains quite separate from it though his presence stimulates the awareness through *Buddhi*. This awareness becomes more and more vivid and simulates more perfectly the consciousness of the *Puruṣa* as it is expressed through the increasingly subtler stages of the *Guṇas* but there can be nothing common between the two, for the former is a pure product of *Prakṛti* while the latter transcends *Prakṛti* altogether. The two are quite distinct. This is what is meant by the phrase *Atyantāsaṃkīrṇayoḥ*.

The second idea which has to be grasped in this *Sūtra* concerns the nature of experience. Since the *Puruṣa* transcends *Prakṛti* altogether and experience is always in the realm of *Prakṛti*, the *Puruṣa* cannot be the experiencer. Experience results when, through *Avidyā*, there is non-distinction or identification between the *Puruṣa* and the conditioned consciousness which is called *Sattva* in this *Sūtra*. Even in ordinary life we find that the more we identify ourselves with our mind and its contents and allow ourselves to get lost in them the greater is the zest of life, while detachment takes the zest out of experiences and converts them into mere awareness. The greater the detachment or *Vairāgya* through discrimination the more perfect is the transformation of *Bhoga* or experience into mere awareness. A *Jīvanmukta* is as much conscious when functioning through a vehicle as the ordinary man but since the element of identification is absent there is no *Bhoga* or tasteful experience. This gradual disengagement of pure consciousness from the *Pratyaya* which is produced by contact with a vehicle is brought about by *Viveka* and *Vairāgya* and when completed leads to *Kaivalya*.

Is then *Kaivalya* a state completely devoid of happiness? Is it a perfectly colourless existence in which there is nothing to compensate for the joys and happiness which we sometimes feel in ordinary life? This is a misconception which frequently troubles those who have studied these questions superficially and is frequently the cause of the repulsion which they sometimes feel towards the *Yogic* ideal of Liberation. To remove this misconception we have merely to ask what is the source of the illusory happiness which we feel in the joyful experiences of our ordinary life and the blissful experiences of the higher life. Of course, the Self whose very nature is bliss. The outer experience is merely an exciting cause. It is the response from within—the source of bliss—which produces the faint reverberations which we feel as joys and pleasures of the lower life. In giving up the joys and pleasures of the lower life we are merely giving up the indirect, feeble and uncertain method of obtaining bliss for the direct method. We give up our hold on the shadow so that we may grasp the substance. Instead of trying vainly to gain blissful experience we become Bliss itself.

As the pure consciousness of the *Puruṣa* is really quite separate and yet appears indistinguishable from awareness in the realm of *Prakṛti*, the question arises how to separate the two in order to gain knowledge of the *Puruṣa*. The method prescribed in this *Sūtra* is *Saṃyama* on the distinction between the purpose hidden behind the *Pratyaya* and the purpose of the *Puruṣa* himself. The *Pratyaya* is for another. It is a product of *Prakṛti* which according to *Sāṃkhya* acts only and always for the *Puruṣa*. The consciousness of the *Puruṣa* is for the *Puruṣa* himself. It has no ulterior motive or purpose, the *Puruṣa* being eternal, changeless and Self-sufficient. This distinction, subtle though it is, can be made the object of *Saṃyama* and it is possible in this manner to resolve the apparently homogeneous *Pratyaya* into its two components, the *Sattva Guṇa* in which the consciousness of the *Puruṣa* is reflected and the consciousness of the *Puruṣa* himself. The problem is not unlike that of distinguishing between a source of light and its reflection in a mirror. Just as there can be several methods of distinguishing between the real object and its reflection so there can be several methods of distinguishing between the reflection of the *Puruṣa* in *Sattva* and the *Puruṣa* himself. The method proposed is one of them and leads to the knowledge of the *Puruṣa* himself as distinguished from his reflection in *Sattva*. When this knowledge is obtained the *Yogi* is in a position to exercise non-instrumental perception hinted at in III-34. As the *Puruṣa* is above the limitations of *Prakṛti* his perception must also be above the limitations of the mind and the sense-organs.

३७. ततः प्रातिभश्रावणवेदनादर्शास्वादवार्ता जायन्ते ।

Tataḥ prātibha-śrāvaṇa-vedanādarśāsvāda-vārtā jāyante.

ततः thence; from it प्रातिभ intuitional श्रावण auditory वेदन tactile आदर्श visual आस्वाद gustatory वार्ता olfactory (knowledge) जायन्ते are born; are produced.

37. Thence are produced intuitional hearing, touch, sight, taste and smell.

Since intuitional perception transcends the mind, and the sense-organs are really the outposts of the mind, it should not be difficult to understand in a general way how the sense-organs are done away with in the exercise of intuitional perception. In the normal course our sensuous cognitions take place through the instrumentality of the sense-organs and we are therefore limited by the limitations inherent in these sense-organs. But when knowledge of the *Puruṣa* has been obtained by performing *Saṃyama* as indicated in the last *Sūtra* these limitations fall away and it is possible for the *Yogi* to perceive everything without the help of the sense-organs. In exercising clairvoyance, etc., the *Yogi* merely extends the scope of the physical sense-organs but in intuitional *Śravaṇa*, etc., he dispenses with the sense-organs altogether and uses his all-embracing general power of perception.

It will help us to understand the nature of intuitional perception if we remember that the *Puruṣa* is the real perceiver (*Draṣṭā*). Whatever knowledge can be acquired on the lower planes through external agencies is present in him already in its totality. Whatever powers and faculties are developed in the course of evolution are present in him potentially from the very beginning and are merely brought out or unfolded from a latent state into activity by the external stimuli provided by *Prakṛti*. It appears that in the earlier stages of evolution it is necessary for the cognitive faculty to be differentiated and to function through separate channels and the sense-organs thus come into being. But after the mind has been evolved to a certain stage and the powers of consciousness have been sufficiently unfolded by direct contact with the *Puruṣa* the cognitive faculty can function as a whole without the aid of the five sense-organs. Intuitional perception is like white light which includes all colours and can therefore bring out the characteristic colours of everything. Sensuous perception is like the colours present in the spectrum which is obtained from white light by diffraction with a prism. When the *Yogi* is able to transcend the prism of the mind he is able to obtain directly all knowledge which he obtained previously through the separate channels of the sense-organs.

There is difference of opinion with regard to the meaning of two words in the *Sūtra*. The first of these is *Pratibhā*. Some commentators seem to think that *Pratibhā* means superphysical cognition and *Prātibha Śravaṇa*, etc., mean merely clairaudience, etc. There does not seem to be any justification for this kind of interpretation, firstly, because the development of these superphysical faculties has been dealt with in other *Sūtras* (III-26, III-42) and secondly, because it should not be necessary for the *Yogi* to obtain at least partial knowledge of the *Puruṣa* to be able to exercise them. *Prātibha Śravaṇa*, etc., are obviously cognitions of a much higher order and from the nature of the context appear to be special powers connected with the *Puruṣa* himself since they appear after the *Yogi* obtains at least partial contact with the pure consciousness of the *Puruṣa*.

The second word which has produced some confusion is *Vārtā*. Although this word is not used now in relation to the sense of smell its use in the present context leaves no doubt that it is this sense for which it stands. If the sense of smell had been an exception to the well-known fivefold sense experiences this fact would have certainly been pointed out. This anomaly shows the inadvisability of interpreting the *Yoga-Sūtras* strictly and rigidly in terms of the current meanings of the words used. They should be interpreted in the light of *Yogic* traditions, the experiences of mystics and occultists and also commonsense, in view of the frequent changes which take place in the meanings of words through the centuries. Philology alone is not a safe guide in these matters.

३८. ते समाधावुपसर्गा व्युत्थाने सिद्धयः ।

Te samādhāv upasargā vyutthāne
siddhayaḥ.

ते they समाधौ in *Samādhi* उपसर्गाः obstacles व्युत्थाने in the state of out-turned-ness सिद्धयः powers.

38. They are obstacles in the way of *Samādhi* and powers when the mind is outward-turned.

The various *Siddhis* which have been described in Section III will naturally be obstacles when the *Yogi* is diving within the deeper layers of his consciousness because they tend to draw consciousness outwards. That is why the mystic fights shy of all such powers. He does not want to have anything to do with *Siddhis* because their exercise creates all kinds of temptations and distractions in his path. But perfection means and includes the power to control all the phenomena of all the planes on which consciousness functions and so the Perfect Man has not only to have direct knowledge of Reality but also knowledge and mastery of all planes on which his consciousness functions. That is why all the *Siddhis* have to be acquired at one stage or another before the stage of Perfection is reached. The Adept has not only all the powers which Section III deals with but also the supreme wisdom which makes the misuse of these powers impossible.

३९. बन्धकारणशैथिल्यात् प्रचारसंवेदनाच्च चित्तस्य परशरीरावेशः ।

Bandha-kāraṇa-śaithilyāt pracāra-saṃ-
vedanāc ca cittasya para-śarīrāveśaḥ.

बन्ध (of) bondage कारण cause शैथिल्यात् on relaxation; on loosening प्रचार (of) passages; channels संवेदनात् from knowledge of च and चित्तस्य of the mind पर (of) another or another's शरीर (into) the body आवेशः entrance.

39. The mind can enter another's body on relaxation of the cause of bondage and from knowledge of passages.

The power of entering the body of another person is a well-known *Siddhi* which occultists sometimes use in their work in the outer world. It should not be confused with obsession which it resembles outwardly. In obsession the entity entering the body is a low type of desire-bound disembodied soul who takes possession of the physical body of his victim forcibly in order to establish some sort of temporary and partial contact with the physical world to satisfy his desires. In the exercise of this power by a *Yogi* of a high order the body of another person is taken possession of, firstly, with the consent and knowledge of the person who is generally a disciple of the *Yogi* and thus in perfect *rapport* with him. In the second place, there is no question of the satisfaction of any personal desire by the *Yogi*. He takes possession of the body of another for the purpose of doing some important and necessary work for the helping of humanity. In most cases the purpose of the *Yogi* can be served by temporarily materializing another artificial body by his *Kriyā Śakti* in the environment in which he wants to do his work. Such an artificial body, known as *Nirmāṇa-kāya*, has, however, certain limitations and it may be more convenient for him to take the body of a disciple for the required period. Under these conditions the disciple steps out of the body and the *Yogi* occupies it. The disciple remains during this period on the higher plane in his subtler vehicle and again occupies his body when it is vacated.

Some people, especially in the West, feel a peculiar abhorrence at this idea of one person occupying the body of another. There is, however, no justification for this kind of feeling if the body is a mere tenement or an instrument for the work of the soul on the physical plane. We do not mind borrowing our friend's house or car temporarily. What is then wrong in the *Yogi* borrowing the body of another person who is prepared to oblige him? This feeling of abhorrence is really due either to our identifying ourselves completely with the physical body or thinking mistakenly that the occupation of another's body in this manner necessarily means dominating his will.

There are two conditions which have to be fulfilled before the *Yogi* is able to exercise this power. The first is the 'relaxation of the cause of bondage'. The bondage here obviously means attachment to life in general and the physical body in particular. The fundamental cause of both is the five *Kleśas* which produce the vehicle of *Karmas* as explained in II-12. This bondage is loosened though not completely destroyed when the *Yogi* has attenuated the *Kleśas* and sufficiently exhausted his *Karmas* through the practice of *Yoga*.

The second condition is that the *Yogi* should have detailed knowledge of the passages or channels along which the centre of mind travels when it enters or leaves the body. Different *Nāḍīs* in the body serve specific purposes and one of these *Nāḍīs* called the *Citta-Vāhā-Nāḍī* serves as a passage for the mental centre when it enters or leaves the body. By mental centre is meant the common centre of the superphysical vehicles through which *Citta* functions. Many people do not realize that the exercise of the *Yogic* powers is based upon detailed and precise knowledge of the physical and superphysical vehicles and rigorous training is necessary in the application of this knowledge for particular purposes. *Yoga* is a Science and its requirements are as exacting as those of physical Science.

४०. उदानजयाज्जलपङ्ककण्टकादिष्वसङ्ग उत्क्रान्तिश्च ।

Udāna-jayāj jala-paṅka-kaṇṭakādiṣv
asaṅga utkrāntiś ca.

उदान (over) one of the five *Prāṇas* or vital airs जयात् by mastery जल water पङ्क mire कण्टकादिषु thorns, etc. असङ्गः non-contact उत्क्रान्तिः levitation च and.

40. By mastery over *Udāna* levitation and non-contact with water, mire, thorns etc.

There are five kinds of *Prāṇa* working in the *Prāṇamaya Kośa*—*Prāṇa*, *Apāna*, *Samāna*, *Udāna* and *Vyāna*. Each of these has a specialized function to perform in the maintenance of the body and control acquired over any one kind means that the corresponding function can be regulated according to the will of the *Yogi*. *Udāna* is obviously connected with the gravitational pull of the earth on the body and by controlling this particular *Prāṇa* it is possible to neutralize this pull. Levitation is a very common phenomenon in *Praṇāyāma* practice and is due to the *Prāṇic* currents flowing in a particular way. If the *Yogi* can neutralize the gravitational pull of the earth and keep his body floating at any desired level he can easily avoid contact with water, mire and thorns etc.

४१. समानजयाज्ज्वलनम् ।

Samāna-jayāj jvalanam.

समान (over) one of the five kinds of *Prāṇas* जयात् by mastery ज्वलनम् blazing (of gastric fire).

41. By mastery over *Samāna* blazing of gastric fire.

The relation of *Samāna Vāyu* with the gastric fire and the digestion of food is well known. Control over *Samāna* will naturally enable the *Yogi* to increase the intensity of the gastric fire to any extent and to digest any amount of food.

That the digestion of food depends upon fire may sound fantastic to people with modern ideas of medical Science. But the word fire is not used here in its ordinary sense. *Agni* is one of the important *Tattvas* which manifests in innumerable ways and the ordinary fire with which we are familiar is only one of these. The function of the gastric fire which is another form of *Agni Tattva* is to stimulate the gastric secretions and thus make the digestion of food possible. *Yogic* Science does not, therefore, contradict the facts of medical Science. It merely takes a more comprehensive view of these natural processes and also includes within its scope the subtler forces and causes which are working behind them.

The interpretation of *Jvalanam* as effulgence does not appear to be correct. In the first place, no one has ever heard of *Yogis* in a luminous condition, and even if one were found in such a condition this could hardly be the result of the deliberate exercise of a *Siddhi*. The traditional halo of light which is seen round the head of very highly advanced spiritual beings is due to the luminosity of their superphysical auras and is not a physical phenomenon.

४२. श्रोत्राकाशयोः संबन्धसंयमाद्दिव्यं श्रोत्रम् ।

Srotrākāśayoḥ saṃbandha-saṃyamād divyaṃ śrotram.

श्रोत्र (of) ear आकाशयोः and space or ether संबन्ध (on) relation संयमाद् by performing *Saṃyama* दिव्यं 'divine'; superphysical श्रोत्रम् hearing.

42. By performing *Saṃyama* on the relation between *Ākāśa* and the ear superphysical hearing.

Sound on the superphysical planes is not essentially different from sound on the physical plane. It is merely a continuation of the same kind of vibrations but finer, the sound vibrations of different planes being related to one another much as the different octaves of music. Anyone who performs *Saṃyama* on the relation between *Ākāśa* and the sense of hearing will become aware of the whole gamut of sound vibrations and be able to hear sounds of the superphysical planes also. *Divyaṃ Śrotram* is nothing but becoming sensitive to the subtler sound vibrations which are beyond the range of the physical ear. *Saṃyama* on any principle or force brings the consciousness of the *Yogi* in touch with the reality underlying that principle or force and thus makes him aware of all the spheres and ranges in which that principle or force operates.

४३. कायाकाशयोः संबन्धसंयमाल्लघुतूलसमापत्तेश्चाकाशगमनम् ।

Kāyākāśayoḥ saṃbandha-saṃyamāt
laghu-tūla-samāpatteś cākāśa-gamanam.

काय (of) the body आकाशयोः (and) space or ether संबन्ध (on) relation संयमात् by performing *Saṃyama* लघु (with) light (opposite of heavy) तूल cotton down समापत्तेः by coalescence of the mind; by (bringing about) rapport च and आकाश space; sky गमनम् going in; passage through.

43. By performing *Saṃyama* on the relation between the body and *Ākāśa* and at the same time bringing about coalescence of the mind with light (things like) cotton down (there comes the power of) passage through space.

Ākāśa-gamanam refers to the well-known *Siddhi* of transferring the body from one place to another via *Ākāśa*. This does not mean, as is generally imagined, flying through the sky bodily as a bird does. It involves resolving the particles of the body into space at one place and then reassembling them at the destination. The physical body is made up of innumerable particles of matter held together by forces of cohesion, these forces being resident in *Ākāśa* the universal medium. In fact, the existence of the body depends upon this relation between the particles of the body and *Ākāśa* from which they are ultimately formed.

If the *Yogi* performs *Saṃyama* on this relation of the physical body with *Ākāśa* he acquires knowledge of these forces of cohesion and the power to manipulate them as he likes. If after gaining this power he brings about coalescence of the mind with a fluffy substance like cotton down he causes the dispersion of the particles of the body and their resolution into *Ākāśa*. *Laghu-Tūla-Samāpatteḥ* is a very expressive phrase which means concentrating the mind on the process by which cotton down is produced from cotton wool, namely, dispersion. This shows that if the *Yogi* exerts his will-power keeping in mind a particular process he can bring about that process provided that he has the capacity to perform *Saṃyama*. To reassemble the particles at the destination all that is necessary is to withdraw the force of will. It was the force of will which kept the particles in a resolved state and as soon as this force is removed the forces of cohesion reassert themselves and the body materializes instantaneously, apparently from nowhere.

The technique of *Ākāśa-gamana* thus depends upon the knowledge of the forces which are responsible for the formation of physical objects from *Ākāśa* and the exertion of will-power in a particular manner. It involves the resolution of the body into *Ākāśa* and the reverse process of rematerialization from *Ākāśa*. But the knowledge is not the ordinary intellectual knowledge such as a scientist has. It is the direct knowledge obtainable only by *Saṃyama* which involves becoming one in consciousness with the object meditated upon. That is the significance of the word *Samāpatteḥ*.

Ākāśa-gamana must be distinguished from the appearance of a materialized body formed by *Kriyā Śakti* at any distant place. In the former case, it is the original physical body of the *Yogi* which is transported to another place by a combined process of dissolution and materialization. In the latter case, the original physical body remains where it was and a second artificial body is temporarily materialized in another place round a *Nirmāṇa Citta* (IV-4). The techniques of the two processes are different and one or the other is adopted according to the needs of the occasion.

४४. बहिरकल्पिता वृत्तिर्महाविदेहा ततः प्रकाशावरणक्षयः ।

Bahir akalpitā vṛttir mahā-videhā; tataḥ
prakāśāvaraṇa-kṣayaḥ.

बहिः outside; external अकल्पिता unimaginable वृत्तिः state (of mind) महाविदेहा (name of a) *Yogic Siddhi* enabling the *Yogi* to remain without a body (here, the mental body) ततः thence; from it प्रकाश (of) light आवरण covering क्षयः wasting away.

44. The power of contacting the state of consciousness which is outside the intellect and is therefore inconceivable is called *Mahā-videhā*. From it is destroyed the covering of light.

If we examine the content of our mind at any moment we shall find in it a combination of two sets of images; one, produced by actual contact with the external world through the sense-organs, the other, the product of our own imagination. These two sets of images are intertwined and constitute our world image at any moment. What is the nature of the image produced by contact with the external world through the sense-organs? What is its origin? If the manifested world around us is the expression of a Reality through Divine Ideation then it is natural to suppose that the world image in our mind is the result of the impact of the Universal Mind on our individual mind. We contact mentally the Universal Mind through our individual mind. The changes which take place in our mind continuously are thus the result of the continuous changes in the Universal Mind as it unfolds itself in the manifested Solar system independently of us. This individualization of the world image by our individual mind limits and distorts the Divine Ideation and only a faint and gloomy image is obtained. The light of the Universal Mind becomes covered, as it were, by our individual mind, and we live our life within the dark prison of our own mind unconscious of the fact that the dark and flitting shadows produced in our mind are the shadows of a tremendous Reality of which we can have no conception as long as our consciousness is confined within the walls of our prison-house. What will happen if we somehow get out of this prison-house? The light of the Universal Mind will burst into our consciousness and we get an all-embracing vision of all those principles and natural laws which we can deal with, only one by one, and in a groping fashion, through the instrumentality of our intellect. This power of getting out of our intellect is called *Mahā-Videhā*, probably because it releases the consciousness into the realm of the Universal Mind which works without a *Deha* or body. The word *Bahir* is used because the Universal Mind is outside the individual mind and the world image in the individual mind has an external source. This all-embracing and vivid image which replaces the dark and partial image of the world process is *Akalpitā* i.e. is outside the range of the intellect. It has an independent reality and is inconceivable. It is a *Vṛtti* because it is a passing state, but a *Vṛtti* of the Universal Mind and not of the extremely limited individual mind.

It will be seen, therefore, that the 'covering of light' in this *Sūtra* is different from the 'covering of light' referred to in II-52. There, the 'covering' referred to the brain which covers the light of the mental world. Here, it refers to the individual mental body which covers the light of the Universal Mind. This latter process takes place at a later stage and at a much higher level. The covering referred to in II-52 is destroyed by *Prāṇāyāma* and prepares the ground for *Dhāraṇā* (II-53). The covering referred to in the present *Sūtra* is destroyed by *Saṃyama*, and on the unfoldment of intuitional perception through knowledge of the *Puruṣa* (III-36). This *Siddhi* enables the *Yogi* not only to transcend the sense-organs (III-37) but also the individual mind for which the sense-organs were created. It is thus complementary to the *Siddhi* referred to in III-37.

४५. स्थूलस्वरूपसूक्ष्मान्वयार्थवत्त्वसंयमाद् भूतजयः ।

Sthūla-svarūpa-sūkṣmānvayārthavattva-
saṃyamād bhūta-jayaḥ.

स्थूल (on) gross (state) स्वरूप real or constant form सूक्ष्म subtle (state) अन्वय all-pervading (state) अर्थवत्त्व subservience to the purpose; function (state) संयमात् by performing *Saṃyama* भूतजयः mastery over the (*Pañca*) *Bhūtas*.

45. Mastery over the *Pañca-Bhūtas* by performing *Saṃyama* on their gross, constant, subtle, all-pervading and functional states.

This *Sūtra* and III-48 are two of the most important and abstruse *Sūtras* in this Section. It will help the student to understand their meaning if we first consider very briefly the fundamental ideas underlying this doctrine of *Pañca-Bhūtas*.

The *Pañca-Bhūtas* are also called *Pañca-Tattvas* and it will help us to understand the nature of the *Pañca-Bhūtas* if we have a clear idea with regard to the meaning of the word *Tattva*. The word *Tattva* as used in the Hindu philosophical systems is one of great and subtle significance. Literally, it means 'that-ness'. The essential quality of a thing which distinguishes it from all other things constitutes its 'that-ness' and so the word *Tattva* stands for the essential qualities which are embodied in different measures in different things. Instead of a quality, a *Tattva* may also mean a principle which is embodied in a number of things in different degrees which acquire on this account a sameness of nature in certain matters though differing in degree and mode of expression. *Tattva* may also refer to a function and 'that-ness' in this case may consist in a group of things having a common function. But this must be a particular function common to a number of things though differing in degree and manner of expression.

It will be seen therefore that *Tattva* is a word of very comprehensive meaning and cannot be translated by any single word in English. Its significance is based really upon the fundamental doctrine of Hindu philosophy according to which the manifested Universe is an emanation of an Ultimate Reality, which pervades and energizes it all the time, everywhere. When the manifested Universe comes into being there must be underlying it a vast number of principles, functions, laws etc. which serve as the foundation for the ever-changing phenomena which constitute the World Process. Without such laws, principles and functions the manifested Universe could not be a Cosmos but would be a chaos which we know it is not. These different fundamental modes of expressions which define the relations of different parts to one another, determine their mutual actions and reactions and ensure a harmonious, ordered and continuous World Process are the *Tattvas* of Hindu philosophy. Though these *Tattvas* are innumerable they are not unrelated to one another, because they are all derived by progressive differentiation from the One Principle which constitutes the very essence of Divine nature. Though they differ from each other and sometimes counteract each other they form an integrated whole in which each *Tattva* is harmonized and balanced by its opposite. When *Pralaya* takes place and the manifested Universe disappears these *Tattvas* are resolved into their Ultimate source to remain there in their balanced and latent state until another Universe is born and the World Process begins again.

The *Pañca-Bhūtas* are five of these innumerable *Tattvas* which have a special function in the manifested Universe, that of relating matter with consciousness. The translation of the word *Bhūtas* as elements, in the sense in which the word element was used formerly (earth, water, air, etc.), has been a great mistake, reducing the whole conception behind this word to an absurd and incomprehensible dogma. The identification of the *Pañca-Bhūtas* with states of matter (solid, liquid, gaseous, etc.) again does not give a correct idea about them though it is certainly an improvement on the previous interpretation. It is not possible to deal at length with the philosophy of the *Pañca-Bhūtas* here but the essential idea behind this doctrine of Hindu philosophy may be put in a nutshell as follows.

The external world is cognized through our five *Jñānendriyas* or sense-organs. We can know the things which exist outside us only as they affect our sense-organs. Now, the things around us have innumerable qualities which are shared by them in different degrees and manners. How can these qualities or attributes which form a jungle of sense impressions be classified scientifically and simply? The Seers who dived through the practice of *Yoga* into the inner and essential nature of all things and whose main objective was to unravel the innermost mystery of life adopted a perfectly scientific and yet very simple method of classifying these qualities. This consisted in dividing them into five groups according as they affected our five *Jñānendriyas*. All the multitudinous qualities through which all objects of the external world are cognized are classified under five heads and these five modes in which all things affect the mind through the five sense-organs are called *Pañca-Bhūtas* or *Pañca Tattvas*. Thus *Tejas* is that all-inclusive quality which in one way or another affects the retina of the eye, *Ākāśa* is that quality which affects the ear and so on.

What more scientific and yet simple classification of qualities could be devised in order to meet the requirements of those who have realized the illusory nature of sensuous perception and are bent on discovering the reality which is hidden behind the phenomenal world? Our theories of matter may change in any way but the essential manner of cognizing objects in the external world cannot change and therefore this method of classification is independent of all theories and discoveries which may come in the future development of scientific knowledge. Those who are in touch with the scientific advancement in this field know how the discoveries of one generation upset the theories of a previous generation and a classification based upon these passing theories and discoveries would always be subject to modification or complete change. But the simple method based on the conception of *Pañca-Bhūtas* will stand unshaken and unaffected amidst all the cataclysmic changes of scientific theories.

Nor can it be said that this classification suffers from the defect of over-simplification. For, it is not a mere rough and ready method of classifying the external world in a crude and arbitrary manner. It is related to the inner nature of things which can be discovered only by the practice of *Yoga* as the few *Sūtras* on this subject clearly indicate. Modern scientific knowledge, though extraordinarily diverse, detailed and precise, suffers from the great defect that it is divorced from knowledge of the inner nature of things with which it deals. It considers matter as a thing apart from mind and consciousness and so its jurisdiction must always remain confined to the surface of things, their superficial appearance and behaviour. *Yogic* philosophy, on the other hand, integrates into one comprehensive whole all aspects of manifestation—matter, mind and consciousness because it has discovered by its special methods that these are intimately related to one another. In fact, the whole theory and practice of *Yoga* is based upon this idea of the interdependence of these three realities of existence and the extraordinary powers which it is possible to acquire through *Yogic* practices shows that the fundamental basis of the *Yogic* doctrine is correct.

This is not the place to go into a detailed discussion with regard to the nature of the *Pañca-Bhūtas*, their relation with the *Indriyas* and the mind but the diagram given in explaining II-54 shows the various factors which are involved, according to *Yogic* psychology, in the process by which the external world is cognized by the mind. It will be seen that the *Pañca-Bhūtas* by their peculiar action affect the *Indriyas* which then transmute the purely physical vibrations into sensations. The sensations are the raw material from which the mind elaborates the world of ideas by a process of integration, reproduction and rearrangement of the component images. But the mind also, according to *Yogic* psychology, is *Jaḍa* (inert) and it is the illumination of the *Buddhi* which imparts to the mechanical work of the mind the element of intelligent understanding. But, as this question has been dealt with thoroughly elsewhere, let us now pass on to the problem with which the present *Sūtra* deals, namely, the mastery of the *Bhūtas*.

The key to the mastery of anything is a correct knowledge of its essential nature. All forces of Nature have been brought under the control of man by the discovery of laws which determine the action of these forces. The mastery of the *Bhūtas* should therefore depend upon the discovery of their essential nature and this is what the *Yogi* aims at in performing *Saṃyama* on the different stages through which they pass in assuming their final form.

If we are to understand what these different stages through which the *Bhūtas* pass in their involution are, we will again have to recall the basic doctrine of the *Yogic* philosophy according to which the whole of the manifested Universe is an emanation of the Self. It is the Self which has become the Not-Self through a progressive involution of a part of Itself. This progressive involution of consciousness accounts for the five stages or aspects of the *Pañca-Bhūtas* referred to in the present *Sūtra* and also shows how it is possible, by reversing the process, to trace them back to their source.

As it is rather difficult to comprehend the five aspects which the *Bhūtas* assume in the five stages of their involution let us consider a simple example to illustrate how a simple outer expression of a thing can have subtler aspects which are hidden from our view. Let us see what stages may be involved in the manifestation of a chemical element like oxygen from the Divine Mind. Since oxygen has to play a definite role in the physical world the first step in its formation should be a conception in the Divine Mind of its function or purpose. This particular function called *Arthavattva* will first require for its fulfilment a particular combination of the three *Guṇas* which lie at the very basis of all manifested objects. This is called the *Anvaya* state because the three *Guṇas* are all-pervading and form the common substratum of all manifested objects. The particular combination of the *Guṇas* from which the element oxygen is derived will require for its next stage in manifestation a particular form such as a modern electronic configuration. This obviously is the *Sūkṣma* or subtle state of the element. A particular combination of electrons and protons with a specific arrangement and motions of the constituent particles constitutes a definite element with a definite set of qualities which characterize the element. These in their totality constitute the *Svarūpa* or real form of the element. These essential qualities are expressed in different ways and varying degrees through different forms of oxygen such as the solid, liquid or gaseous oxygen or through compounds in which oxygen enters in combination with different elements. This is the *Sthūla* or gross state of the element.

We see thus how, on the basis of our ordinary knowledge, we can conceive of certain hidden aspects or states of such a common substance like oxygen. A similar though not so easily comprehensible series of five states or aspects is present in the case of the five *Bhūtas* through which we cognize the external world. It is true that the *Bhūtas* are not elements but principles but since these principles find expression through the medium of matter and energies of various kinds their different states or aspects may be considered to be somewhat analogous to those of the elements.

It should not be imagined, however, that a mere intellectual comprehension of these five states of the *Pañca-Bhūtas*, however clear and precise it may be, will enable anybody to acquire mastery over them. An intellectual comprehension obtained through intellectual processes, as pointed out before, is utterly different from the direct knowledge gained in *Samādhi* by performing *Saṃyama*. The latter kind of knowledge is obtained by becoming one in consciousness with the thing or principle and, therefore, carries with it powers which are inherent in that thing or principle. In *Samādhi* we come into touch with the reality of the object meditated upon, while in intellectual comprehension we merely contact the blurred and distorted image produced by the object in our mind. The difference between the two is the difference between a substance and its shadow.

४६. ततोऽणिमादिप्रादुर्भावः कायसंपत् तद्धर्मानभिघातश्च ।

Tato 'ṇimādi-prādurbhāvaḥ kāya-sampat taddharmānabhighātaś ca.

ततः thence; from it अणिमादि (of) *Aṇiman*, etc., the group of eight *Siddhis* of which *Aṇiman* is one प्रादुर्भावः appearance कायः (of) the physical body संपत् perfection; wealth तत् of them (of the *Pañca-Bhūtas*); धर्म attributes; functions अनभिघातः non-obstruction; not-overcoming (of the *Yogi's* body) च and.

46. Thence, the attainment of *Aṇimān* etc., perfection of the body and the non-obstruction of its functions (of the body) by the powers (of the elements).

This *Sūtra* gives the three results of the mastery of the *Pañca-Bhūtas*. The first is the appearance of the well-known group of eight high occult powers known as *Mahā-Siddhis*. These are *Aṇiman*, *Mahiman*, *Laghiman*, *Gariman*, *Prāpti*, *Prākāmya*, *Īśatva* and *Vaśitva*. The second result of *Bhūta-Jaya* is the perfection of the physical body which is described in the next *Sūtra*. The third result is the immunity from the natural action of the *Pañca-Bhūtas*. Thus the *Yogi* can pass through fire without being burnt. His physical body can enter the solid earth just as an ordinary person can enter water.

These powers attained by mastery over the *Bhūtas* appear most extraordinary and almost unbelievable. But they are known to be real as the *Yogic* tradition of thousands of years and the experiences of those who are in touch with high class *Yogis* show. The previous discussion on the nature of the *Pañca-Bhūtas* and the way they are mastered will give some indication as to how such extraordinary results can follow from such a mastery. The whole of the phenomenal world is a play of the *Pañca-Bhūtas* and anyone who has acquired complete control over them naturally becomes master of all natural phenomena. The student will recall that the *Anvaya* state of the *Pañca-Bhūtas* is related to the three *Guṇas* which lie at the very basis of the manifested Universe. Mastery of the *Pañca-Bhūtas* thus means becoming one with the Divine Consciousness upon which manifestation is based and therefore gaining the capacity to exercise Divine powers which are inherent in that Consciousness. This does not mean that such a *Yogi* can do whatever he likes. He has still to work within the framework of natural laws, but his knowledge is so vast and his powers, therefore, so extraordinary that he appears capable of doing anything.

More important than the extraordinary nature of these powers is the question of the nature of this manifested Universe which the existence of such powers raises. What is the essential nature of the Universe in which such powers can be exercised? The mystery of life, matter and consciousness appears to deepen and acquire a new significance and we seem almost forced to the conclusion that all phenomena, even those which seem to have a solid material basis, are a play of consciousness. The *Vedāntic* doctrine 'Verily, all is *Brahman*' seems to be the only plausible explanation.

४७. रूपलावण्यबलवज्रसंहननत्वानि कायसंपत् ।

Rūpa-lāvaṇya-bala-vajra-saṃhananatvāni
kāya-saṃpat.

रूप beauty लावण्य fine complexion; gracefulness बल strength -वज्रसंहननत्वानि adamantine-hardness; extra-ordinary cohesion काय (of) the physical body संपत् perfection.

47. Beauty, fine complexion, strength and adamantine hardness constitute the perfection of the body.

This *Sūtra* defines the perfection of the body referred to in the previous *Sūtra*. The mastery of the *Bhūtas* will naturally lead to the body acquiring all these qualities because they depend upon the action of the *Bhūtas*. Anyone who is a master of the *Bhūtas* can regulate the processes taking place in the body. Besides, when the distortions caused by accumulated *Karma* are removed the body tends to conform naturally to the archetype of the human form which is exquisitely beautiful and has the above-mentioned attributes.

Let us not forget that the ugliness and imperfections in the physical body which we see around us are the result of the disharmonies and obstructions and *Karmas* which are inherent in the earlier stages of evolution. When these are removed on attaining perfection, the imprisoned splendour breaks forth even through the physical body which is the grossest of our vehicles.

४८. ग्रहणस्वरूपास्मितान्वयार्थवत्त्वसंयमादिन्द्रियजयः ।

Grahaṇa-svarūpāsmitānvayārthavattva-
saṃyamād indriya-jayaḥ.

ग्रहण (on) power of cognition; apprehension स्वरूप real nature; अस्मिता egoism अन्वय all-pervasiveness अर्थवत्त्व subservience to the purpose; function संयमात् by performing *Saṃyama* इन्द्रियजयः mastery over the sense-organs.

48. Mastery over the sense-organs by performing *Saṃyama* on their power of cognition, real nature, egoism, all-pervasiveness and functions.

This *Sūtra* is complementary to III-45 and what has been said with regard to *Bhūtas* in connection with the former also applies, to some extent, to *Indriyas* in the latter. The successive five stages on which *Saṃyama*, in relation to the sense-organs, has to be performed in order to gain complete mastery over them correspond to the five stages in the case of the *Bhūtas*. But the student will notice that the stages called *Sthūla* and *Sūkṣma* in the case of *Bhūtas* are replaced by *Grahaṇa* and *Asmitā* respectively in the case of the *Indriyas*.

The first stage in the case of the *Indriyas* is the power of cognition. The exercise of every sense-organ begins with the response of the organ to an external stimulus which is provided by the *Pañca-Bhūtas*. The mechanism through which such response takes place and the result of the response are, of course, different in the case of the five sense-organs as shown in dealing with III-45. So *Saṃyama* for the mastery of the *Indriyas* begins with the specific power of cognition which resides in the particular sense-organ. Then comes the real nature of the sense which, of course, is the particular type of sensation which results and which is called *Tanmātra*. Now, mere sensation by itself does not complete the process of sensing. The sensations must be individualized, as it were, before they can be used by the mind for constructing its mental images. Without the joining of this ' I '-ness with the sensation it remains merely a sensuous phenomenon and does not become an act of sensing. The mind cannot under these circumstances integrate the five sensations obtained through the separate channels into composite mental images. And what is at the basis of this individualized sensation? Is it not a mode of motion, a peculiar combination of the *Guṇas*? That is the all-pervading aspect of the *Indriyas* which corresponds with the all-pervading aspect of the *Bhūtas*. At this level both the *Bhūtas* and *Indriyas* are merely particular combinations of the three *Guṇas*. But behind every particular combination of the *Guṇas* there is a function which that combination is meant to fulfil. This is the last, *Arthavattva* stage corresponding with the *Arthavattva* stage of the *Bhūtas*.

It will be seen, therefore, that both the *Bhūtas* and *Indriyas* are initially merely functions in the Divine Mind. The exercise of these functions is made possible by the selection of particular combinations of *Guṇas* both for the *Bhūtas* and the *Indriyas*. One set of combination becomes the stimulator in the form of the

Bhūtas and another set of combination becomes the mechanism of stimulation in the form of the *Indriyas* and the sensations which are the raw materials for the mind are the result of the interaction of the two. The one consciousness which is whole and integral thus divides into two streams in order to provide this subjective-objective play of manifestation—this *Līlā* of *Bhagavān*.

४९. ततो मनोजवित्वं विकरणभावः प्रधानजयश्च ।

Tato manojavitvaṃ vikaraṇa-bhāvaḥ
pradhāna-jayaś ca.

ततः thence; from it मनोजवित्वं fleetness or speed like that of the mind; विकरणभावः condition of being independent of instruments; un-instrumental state प्रधानजयः conquest of *Pradhāna*, i.e. *Prakṛti* च and.

49. Thence, instantaneous cognition without the use of any vehicle and complete mastery over *Pradhāna*.

Just as the mastery of the *Bhūtas* brings about three results, in the same way, the mastery of the *Indriyas* enables the *Yogi* to acquire two *Siddhis* of the most comprehensive character. The first of these is the capacity to perceive anything in the realm of *Prakṛti* without the help of any organized vehicle of consciousness. Perception, in the usual course, always takes place through the instrumentality of the sense-organs whether these belong to the physical body or to the superphysical vehicles of consciousness. When the *Yogi* has obtained mastery over the sense-organs through *Saṃyama* he can dispense with the aid of instruments in perceiving anything in the manifested Universe. The non-instrumental perception is direct and instantaneous. This means that the *Yogi* has to direct his consciousness to any place or thing and he becomes instantaneously aware of everything which he wants to know.

The student will notice how the enormous limitations which characterize ordinary perception through the sense-organs of the physical body fall away progressively as the *Yogi* makes progress on the path of Self-realization. The consciousness of the ordinary man is confined rigidly within the physical body and the range of his perceptive power is limited by the capacity of its sense-organs, though this capacity can be enlarged greatly through the use of the physical instruments like the microscope, telescope, etc. When the *Yogi* develops the senses of the superphysical vehicles through the practice of *Yoga* the range of his perceptive powers is increased enormously as indicated in III-26. A further increase in the range and depth of his perceptive powers takes place when the capacity for *Prātibha* perception is born as indicated in III-37. In this type of perception it is not the sense-organs of the subtler vehicles but the spiritual faculty of intuition which is used. This faculty works within the realm of *Prakṛti* though without the aid of sense-organs of any kind. In the stage to which the present *Sūtra* refers even this spiritual faculty is transcended and the *Puruṣa* perceives by his own, over-all and all-inclusive power of perception. He has conquered the illusion which *Prakṛti* imposes on his consciousness and the whole of her vast realm lies before him like an open book.

The second result or rather aspect of *Indriya-Jaya* is the mastery of *Pradhāna*. In transcending the limitations of instrumental perception the *Puruṣa* has really transcended *Prakṛti* and is, therefore, now master of *Prakṛti*. The secret of mastering anything completely lies in transcending it. *Karma* is mastered when we pass beyond its operation. The physical body is mastered completely when we can pass out of it at will and use it as a mere vehicle of consciousness.

From the results which follow the mastery of *Bhūtas* and *Indriyas* it should be clear that these words do not refer only to the *Bhūtas* and *Indriyas* as they function on the physical plane but as they function on all the planes. For there is cognition through the sense-organs also on the superphysical planes, though the mechanism of cognition differs from plane to plane. The *Bhūtas* and *Indriyas* are, therefore, to be taken as principles which are applicable to the phenomena of cognition on all the planes. As consciousness penetrates from one plane into another the essential process of cognition remains the same, only the mechanism changes from plane to plane. The *Bhūtas* change, the *Indriyas* change and the *Draṣṭā* changes (the *Draṣṭā* on each plane being the *Puruṣa* encased in all the vehicles not yet transcended) but the mutual relationship of the three remains the same. That is why the words used in *Yogic* philosophy for the trio are of a most general nature: *Grāhya*, *Grahaṇa* and *Grahītṛ*. It will be seen, therefore, that the cognition of the Not-Self by the Self on the physical plane is the lowest manifestation of this process of cognition involving the subject-object relationship and the process becomes more and more subtle until the *Bhūtas* and *Indriyas* are completely mastered and the *Puruṣa* becomes independent of *Prakṛti*.

Another important point which should be borne in mind is that the phrase *Vikaraṇa Bhāva* means not only cognition without the use of any instrument but also action without the use of any instrument. In attaining the power of cognition without any instrument the *Yogi* transcends the *Jñānendriyas*. In attaining the power of action without any instrument he transcends the *Karmendriyas*. The former power without the latter would reduce the *Puruṣa* to the status of an impotent spectator and this would be inconsistent with the whole trend of thought upon which the philosophy of *Yoga* is based. In the progress of the *Yogi* knowledge and power go together and the attainment of knowledge with regard to any force or principle confers upon him the corresponding power to use or manipulate that force or principle according to his will. Most of the third Section of the *Yoga-Sūtras* is devoted to the development of powers of various kinds and it is absurd to suppose that the *Yogi* who has been developing knowledge and power, side by side, is denuded of power at the last stage, all of a sudden, and becomes a mere spectator in the drama which is being played around him. Apart from the irrationality of this idea it is at complete variance with the role which Adepts in *Yoga* play in the manifested Universe and with other facts known to practical Occultism. In thus attributing to the *Puruṣa* the dual role of *Draṣṭā* and *Kartā* (Spectator and Actor) the *Yogic* philosophy differs fundamentally from the orthodox *Sāṃkhya* doctrine.

५०. सत्त्वपुरुषान्यताख्यातिमात्रस्य सर्वभावाधिष्ठातृत्वं सर्वज्ञातृत्वं च ।

Sattva-puruṣānyatā-khyāti-mātrasya sarva-bhāvādhiṣṭhātṛtvaṃ sarvajñātṛtvaṃ ca.

सत्त्व one of three *Gunas* which is at the basis of the principle of perception; refined *Buddhi* पुरुष the individual Self अन्यता distinction; difference ख्याति awareness मात्रस्य only सर्व (over) all भाव states or forms of existence अधिष्ठातृत्वं supremacy सर्व-ज्ञातृत्वं omniscience च and.

50. Only from the awareness of the distinction between *Sattva* and *Puruṣa* arise supremacy over all states and forms of existence (omnipotence) and knowledge of everything (omniscience).

Vikaraṇa Bhāva which is gained by *Indriya-Jaya* (III-49) gives the power to exercise perception and to manipulate all the forces working within the realm of *Prakṛti* without the aid of any instrument. But it does not confer on the *Yogi* Omniscience and Omnipotence. This can be attained only on becoming fully aware, through *Saṃyama*, of the distinction between *Sattva* and *Puruṣa*. *Vikaraṇa Bhāva* is, however, a prerequisite for the development of Omnipotence and Omniscience because these are unlimited and cannot function through an instrument which is by its very nature limited. It is only on the foundations of *Vikaraṇa Bhāva* that the infinite superstructure of Omniscience and Omnipotence can rest.

It should also be noted that the mastery of *Pradhāna* referred to in III-49 can be attained merely by the separation of the *Dṛśyam* (II-18) from the *Draṣṭā* (II-20). But in this seeing the *Dṛśyam* apart from Himself the *Draṣṭā* is still seeing and is thus identified with *Sattva Guṇa* which is the very basis of perception. As long as this identification remains he is limited because the *Sattva Guṇa* is also within the realm of *Prakṛti*. He cannot, therefore, exercise Omnipotence and Omniscience. It is only when he is able to realize himself as separate from the power of seeing or *Sattva* that he goes completely out of the realm of *Prakrti* and can exercise Omnipotence and Omniscience. The *Grahītr* must realize himself separate not only from *Grāhya* but also from *Grahaṇa* to become quite free from limitation.

This *Sūtra* also confirms the view expressed in dealing with the previous *Sūtra* that the *Puruṣa* has the dual role of Spectator and Actor. He not only gains more and more knowledge but also exercises the powers which that knowledge confers. He not only becomes Omniscient but also Omnipotent. The fact that the two functions are referred to separately in this *Sūtra* seems to leave no doubt on this point. Why then does there appear to be a constant emphasis on the cognitive aspect in the *Yoga-Sūtras* and the volitional aspect is rarely mentioned? Obviously, because power is a correlate of knowledge and is for all practical purposes included in the knowledge of the type which the *Yogi* acquires.

The student would do well to compare this *Sūtra* with III-36. The method prescribed in the former leads to Omniscience and Omnipotence while that in III-36 leads only to the development of *Pratibha* hearing, seeing, etc. (III-37). The difference in the results which follow is due to the fact that knowledge of the *Puruṣa* referred to in III-36 is partial while that referred to in III-50 is complete. In the total eclipse of the Sun, only a part of the Sun comes out of the shadow in the beginning but this portion becomes larger and larger until the Sun is quite out of the shadow cast by the moon. These two stages will serve to throw some light on the partial and complete separation of the *Puruṣa* from *Prakṛti* referred to in the two *Sūtras*.

५१. तद्वैराग्यादपि दोषबीजक्षये कैवल्यम् ।

Tad-vairāgyād api doṣa-bīja-kṣaye kaivalyam.

तद्-वैराग्यात् from non-attachment to that (*Siddhi* referred to in previous *Sūtra*) अपि even दोष (of) bondage; defect बीज seed क्षये on the destruction कैवल्यम् Liberation.

51. By non-attachment even to that, on the very seed of bondage being destroyed, follows *Kaivalya*.

When Omniscience and Omnipotence have developed as a result of awareness of the subtle distinction between the *Puruṣa* and *Sattva* the *Yogi* has gone out of the sphere of *Prakṛti*, but if there is attachment to these transcendent powers which can be exercised only in the realm of *Prakṛti* he is still dependent upon *Prakṛti* in a way and therefore subservient to her. Mastery over a thing does not necessarily mean independence from that thing and as long as there is dependence there is bondage. A man who loves a woman can have her completely in his power and yet be a slave to her. In this case it is the attachment to her which is the cause of his bondage and unless this attachment is destroyed he is not free and, therefore, his power over her is limited. In the same way, Omnipotence and Omniscience mean mastery over *Prakṛti* but unless the *Yogi's* attachment to these is destroyed he is dependent upon her and therefore not quite free. And since *Kaivalya* is a state of complete freedom it can be attained only after this kind of attachment has been destroyed by *Vairāgya*. The *Yogi* must not have the slightest attachment or attraction for these powers even though he may have to exercise them.

It is obvious, therefore, that the journey towards *Kaivalya* is a process of attaining higher and higher states of knowledge and power and then discarding them in turn for the ultimate goal. Attachment to any state, however high it may be, means not only stoppage of further progress but also the possibility of falling headlong from the dizzy height which has been reached. The traveller must press forward relentlessly until the final goal is reached and he is free from this danger.

५२. स्थान्युपनिमन्त्रणे सङ्गस्मयाकरणं पुनरनिष्टप्रसङ्गात् ।

Sthāny-upanimantraṇe saṅga-smayā-
karaṇaṃ punar aniṣṭa-prasaṅgāt.

स्थानि[न्] (by) the local authority; the superphysical entity in charge of the world or plane; powers of spaces उपनिमन्त्रणे on being invited सङ्ग attachment; pleasure स्मय wonder; pride; smile of complacence अकरण avoidance; no action of पुन: again अनिष्ट (of) the undesirable; the evil प्रसंगात् because of the recurrence or revival.

52. (There should be) avoidance of pleasure or pride on being invited by the super-physical entities in charge of various planes because there is the possibility of the revival of evil.

It was pointed out in the previous *Sūtra* that attachment to Omniscience and Omnipotence contains the seeds of bondage which must be destroyed by *Vairāgya* before *Kaivalya* can be attained. This *Sūtra* points out that attachment to these is not only a source of bondage but also a source of danger. The *Yogi* occupying such an exalted position is always tested by the Powers in charge of the various departments or planes of Nature and if he yields to their seductions owing to lack of complete non-attachment he is sure to bring about his downfall. Being subjected to such temptations is the lot of all highly advanced *Yogis* and references of this nature are found in the life of all great spiritual teachers such as the Christ or the Buddha. The actual mode of tempting may not be as depicted in the colourful stories of their lives but that they had to pass through trials of this nature appears to be certain.

It should not, however, be imagined that such temptations come only to those who are very highly advanced spiritually. The moment a *Yogi* attains to any measure of real power he becomes an object of attack and has to be on his guard all the time. The nature of the temptations will naturally depend upon his particular weaknesses and the stage of his development. While the beginner trying to break into the next super-physical plane may be tempted merely by elementals, those who have attained to high states of knowledge and power become the object of attack by great *Devas* in charge of the various departments of Nature. The higher the stage the subtler is the temptation and the greater is the degree of *Vairāgya* needed to counteract the temptation.

Nor must it be supposed that this constant tempting by these Powers is the result of malice on their part. Their work should be taken as a beneficent force working in Nature which tests us at every step so that we may be able to remove our weaknesses and may be able to advance steadily towards our goal. The student should try to imagine what would happen if there were no such agencies at work. Those who are treading the path of Self-realization would remain unconscious of their weaknesses, tied down to the lower stages and unable to advance further. The sword of temptation which searches out and strikes our weaknesses certainly causes us temporary suffering and anguish but it also gives us an opportunity for removing those weaknesses and thus frees us for advancing further on the Path.

५३. क्षणतत्क्रमयोः संयमाद्विवेकजं ज्ञानम् ।

Kṣaṇa-tat-kramayoḥ saṃyamād vivekajaṃ jñānam.

क्षण (on) moment तत्-क्रमयोः (and) its order, succession संयमात् by performing *Saṃyama* विवेकजं born of awareness of Reality ज्ञानम् knowledge.

53. Knowledge born of awareness of Reality by performing *Saṃyama* on moment and (the process of) its succession.

This *Sūtra* should be studied along with IV-33 in discussing which the *Yogic* theory of *Kṣaṇa* and nature of time has been explained. *Kṣaṇa-Tat-Kramayoḥ* is the process by which the eternal Reality which transcends time is projected in manifestation in terms of time. This obviously is the last veil of illusion which must be pierced before the *Yogi* can attain *Kaivalya*. The technique of piercing this final veil is the same as in the case of others—*Saṃyama*. The knowledge which is gained as a result of performing *Saṃyama* on the process of time is the highest kind of knowledge which can be attained—even higher than Omniscience referred to in III-50. It is called *Vivekajaṃ-Jñānam* 'knowledge born of the awareness of Reality'. The word *Viveka* is generally translated into English by the word 'discrimination' but the use of this word in the present context is not appropriate. The word 'discrimination' is used ordinarily for that process of spiritual discernment which enables us to detect the illusions of life and to discover the relative reality hidden behind them. But the word *Viveka* in the present context stands for the full awareness of the Ultimate Reality. Essentially the process is the same in both the cases and involves passing from a less real to a more real state of consciousness but the difference in degree is so tremendous that the use of the rather vague word 'discrimination' for this final 'discovery' may not give an adequate conception of the change which is involved. It is, therefore, better to translate the phrase *Vivekajaṃ-Jñānam* by 'awareness of the Ultimate Reality' because the use of the word knowledge in connection with this exalted state of consciousness does not seem to be proper. A state of consciousness which transcends Omniscience itself cannot be called knowledge. It is better to use for it the phrase given above.

५४. जातिलक्षणदेशैरन्यतानवच्छेदात् तुल्ययोस्ततः प्रतिपत्तिः ।

Jāti-lakṣaṇa-deśair anyatānavacchedāt
tulyayos tataḥ pratipattiḥ.

जाति (by) class लक्षण characteristic देशैः place; position अन्यता (of) separateness; difference अनवच्छेदात् because of the absence of definition तुल्ययोः of the two equals ततः from it प्रतिपत्तिः understanding; knowledge (of distinction).

54. From it (*Vivekajaṃ-Jñānam*) knowledge of distinction between similars which cannot be distinguished by class, characteristic or position.

The fact that *Vivekajaṃ-Jñānam* transcends Time leads to the attainment of a peculiar, and from the intellectual point of view, an interesting power. The significant word in this *Sūtra* is *Pratipattiḥ*. What does it mean? *Samāpattiḥ* is the fusion of two things apparently separate. *Pratipattiḥ* is the resolution of two things originally fused or inseparable. Now, what is the *Yogi* to do if he has to distinguish between two things which are indistinguishable by the ordinary methods, namely, by differences of class, characteristic or position?

To have some idea of the method which can be adopted in solving such a problem it is necessary to remember that if two things are exactly similar and occupy the same position it means that they appear and disappear alternately in that position. And under these circumstances the time factor alone can distinguish between them. You will have to subject them to a time analysis of greater resolving power than the frequency with which they replace each other in the same position. But the frequency with which two things can replace each other in this manner has a limiting value and that is the frequency with which *Kṣaṇas* or moments succeed each other. Therefore, anyone who can go beyond the process of time referred to in the last *Sūtra* should be in a position to distinguish between two such things.

The other powers of the *Yogi* will enable him to distinguish between two things apparently similar. This *Sūtra* is concerned not with such ordinary similarities but with similarities of a very subtle nature which baffle even Omniscience. For this *Siddhi*, as the context shows, comes last of all when even time is transcended and the *Yogi* is established in the Eternal Reality which transcends all limitations and illusions.

५५. तारकं सर्वविषयं सर्वथाविषयमक्रमं चेति विवेकजं ज्ञानम् ।

Tārakaṃ sarva-viṣayaṃ sarvathā-viṣayam
akramaṃ ceti vivekajaṃ-jñānam.

तारकं transcendent; that which helps to 'cross over' (the ocean of existence) सर्वविषयं cognizing all objects at once or simultaneously सर्वथाविषयम् pertaining to all objects whatsoever in the past, present and future; pertaining to all objects and processes and in all time and all space अक्रमं successionless; orderless; transcending the World Process च and इति finish; end of anything (here subject) विवेकजं ज्ञानम् knowledge born of the awareness of Reality.

55. The highest knowledge born of the awareness of Reality is transcendent, includes the cognition of all objects simultaneously, pertains to all objects and processes whatsoever in the past, present and future and also transcends the World Process.

III-53 dealt with the method of obtaining the highest knowledge which is the ultimate objective of *Yoga*. This *Sūtra* defines the nature of this knowledge. In the first place, it is transcendent, i.e., it transcends all forms of knowledge within the sphere of phenomenal existence. It is the knowledge or rather full awareness of Reality while all other forms of knowledge, even those pertaining to the highest levels of consciousness are in the realm of Relativity. The word *Tārakaṃ* also means that which enables the *Yogi* to cross over *Bhava Sāgara* or the ocean of conditioned existence. The soul which is involved in the limitations and illusions of conditioned existence is liberated completely from these on the attainment of *Tāraka-Jñāna*.

In the second place, this knowledge is *Sarva-Viṣayaṃ*. This means not only embracing all objects but having all objects in consciousness simultaneously. *Sarvathā-Viṣayaṃ* means knowledge pertaining to the past, present and future. Just as *Sarva-Viṣayaṃ* has reference to space so *Sarvathā-Viṣayaṃ* has reference to time. So *Vivekajaṃ-Jñānam* includes everything within the realm of time and space, i.e., all things which are within the World Process.

In the third place, *Vivekajaṃ-Jñānam* is *Akramaṃ*, i.e., transcends the World Process which produces time. In the world of the Relative which is subject to the World Process, things take place one after another and it is this which produces the impression of past, present and future. In the world of Reality which is beyond the World Process time cannot exist and this timeless condition is called the Eternal. This is not a mere interesting hypothesis. Time according to the highest occultists and mystics has no real existence. It is merely an impression produced in consciousness by the succession of phenomena which are produced by the World Process. When, therefore, the *Yogi* transcends the World Process he also conquers the illusion of time. This is the most fundamental illusion in which his consciousness is involved and is therefore, naturally, the last to disappear as pointed out in IV-33.

The fact that *Vivekajaṃ-Jñānam* is *Sarva-Viṣayaṃ*, *Sarvathā-Viṣayam* and *Akramaṃ* at the same time, means that the world of the Real is not something apart from the world of the Relative. Passing into the world of the Real does not therefore mean leaving the world of the Relative behind. It means seeing the world of the Relative in its true nature and correct perspective and living in that world in the light of the Real. Established in his true Self the Self-realized *Yogi* can live and work in the world of the Relative, using all the powers which *Prakṛti* has placed at his disposal but without being in the least affected by the illusions which she creates for those who have not yet mastered her.

The student will see that III-55 gives with marvellous lucidity and in a few words the essential characteristics of the Eternal Reality which is the goal of *Yogic* training and discipline. Of course, he will not be able to have from this intellectual statement the slightest idea with regard to the actual nature of the experience of this Reality but he will be able to see that it is something tremendous and worth striving after. The word *Iti* merely indicates the close of the subject (*Siddhis*) which was being dealt with.

५६. सत्त्वपुरुषयोः शुद्धिसाम्ये कैवल्यम् ।

Sattva-puruṣayoḥ śuddhi-sāmye kaivalyam.

सत्त्वपुरुषयोः of *Sattva* and *Puruṣa* शुद्धि (of) purity साम्ये on equality कैवल्यम् Liberation.

56. *Kaivalya* is attained when there is equality of purity between the *Puruṣa* and *Sattva*.

This *Sūtra* completes the idea already dealt with partly in III-36 and III-50. In III-36 it was pointed out that *Sattva* and

Puruṣa though ordinarily indistinguishable are quite distinct and it is possible to know the *Puruṣa* apart from *Sattva*. In III-50 it was made clear that it is only on knowing the *Puruṣa* completely apart from *Sattva* that the limitations which *Prakṛti* places on the knowledge and power of the *Puruṣa* can be destroyed. But this realization of the utterly distinct nature of the *Puruṣa* and *Sattva* cannot take place suddenly. It proceeds by states and with each clearer realization of the distinct nature of the *Puruṣa* and *Sattva* the *Yogi* approaches nearer to his goal of complete freedom from limitations and illusions.

It should be noted that the purification of *Sattva* means in effect this progressive realization on the part of the *Yogi* and not some substantial change in his nature, and the increasing awareness of Reality which accompanies this realization is also not connected with any substantial change. It is a matter of realization only. That is why it is called *Vivekajaṃ-Jñānam*. The purification of *Sattva* and *Puruṣa* becomes equal when the *Yogi* has realized fully the distinction between the *Puruṣa* and *Sattva*. The *Sattva* or perception of the *Yogi* is free from the illusion of apparent identity of the *Puruṣa* and *Sattva* and the Self-realization of the *Puruṣa* is free from any self-identification with the *Sattva*.

When the conditions mentioned above are present the presence of *Sattva* does not interfere with the Self-realization of the *Yogi*. He may remain within the realm of *Prakṛti* and yet be in full realization of his Eternal nature. From this *Sūtra* it is clear that *Kaivalya* does not necessarily mean the separation of *Puruṣa* and *Prakṛti*. If the *Sattva* has been purified to the necessary extent the *Puruṣa* can function through *Prakṛti* in full realization of his Real nature, and always free. Thus, it is the realization of his *Svarūpa* in the fullest degree which is the characteristic and indispensable condition of *Kaivalya* and not the separation from *Prakṛti*. The 'isolation' of *Kaivalya* is thus subjective and not necessarily objective. The vehicles that have been built up and perfected by him in the realm of *Prakṛti* can then be used by him for any kind of work without egoism and without any illusions. Such are the perfected men of humanity, the Adepts of *Yoga* who are the masters of this Sacred Science and who guide humanity in its progress towards perfection.

SECTION IV

KAIVALYA PĀDA

KAIVALYA PĀDA

१. जन्मौषधिमन्त्रतपःसमाधिजाः सिद्धयः ।

Janmauṣadhi-mantra-tapaḥ-samādhi-jāḥ siddhayaḥ.

जन्म birth औषधि drugs मन्त्र incantation; a group of words whose constant repetition produces specific results तपः austerities; purificatory actions; penance समाधि trance; -जाः born of; are the result of सिद्धयः attainments; occult powers.

1. The *Siddhis* are the result of birth, drugs, *Mantras*, austerities or *Samādhi*.

Section IV of the *Yoga-Sūtras* provides the theoretical background for the technique of *Yoga* which has been dealt with in the previous three Sections. It deals with the various general problems which form an integral part of the *Yogic* philosophy and which must be clearly understood if the practice of *Yoga* is to be placed on a rational basis. The practice of *Yoga* is not a sort of floundering in the Unknown for attaining a vague spiritual ideal. *Yoga* is a Science based upon a perfect adaptation of well-defined means to an unknown but definite End. It takes into account all the factors which are involved in the attainment of its objective and provides a perfectly coherent philosophical background for the practices which are its more essential part. It is true that the doctrines which constitute this theoretical background will hardly appear rational or intelligible to people who are not familiar with this subject but that is true of any kind of knowledge which deals with problems of an unfamiliar nature. It is only those who have given considerable thought to this subject and are familiar at least with the elementary doctrines of the *Yogic* philosophy who can be expected to appreciate the grand and almost flawless line of reasoning which underlies the apparently disconnected topics dealt with in Section IV.

As this Section deals with many difficult topics which are apparently unconnected, it will perhaps help the student to grasp the underlying thread of reasoning running throughout the Section if a synopsis of the whole Section is given at the beginning. This will inevitably involve some repetition of ideas but such a bird's-eye view will be definitely helpful in understanding this rather abstruse aspect of *Yogic* philosophy.

SYNOPSIS

Sūtra 1: This enumerates the different methods of acquiring *Siddhis*. Of the five methods given only the last based upon *Samādhi* is used by advanced *Yogis* in their work because it is based upon direct knowledge of the higher laws of Nature and is, therefore, under complete control of the will. The student must have noticed that all the *Siddhis* described in the previous Section are the result of performing *Saṃyama*. They are the product of evolutionary growth and thus give mastery over the whole range of natural phenomena.

Sūtras 2-3: These two *Sūtras* hint at the two fundamental laws of Nature which govern the flux of phenomena constituting the world of the Relative. An understanding of these two laws is necessary if we are to form a correct estimate of the functions and limitations of *Siddhis*. The student should not run away with the impression that it is possible for the *Yogi* to do anything he likes because he can bring about many results which appear miraculous to our limited vision. The *Yogi* is also bound by the laws of Nature and as long as his consciousness functions in the realms of Nature, it is subject to the laws which govern these realms. He has to work out his liberation from the realm of *Prakṛti* but he can do so only by obeying and utilizing the laws which operate in her realm.

Sūtras 4-6: The *Yogi* brings from his past lives, like everyone else, an enormous number of tendencies and potentialities in the form of *Karmas* and *Vāsanās*. These exist in his subtler vehicles in a very definite form and have to be worked out or destroyed before *Kaivalya* can be attained. These *Sūtras* refer to these individual vehicles which are of two types—those which are the product of evolutionary growth during successive lives and those which the *Yogi* can create by the power of his will. Before one can understand the methods adopted for the destruction of *Karmas* and *Vāsanās* he should have some knowledge of the mental mechanisms through which these tendencies function.

Sūtras 7-11: These deal with the *modus operandi* by which the impressions of our thoughts, desires and actions are produced and then worked out during the course of successive lives in our evolutionary growth. The problem for the *Yogi* is to stop adding to these accumulated impressions by learning the technique of *Niṣkāma Karma* and desirelessness and to work out those potentialities which have already been acquired in the quickest and most efficient manner. The destruction of the subtler or dormant *Vāsanās* depends ultimately upon the destruction of *Avidyā* which is the cause of attachment to life.

Sūtras 12-22: After dealing with the vehicles of the mind (*Citta*) and the forces (*Vāsanās*) which bring about incessant transformations (*Vṛttis*) in these vehicles Patañjali discusses the theory of mental perception, using the word ' mental ' in its most comprehensive sense. According to him two entirely different kinds of elements are involved in mental perception. On the one hand, there must be the impact of the object upon the mind through their characteristic properties and, on the other, the eternal *Puruṣa* must illuminate the mind with the light of his consciousness. Unless both these conditions are simultaneously present there can be no mental perception because the mind itself is inert and incapable of perceiving. It is the *Puruṣa* who is the real perceiver though he always remains in the background and the illumination of the mind with the light of his consciousness makes it appear as if it is the mind which perceives. This fact can be realized only when the mind is entirely transcended and the consciousness of the *Puruṣa* is centred in his own *Svarūpa* in full awareness of Reality.

Sūtra 23: This throws a flood of light on the nature of *Citta* and shows definitely that the word *Citta* is used by Patañjali in the most comprehensive sense for the medium of perception at all levels of consciousness and not merely as a medium of intellectual perception as commonly supposed. Wherever there is perception in the Relative realm of *Prakṛti* there must be a medium through which that perception takes place and that medium is *Citta*. So that even when consciousness is functioning on the highest planes of manifestation, far beyond the realm of the intellect, there is a medium through which it works, however subtle this medium may be, and this medium is also called *Citta*.

Sūtras 24-25: These two *Sūtras* point out the nature of the limitations from which life suffers even on the highest planes of manifestation. The *Puruṣa* is not only the ultimate source of all perception as pointed out in IV-18 but he is also the motive power or reason of this play of *Vāsanās* which keep the mind in incessant activity. It is for him that all this long evolutionary process is taking place although he is always hidden in the background. It follows from this that even in the exalted conditions of consciousness which the *Yogi* might reach in the higher stages of *Yoga* he is dependent upon something distinct and separate, though within him. He cannot be truly Self-sufficient and Self-illuminated until he is fully Self-realized and has become one with the Reality within himself. It is the realization of this fact, of his falling short of his ultimate objective, which weans the *Yogi* from the exalted illumination and bliss of the highest plane and makes him dive still deeper within himself for the Reality which is the consciousness of the *Puruṣa*.

Sūtras 26-29: These *Sūtras* give some indication of the struggle in the last stages before full Self-realization is attained. This struggle culminates ultimately in *Dharma-Megha-Samādhi* which opens the door to the Reality within him.

Sūtras 30-34: These *Sūtras* merely indicate some of the consequences of attaining *Kaivalya* and give a hint about the nature of the exalted condition of consciousness and freedom from limitations in which a fully Self-realized *Puruṣa* lives. No one, of course, who has not attained *Kaivalya* can really understand what this condition is actually like.

After taking a bird's-eye view of the Section let us now deal with the different topics one by one. In the first *Sūtra* Patañjali gives an exhaustive list of methods whereby occult powers may be acquired. Some people are born with certain occult powers such as clairvoyance etc. The appearance of such occult powers is not quite accidental but is generally the result of having practised *Yoga*, in some form or another, in a previous life. All special faculties which we bring over in any life are the result of efforts which we have made in those particular directions in previous lives and *Siddhis* are no exception to this rule. But the fact that a person has practised *Yoga* and developed these powers in previous lives does not mean necessarily that he shall be born with those powers in this life. These powers have generally to be developed afresh in each successive incarnation unless the individual is very highly advanced in this line and brings over from previous lives very powerful *Saṃskāras*. It is also necessary to remember in this connection that some people whose moral and intellectual development is not very highly advanced are sometimes born with certain spurious occult powers. This is due to their dabbling in *Yogic* practices in their previous lives as explained in I-19.

Psychic powers of a low grade can often be developed by the use of certain drugs. Many *Fakirs* in India use certain herbs like *Gānjā* for developing clairvoyance of a low order. Others can bring about very remarkable chemical changes by the use of certain drugs or herbs, but those who know these secrets do not generally impart them to others. Needless to say that the powers obtained in this manner are not of much consequence and should be classed with the innumerable powers which modern Science has placed at our disposal.

The use of *Mantras* is an important and potent means of developing *Siddhis* and the *Siddhis* developed in this manner may be of the highest order. For, some of the *Mantras* like *Praṇava* or *Gāyatrī* bring about the unfoldment of consciousness and there is no limit to such unfoldment. When the higher levels of consciousness are reached as a result of such practices the powers which are inherent in those states of consciousness begin to appear naturally, though they may not be used by the devotee. Besides the natural development of *Siddhis* in this manner, there are specific *Mantras* for the attainment of particular kinds of objectives and when used with knowledge in the right manner bring about the desired results with the certainty of a scientific experiment. The *Tantras* are full of such *Mantras* for obtaining very ordinary and sometimes highly objectionable results. The reason why the ordinary man cannot get the desired results by simply following the directions in the books lies in the fact that the exact conditions are deliberately not given and can be obtained only from those who have been regularly initiated and have developed the powers. Of course, the true *Yogi* regards all such practices with contempt and never goes near them.

Tapas is another well-recognized means of obtaining *Siddhis.* The *Purāṇas* are full of stories of people who obtained all kinds of *Siddhis* by performing austerities of various kinds and thus propitiating different deities. Those stories may or may not be true but that *Tapas* leads to the development of certain kinds of occult powers is a fact well known to all students of *Yoga.* The important point to be noted in this connection is that the *Siddhis* acquired by this method, unless they are the result of the general unfoldment of consciousness by the practice of *Yoga,* are of a restricted nature and do not last for more than one life. And it frequently happens that the person who acquires such a *Siddhi,* being morally and spiritually undeveloped, misuses it, thus not only losing the power but bringing upon himself a lot of suffering and evil *Karma.*

The last and the most important means of developing *Siddhis* is the practice of *Saṃyama.* The major portion of Section III deals with some of the *Siddhis* that may be developed in this manner. The list of *Siddhis* referred to in that Section is not exhaustive but the more important ones are given. They should be taken merely as representative of an almost innumerable class to which references are found in *Yogic* literature.

One fact has, however, to be noted in this connection. The *Siddhis* which are developed as a result of the practice of *Saṃyama* belong to a different category and are far superior to those developed in other ways. They are the product of the natural unfoldment of consciousness in its evolution towards perfection and thus become permanent possessions of the soul, although a little effort may be needed in each new incarnation to revive them in the early stages of *Yogic* training. Being based upon knowledge of the higher laws of Nature operating in her subtler realms they can be exercised with complete confidence and effectiveness, much in the same way as a trained scientist can bring about extra-ordinary results in the field of physical Science.

२. जात्यन्तरपरिणामः प्रकृत्यापूरात् ।

Jāty-antara-pariṇāmaḥ prakṛty-āpūrāt.

जात्यन्तर into another class, species or kind परिणामः change; transformation प्रकृति Nature which makes, acts, creates; natural tendencies or potentialities आपूरात् by the filling up or overflow.

2. The transformation from one species or kind into another is by the overflow of natural tendencies or potentialities.

The word *Jāti* is generally used in *Saṃskṛta* for class, species etc., but in the context in which it is used here it is obvious that it has to be interpreted in a much wider sense. It is only then that the profound significance of the *Sūtra* reveals itself and can be understood in terms of modern scientific thought.

It is difficult to grasp the underlying idea of this *Sūtra* from its mere translation and it will, therefore, be necessary to explain its real significance in some detail. *Jāty-Antara-Pariṇāma* means a transformation involving a fundamental change of nature, or substance such as genus or chemical composition and not merely a change of state or form. Thus when water is changed into ice it is merely a change of state and does not involve an essential change of substance. When a bangle made of gold is changed into a necklace, again, there is no fundamental change but merely a change of form. But when hydrogen is changed into helium, or uranium is changed into lead, it is a fundamental change of substance and comes under *Jāty-Antara-Pariṇāma*. Now, the *Sūtra* lays down that all such changes involving fundamental differences can take place only when there is present in the substance the potentiality for the change under the specified conditions. *Prakṛty-āpūrāt* is a beautiful and pregnant phrase for expressing a very comprehensive scientific law. Literally, it means 'by the flow of *Prakṛti*'; but let us try to understand in terms of modern Science what the real significance of this phrase is. It will be best to take a few facts from our common experience to illustrate the working of this law. If we take a dry mass of wood and apply a burning match to it, the wood immediately takes fire and a whole timber yard may be reduced to ashes in a short time. But if we apply a burning match to a heap of bricks and mortar nothing happens. Why? Because, wood has in it the potentiality of combining with the oxygen of the air with the liberation of a great amount of heat and a number of volatile products and as the reaction is self-propagating involving a sort of 'chain reaction' a mere spark is enough to reduce the whole mass of wood to ashes. But in the case of bricks and mortar there is no potentiality to react in this manner and, therefore, when the match is applied nothing happens. Change, in such a case, therefore, takes place according to the potentialities existing in the material and follows the tendency of natural forces under the given conditions. If the conditions change, the tendencies may also change and an entirely new kind of change may be brought about. For example, the wood may be subjected to the action of certain chemical substances and converted into charcoal. Let us take another example. A breeder can evolve a new species of dog by the appropriate crossing of different kinds of dogs but he cannot produce a new species of cat in this manner. The potentiality for the production of a new species of cat does not exist in the latter case. Here again, therefore, we are bound by limitations set by natural tendencies and potentialities and cannot go against them. It is true that if we have the necessary knowledge we can, by the introduction of new factors, bring about changes which appeared impossible before, but that does not mean that we have violated the fundamental law of Nature referred to above.

३. निमित्तमप्रयोजकं प्रकृतीनां वरणभेदस्तु ततः क्षेत्रिकवत् ।

Nimittam aprayojakaṃ prakṛtīnāṃ varaṇa-
bhedas tu tataḥ kṣetrikavat.

निमित्तम् incidental cause अप्रयोजकं non-urging; not directly causing प्रकृतीनाम् of natural tendencies; of predisposing causes वरण obstacle भेद: piercing through; removal तु verily; on the other hand तत: from that क्षेत्रिकवत् like the farmer.

3. The incidental cause does not move or stir up the natural tendencies into activity; it merely removes the obstacles, like a farmer (irrigating a field).

The idea embodied in IV-2 is further elaborated in IV-3. Transformation from one kind into another takes place, as we have seen, according to the resultant effect of all forces involved. Everything has the potentiality of changing in a number of directions and by bringing to bear upon it different kinds of forces, we can make it change in one or another of the directions as illustrated in the following diagram.

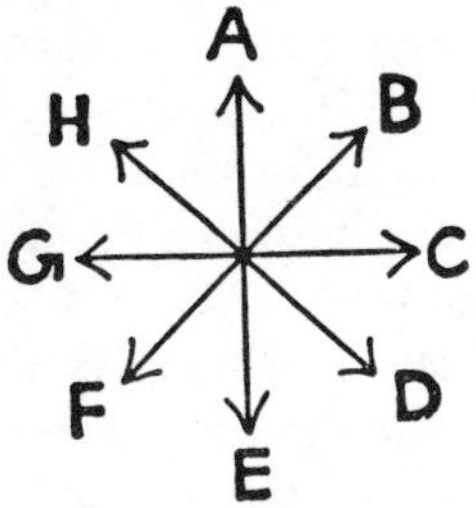

FIG. 11

If we have a beaker full of sugar solution we can change the sugar into alcohol by inoculating the solution with a certain kind of ferment, we can change it into a mixture of glucose and fructose by adding hydrochloric acid, we can change it into carbon by adding strong sulphuric acid and so on. All these different kinds of changes can be brought about by producing different conditions, by applying different kinds of stimuli for the manifestation of different potentialities. But the potentialities for all these changes already exist in the sugar solution. We cannot, for instance, change the sugar into mercury because there is no potentiality, in the chemical sense, for sugar to change into mercury.

The incidental or existing cause which seems outwardly to bring about the change is not the real cause of the change. The change is really brought about by the predisposing causes determined by the nature of potentialities existing in the things undergoing change. What the incidental cause does is merely to determine in which direction change will take place and thus to direct the flow of natural forces in that particular direction.

The respective role of the exciting and predisposing causes in bringing about all kinds of changes in Nature is then further made clear by the use of a very apt simile " like a farmer ". Anyone who has observed a farmer directing the current of water into different parts of a field will see at once how closely such a process resembles the action of natural forces being directed by one or the other of the outward causes which seem to bring about different kinds of changes. He removes a little earth here and the water begins to flow in one furrow. Then he closes up the gap and makes a breach at another place and the water begins to flow in another direction. The removal of a little earth from one particular spot does not produce the current of water. It merely removes an obstacle in the path of the water and determines the direction of the current.

The great natural law embodied in the above two *Sūtras* is applicable not only to physical phenomena but to all kinds of phenomena in the realm of *Prakṛti*. For example, the nature of our actions, good or bad, does not make our life. It merely determines the direction of our future lives. The current of our life must flow on incessantly, its direction being continually determined by our actions, thoughts and feelings.

The student may well ask: " What has this law to do with *Yoga*? " Everything. As has been pointed out before, the *Yogi* has to work out his liberation with the help of the laws which operate in the realm of *Prakṛti* and he, therefore, ought to have a clear idea of this fundamental law which determines the flux of phenomena taking place around him and within him. As he has to destroy completely, and for ever, certain deep-seated tendencies in his nature he ought to know their root causes which give rise to different forms of those tendencies. He ought to know that mere suppression of a tendency does not mean its removal. It will lie low in a potential form for an indefinite period and then again raise its head when suitable conditions present themselves. It is no use merely removing the exciting causes. The predi posing causes must be removed. The modern tendency is to deal only with the superficial causes and to get over the present difficulties somehow. This leads us nowhere and continually brings before us the old troubles in new and different forms.

४. निर्माणचित्तान्यस्मितामात्रात् ।

Nirmāṇa-cittāny asmitā-mātrāt.

निर्माण created; artificial चित्तानि minds अस्मिता egoism; 'I-am-ness'; sense of individuality मात्रात् from alone.

4. Artificially created minds (proceed) from 'egoism' alone.

The two previous *Sūtras* should prepare the ground for understanding the *modus operandi* of the method by which any number of additional 'minds' can be artificially produced by the highly advanced *Yogi*. *Citta*, as pointed out in I-2, is the universal principle which serves as a medium for all kinds of mental perceptions. But this universal principle can function only through a set of vehicles working on the different planes of the Solar system. These vehicles of consciousness, or *Kośas* as they are called, are formed by the appropriation and integration of matter belonging to different planes round an individual centre of consciousness and provide the necessary stimuli for mental perceptions which take place in consciousness. Patañjali has used the same word, *Citta*, for the universal principle which serves as a medium for mental perception as well as the individual mechanism through which such perception takes place. It is necessary to keep this distinction in mind because one or the other of the two meanings is implied by the same word—*Citta*—at different places.

Since the object of Section IV is partly to elucidate the nature of *Citta*, the question of the creation of 'artificial minds' has been dealt with by Patañjali in this Section. There is, of course, a 'natural mind', if we may use such a phrase, through which the individual works and evolves in the realms of *Prakṛti* during the long course of his evolutionary cycle. That mind, working through a set of vehicles, is the product of evolution, carries the impressions of all experiences through which it has passed in successive lives and lasts till *Kaivalya* is attained. But, during the course of the *Yogic* training when the *Yogi* has acquired the power of performing *Saṃyama* and manipulating the forces of the higher planes, especially *Mahat-Tattva*, it is possible for him to create any number of mental vehicles by duplication, vehicles which are an exact replica of the vehicle through which he normally functions. Such vehicles of consciousness are called *Nirmāṇa-Cittāni* and the question arises: 'How are these "artificial minds" created by the *Yogi*?' The answer to this question is given in the *Sūtra* under discussion.

Such artificial minds with their appropriate mechanism are created from '*Asmitā* alone'. *Asmitā* is, of course, the principle of individuality in man which forms, as it were, the core of the individual soul and maintains in an integrated condition all the vehicles of consciousness functioning at different levels. It is this principle which on identification with the different vehicles, produces egoism and other related phenomena which have been dealt with thoroughly in II-6. This principle is called *Mahat-Tattva* in Hindu philosophy and it is through its agency that artificial minds can be created. The advanced *Yogi* who can control the *Mahat-Tattva* has the power of establishing any number of independent centres of consciousness for himself and as soon as such a centre is established an 'artificial mind' automatically materializes round about it. This is an exact replica of the 'natural mind' in which he functions normally and remains in existence as long as he wills it to be maintained. The moment the *Yogi* withdraws his will from the 'artificial mind' it disappears instantaneously.

It is worthwhile noting the significance of the word 'alone' in the *Sūtra*. The significance, of course, is that the creation of an 'artificial mind' does not require any other operation except that of establishing a new centre of individuality. The precipitation of an 'artificial mind' round about this centre is brought about automatically by the forces of *Prakṛti* because the capacity of gathering a 'mind' round itself is inherent in the *Mahat-Tattva.* There is nothing extraordinary or incredible in such materializations and similar phenomena take place even on the physical plane. What happens when we place a tiny seed in the ground? The seed, by the potential power which is inherent in it, immediately begins to work upon its surroundings and gradually elaborates a tree from the matter appropriated from its environment. The flow of natural forces brings about all the necessary changes needed for this development. Do we know the secret of this power? No! But still it exists and we see its action all around us in every sphere of life. What is, therefore, incredible or miraculous in a centre established in the *Mahat-Tattva* gathering a *Citta* or 'mind' round itself by the automatic action of natural forces (*Prakṛti-Āpūrāt*)? The only difference is that of time. While the tree takes considerable time to grow, the production of the 'artificial mind' seems to take place instantaneously. But time is a relative thing and its measure varies according to the plane upon which it functions.

The automatism which is involved in the creation of 'artificial minds' cannot be adequately understood unless we have a clear grasp of the natural law enunciated in IV-2-3. This, no doubt, partly accounts for the insertion of these two *Sūtras* before the problem of 'artificial minds' is dealt with by the author.

५. प्रवृत्तिभेदे प्रयोजकं चित्तमेकमनेकेषाम्।

Pravṛtti-bhede prayojakaṃ cittam ekam anekeṣām.

प्रवृत्ति activity; pursuit भेदे in the difference प्रयोजकम् directing; moving चित्तम् mind एकम् one अनेकेषाम् of many.

5. The one (natural) mind is the director or mover of the many (artificial) minds in their different activities.

If the *Yogi* can duplicate his 'mind' at different places the question arises: 'How are the activities of these "artifical minds" thus created, co-ordinated and controlled?' According to this *Sūtra* the activities and functions of the 'artificial minds'—whatever their number—are directed and controlled by the one 'natural mind' of the *Yogi*. The 'artificial minds' are merely the instruments of the one 'natural mind' and obey it automatically. Just as the activities of the hands and other organs working in the physical body are co-ordinated by the brain and are directly under its control, in the same way the activities of the 'artificial minds' are co-ordinated and controlled by the Intelligence working in and through the 'natural mind'. Of course, this Intelligence working through the 'natural mind' is none else but the *Puruṣa* whose consciousness illuminates and energizes all the vehicles. It should also be noted that the 'artificial minds' act not only as instruments of the 'natural' mind but also, as it were, the outposts of its consciousness. *Pravṛtti* includes both kinds of activities, those corresponding to *Jñānendriyas* and *Karmendriyas*, the receptive and operative functions of consciousness.

६. तत्र ध्यानजमनाशयम् ।

Tatra dhyānajam anāśayam.

तत्र of them ध्यानजम् born of meditation अनाशयम् free from *Saṃskāras* or impressions; germless.

6. Of these the mind born of meditation is free from impressions.

To all outer appearances the 'artificial minds' are exact replicas of the 'natural mind' but they differ from it in one fundamental respect. They do not carry with them any impressions, *Saṃskāras* or *Karmas* which are an integral part of the 'natural mind'. The 'natural mind' is the product of evolutionary growth and is the repository of the *Saṃskāras* of all the experiences which it has passed through during the course of successive lives. These *Saṃskāras* in their totality are referred to as *Karmāśaya* 'the vehicle of *Karmas*' and have been dealt with in II-12. The 'artificial minds' created by the will-power of the *Yogi* are free from these impressions and one can easily see why this should be so. They are merely temporary creations which disappear as soon as the work for which they are created is finished. A business firm may be obliged to open a temporary branch in some locality for a particular purpose. Although business is transacted at the office of the new branch all accounts etc. are kept at the head office. The temporary office is merely an outpost of the head office and has really no independent status. The assets and liabilities belong to the head office. A somewhat similar relationship exists between the 'artificial minds' and the one 'natural mind'.

७. कर्माशुक्लाकृष्णं योगिनस्त्रिविधमितरेषाम् ।

Karmāśuklākṛṣṇaṃ yoginas tri-vidham itareṣām.

कर्म action अशुक्ल not white अकृष्णम् not black योगिनः of a *Yogi* त्रिविधम् threefold इतरेषाम् of others.

7. *Karmas* are neither white nor black (neither good nor bad) in the case of *Yogis*, they are of three kinds in the case of others.

The next topic which Patañjali takes up is the question of gaining freedom from the bondage of *Karma* which is a *sine qua non* for the attainment of *Kaivalya*. The subject of *Karma* has already been dealt with in II-12-14 and is taken up again here. In Section II the problem was discussed from a different angle—in relation to *Kleśas*—and it was shown how the *Kleśas* are the underlying cause of *Karmas* which in their turn produce pleasant or unpleasant conditions in this or future lives according as they are good or bad. But here, in Section IV, the subject has been taken up again and is dealt with from an entirely different point of view—with the object of showing how the *Yogi* may get rid of the *Karmāśaya*—the vehicle of *Karma*—which contains the accumulated *Saṃsakāras* of all the previous lives and which binds the soul to the wheel of birth and death. Unless and until all these *Saṃskāras* are destroyed or rendered inoperative no freedom from the bondage of *Prakṛti* is possible even though the *Yogi* may have reached an advanced state of illumination. The force of his *Saṃskāras* will pull him back again and again and prevent him from reaching the ultimate goal.

IV-7 gives a classification of *Karma* as well as indicates the means of avoiding the formation of new *Karma*. *Karmas* are neither black nor white in the case of those who are *Yogis*, they are of three kinds in the case of ordinary people. Black and white obviously describe the two kinds of *Karmas* which produce painful and pleasurable fruits referred to in II-14. The third kind of *Karmas* are those which are of mixed character. For example, many actions which we do have different effects upon different people. They benefit some and harm others and consequently produce *Karmas* of mixed character.

The word *Yogi* in this *Sūtra* means not only one who is practising *Yoga* but also one who has learnt the technique of *Niṣkāma Karma*. He does all his actions in a state of at-one-ment with *Īśvara* and does not, therefore, produce any personal *Karma*. The theory of *Niṣkāma Karma* is an integral part of Hindu philosophical thought and is well known to all students of *Yoga*. It is not, therefore, necessary to discuss it here in detail, but the broad central idea underlying it may be given. According to this doctrine personal *Karma* results from the performance of an ordinary action because the guiding force or motive of the action is personal desire—*Kāma*. We do our actions identifying ourselves with our ego who sees the fulfilment of his own desires and naturally reaps the fruits in the form of pleasurable and painful experiences. When an individual can dissociate himself completely from his ego and performs action *in complete identification with the Supreme Spirit* which is working through his ego, such an action is called *Niṣkāma* (without desire). It does not naturally produce any personal *Karma* and consequently does not bring any fruit to the individual.

It is necessary to note, however, that it is *conscious and effective* dissociation from the ego which neutralizes the operation of the law of *Karma* and not a mere thought or intention or wish on the part of the individual. So real *Niṣkāma Karma* is possible only to highly advanced *Yogis* who have risen above the plane of desires. Many well-meaning people trying to lead the religious life imagine that merely by wishing to be desireless or thinking of dissociating themselves from their ego, superficially dedicating their actions to God, will free them from the binding action of *Karma*. This is a mistake though it is true that persistent efforts of this kind will naturally pave the way for acquiring the right technique. As well may a person hope to free himself from the law of gravitation by thinking of rising in the air. What is needed, as has been pointed out above, is a real, conscious identification with the Divine within us and freedom from any taint of personal motive. To the extent that the action is so tainted will it produce *Kārmic* effect with its binding power over the individual.

When the technique of *Niṣkāma Karma* has been learnt and applied to all actions, no personal *Karma* is incurred by the *Yogi* even though he may be busily engaged in the affairs of the world as an agent of the Divine Life within him. All his *Karmas* are 'consumed in the fire of Wisdom' in the words of the *Bhagavad-Gītā*. But what about the *Karmas* that he has already accumulated in his present and past lives? He ceases to add any new *Saṃskāras* to the accumulated stock, but an enormous number of *Saṃskāras* are already there in his *Karmāśaya* which must be exhausted before Liberation is attained. He cannot, simply by willing, make these *Saṃskāras* disappear. He must wait patiently till they have been completely exhausted and he has paid up the last pie of his debt. It is, therefore, natural that the exhaustion of his *Karmas* which bind him to other souls should be a long drawn-out process extending probably over many lives. It is true that he has been paying heavy instalments of his *Kārmic* debts since he has taken to the path of *Yoga*. It is also true that as he advances on the path of *Yoga* and is able to function on the higher planes new powers come to him which enable him to expedite this process. For example, he can make 'artificial minds' and 'artificial bodies' (*Nirmāṇakāyās*) and through them pay off simultaneously his debts to people who are scattered far and wide in time and space. Still, with these new powers and facilities for hastening the *Kārmic* process at his disposal he is bound by the laws of *Prakṛti* and has to work within the framework of these laws. And this naturally requires time and wise and careful adaptation of means to ends.

८. ततस्तद्विपाकानुगुणानामेवाभिव्यक्तिर्वासनानाम् ।

Tatas tad-vipākānuguṇānām evābhi-
vyaktir vāsanānām.

ततः thence तद्-विपाक their ripening; fruition अनुगुणानाम् accordant; correspondent; favourable एव only अभिव्यक्तिः manifestation वासनानाम् of potential desires; of tendencies.

8. From these only those tendencies are manifested for which the conditions are favourable.

What has been said above about the nature of *Niṣkāma Karma* must have brought home to the student that it is desire or personal attachment which is the motive power of action in the case of ordinary people and which produces the *Saṃskāras* both in the form of tendencies and potentialities as well as *Karmas* which bring pleasant or painful experiences.

The forces set in motion by our thoughts, desires and actions are of a complex nature and produce all kinds of effects which it is difficult to classify completely. But all these leave some kind of *Saṃskāra* or impression which binds us in one way or another for the future. Thus our desires produce potential energy which draws us irresistably to the environment or conditions in which they can be satisfied. Actions produce tendencies which make it easier for us to repeat similar actions in future and if they are repeated a sufficient number of times may form fixed habits. In addition, if our actions affect other people in some way they bind us to those people by *Kārmic* ties and bring pleasant or unpleasant experiences to ourselves. Our thoughts also produce *Saṃskāras* and result in desires and actions in accordance with their nature.

If, however, we analyse these different kinds of mental and physical activities we shall find that at their base there are always desires of one kind or another which drive the mind and result in these thoughts and actions. Desire in its most comprehensive sense is thus a more fundamental factor in our life than our thoughts and actions because it is the hidden power which drives the mind and body in all kinds of ways for the satisfaction of its own purposes. The mind is thus mostly an instrument of desires and its incessant activity results from the continuous pressure of these desires upon it. Of course, 'desire' is not an apt word for the subtle power which drives the mind at its higher levels and which binds consciousness to the glorious realities of the spiritual planes. The word used in *Saṃskṛta* for this power which works at all levels of the mind is *Vāsanā*. Just as *Citta* is the universal medium for the expression of the mind principle, so *Vāsanā* is the universal power which drives the mind and produces the continuous series of its transformations which imprison consciousness. In fact, the word *Vāsanā* used in the present context is of a still more comprehensive significance, for it not only indicates the principle of desire in its widest sense but also the tendencies and *Karmas* which this principle generates on the different planes. For desire and the *Karmas* or tendencies which it produces form a vicious circle in which causes and effects are intertwined and it is difficult to separate them. So the use of the word *Vāsanā* for both is quite justifiable.

Since different types of *Vāsanās* require differerent kinds of conditions and environment for their manifestation, it is quite obvious that they cannot find expression in any haphazard manner but must follow a certain sequence determined by the different types of environments and conditions through which the individual passes in the successive incarnations. And this is what IV-8 points out. If a person has a strong desire for being a champion athlete when he has inherited a weak and diseased body his desire cannot naturally be fulfilled in that life. If an individual A has strong *Kārmic* ties with another individual B who is not in incarnation at the time and those ties require physical expression they will naturally remain in abeyance for the time being and can be worked out only when both are present in physical incarnation at the same time. It will be seen, therefore, that only a limited number of *Vāsanās*, whether in the form of desire or *Karmas*, can find expression in a particular incarnation, firstly, because the span of human life is more or less limited, and secondly, because the conditions for the expression of different kinds of *Vāsanās* are frequently incompatible. That portion of the accumulated stock of *Vāsanās* (*Sancita Karma*) which can find expression and is ready to be precipitated in one particular incarnation is known as *Prārabdha Karma* of the individual. The life of an ordinary individual is confined within the framework thus made for him and his freedom to alter its main trends is extremely limited. But a man of exceptionally strong will, and especially a *Yogi* whose knowledge and powers are extraordinary, can make considerable changes in the plan of life thus marked out for him. In fact, the more the *Yogi* advances on the path of *Yoga* which he is treading the greater is his hand in determining the pattern of his lives, and when he is on the threshold of *Kaivalya* he is practically the master of his destiny.

In spite of the comprehensive sense in which the word *Vāsanā* is used it should be noted that emphasis in this *Sūtra* is on that aspect of *Vāsanā* which is expressed in the form of tendencies of which *Karmas* are merely secondary effects.

९. जातिदेशकालव्यवहितानामप्यानन्तर्यं स्मृतिसंस्कारयोरेकरूपत्वात्।

Jāti-deśa-kāla-vyavahitānām apy ānantar-
yaṃ smṛti-saṃskārayor ekarūpatvāt.

जाति (by) class देश (by) locality काल (by) time व्यवहितानाम् separated; divided अपि even आनन्तर्यम् sequence; non-interruption; immediate succession स्मृति-संस्कारयोः of memory and impressions एकरूपत्वात्-because of the sameness in appearance or form.

9. There is the relation of cause and effect even though separated by class, locality and time because memory and impressions are the same in form.

The seemingly irrational and disjointed manner in which *Vāsanās* have to work out in the successive incarnations may give rise to a philosophical difficulty in the mind of the student and Patañjali proceeds to remove this difficulty in this *Sūtra.* It happens very frequently that one personality of an individual does some particular action but because the *Karma* of that action cannot be worked out by that personality owing to the absence of the necessary conditions, it has to be worked out by another personality of the same individual in a later life. And this second personality has no memory of the particular action for which it is undergoing that experience. Of course, if this experience is pleasurable no question arises in the mind of the second personality as to the justice of the undeserved good luck. But if the experience is painful there is felt a grievance against Fate for the undeserved pain or suffering. A tremendous amount of this kind of resentment against 'undeserved' suffering poisons the minds of people who are ignorant of the Law of *Karma* and its mode of working and a wider understanding of this Law will do much to make people see things in their true light and to take the experiences of life as they come with patience and without bitterness.

Coming back to the philsophical difficulty we may ask: 'Why should the second personality in the later life suffer for the wrongs done by the first personality in the previous life, and if it has to, how can the law of *Karma* be called just?' The answer to this question is given in the *Sūtra* we are dealing with. Of course, in expounding a philosophical system or scientific technique in the *Sūtra* form much is left to the intelligence of the student who is supposed to be familiar with the general doctrines upon which the philosophy or science is based. Only the essential ideas which form, as it were, the steel frame of the mental structure are given and even these are stated as conscisely as possible. The doctrine of reincarnation which is an integral part of

Yogic philosophy and which is taken for granted by Patañjali implies that the chain of personalities in the successive incarnations are temporary expressions of a higher and more permanent entity who is called by different names in different schools of thought such as the *Jīvātmā* or the Immortal Ego or the individuality. It is this *Jīvātmā* who really incarnates in the different personalities and the latter may be considered to be more or less outposts of his consciousness in the lower worlds during the period of the incarnations.

Now, the important point to note here is that the over-all memory embracing all the successive lives resides in the 'mind' of the *Jīvātmā* and the different personalities which succeed one another do not share the over-all continuous memory. Their memory is confined only to the particular experiences gone through by them in each separate incarnation. This continuous memory embracing the chain of lives is due to the fact that the *Saṃskāras* of all the experiences gone through in these lives are present in the permanent higher vehicles of the *Jīvātmā*. Just as the contact of the needle with the impressions on the gramophone record reproduces sound, just as the contact of the mind with the physical brain reproduces memory of experiences gone through in this life, in the same way, the contact of the higher consciousness with the *Saṃskāras* or impressions in the higher vehicles of the *Jīvātmā* reproduces memories corresponding to the *Saṃskāras* contacted. The vehicle which is the repository of all these *Saṃskāras* is called '*Kāraṇa Śarīra*' in *Vedāntic* terminology because it is the repository of all the germs of future experiences.

It will be seen from what has been said above how the experiences and the corresponding memories of the different personalities scattered in different conditions of class, time and space are integrated in the consciousness of the *Jīvātmā* who has passed through all the experiences and is the real sower and reaper of the *Karmas* accruing from them. Seen in this light, reaping the bitter fruits by a personality for the wrongs done by another personality which has gone before does not involve any injustice because the different personalities are expressions, under different conditions, of the same entity though they may not be aware of the fact in their physical consciousness. A particular personality

(*Jīva*) is not aware of the whole series of experiences and *Saṃskāras* but the *Jīvātmā* is, and in the long uninterrupted series of actions and reactions sees the natural working out of the law of *Karma* and no favouritism or injustice whatsoever. We do not grumble when we find that the unpleasant experiences which we have to go through are the direct result of our own folly or wrong-doing. And neither does the *Jīvātmā* before whose vision all the past lives lie like an open book.

The manner in which the over-all memory of the *Jīvātmā* enables him to see the perfect working out of causes and effects even though they are scattered over different lives in an irregular manner can be illustrated by a simple diagram given below:

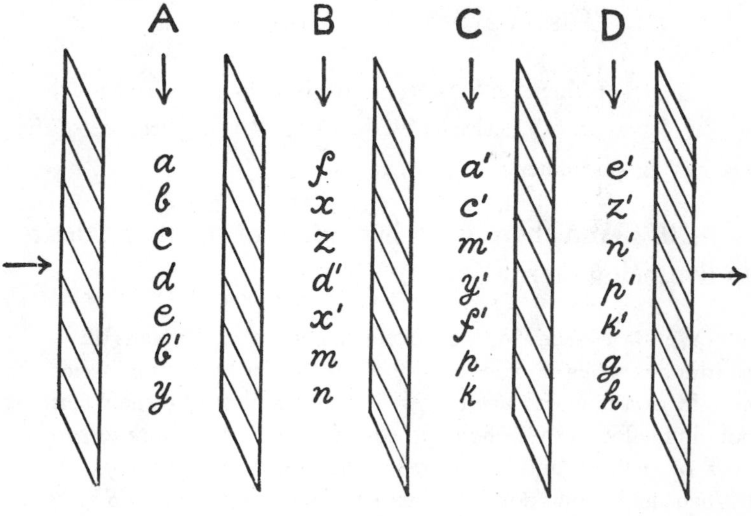

FIG. 12

a, b, c, d, etc. represent the different causes set going by a particular *Jīvātmā* in four lives represented by compartments A, B, C and D and a′ b′ c′ d′, etc. the corresponding *Kārmic* effects which ensue in the same or a subsequent life. If these letters are distributed in the four separate compartments in an irregular manner only keeping in mind that each effect *follows* its corresponding cause then it will not be possible for anyone whose vision is confined to only one compartment to correlate all the causes and the effects which are precipitated when the appropriate conditions present themselves either in the same life or in subsequent lives. But if anyone looks at the letters from a distance so that all the letters in the different compartments are visible simultaneously then every effect can be traced to its corresponding cause, and in spite of the irregular mixing up of the causes and effects in the different compartments, the law of cause and effect is seen to be strictly obeyed.

१०. तासामनादित्वं चाशिषो नित्यत्वात् ।

Tāsām anāditvaṃ cāśiṣo nityatvāt.

तासाम् of them अनादित्वम् no beginning च and; also आशिषः of the (current of) desire or will to live नित्यत्वात् because of the eternity or permanence.

10. And there is no beginning of them, the desire to live being eternal.

We have seen in the previous *Sūtra* that human life is a continuous series of experiences brought about by setting in motion certain causes which are followed sooner or later by their corresponding effects, the whole process thus being an uninterrupted play of actions and reactions. The question naturally arises: 'When and how does this process of accumulating *Saṃskāras* begin and how can it be ended?' We are bound to the wheel of births and deaths on account of *Vāsanās* which result in experiences of various kinds and these in their turn generate more *Vāsanās*. We seem to be facing one of those philosophical riddles which seem to defy solution. The answer given by Patañjali to the first part of the question posed above is that this process of accumulating *Saṃskāras* cannot be traced to its source because the 'will to live' or the 'desire to be' does not come into play with the birth of the human soul but is characteristic of all forms of life through which consciousness has evolved in reaching the human stage. In fact, the moment consciousness comes into contact with matter with the birth of *Avidyā* and the *Kleśas* begin to work, *Saṃskāras* begin to form. Attractions and repulsions of various degrees and kinds are present even in the earliest stages of evolution—mineral, vegetable and animal—and an individual who attains the human stage after passing through all the previous stages brings with him all the *Saṃskāras* of the stages through which he has passed, though most of these *Saṃskāras* lie dormant in a latent condition. Animal traits are recognized even by Western psychology as present in our sub-conscious mind, and the occasional emergence of these traits belonging to the lower stages is due to the presence within us of all the *Saṃskāras* which we have gathered in our evolutionary development. That is why, as soon as the control of the Higher Self temporarily disappears or slackens owing to heightened emotional disturbances or other causes, human beings begin to behave like beasts or even worse than beasts. That, incidentally, shows the necessity of keeping a rigid control over our mind and emotions because once this is completely lost there is no knowing what undesirable *Saṃskāras* which have been lying dormant through the ages may become active and make us do things for which we may have to repent afterwards. History provides many instances of the recrudescence of such traits in human beings and the temporary reversion to the animal stage. It is true that the human, animal, vegetable and mineral kingdoms are clearly defined and are separate stages of evolution and there can be no retrogression, from one kingdom to another, but as far as *Saṃskāras* are concerned they may be considered to be continuous and the human stage may be considered as the summation and culmination of the previous stages.

As evolution progresses, *Vāsanās* become more and more complicated and in the human stage assume a bewildering variety and complexity owing to the introduction of the mental element. The intellect, though it is the servant and instrument of desire to a certain extent, plays in its turn an important part in the growth of the desire nature and the highly complicated and various desires of the modern civilized man bear an interesting contrast to the comparatively simple and natural desires of the primitive man.

As evolution progresses still further and with the practice of *Yoga* subtler levels of consciousness are contacted, desires become more and more refined and subtle and thus more difficult to detect and transcend. But even the subtlest and most refined desire which binds consciousness to the bliss and knowledge of the highest spiritual planes differs only in degree and is really a refined form of the primary desire—' will to live ' which is called *Āśiṣaḥ*. It will be seen that it is not possible to destroy *Vāsanās* and thus put an end to the life process by tackling them on their own plane. Even *Niṣkāma Karma* when practised perfectly can only stop generating new personal *Karma* for the future. It cannot destroy the root of *Vāsanā* which is inherent in manifested life. As *Viveka* and *Vairāgya* develop, the active *Vāsanās* become more and more quiescent but their *Saṃskāras* remain and like seeds can burst forth into active form whenever favourable conditions present themselves and appropriate stimuli are applied to the mind.

११. हेतुफलाश्रयालम्बनैः संगृहीतत्वादेषामभावे तदभावः ।

Hetu-phalāśrayālambanaiḥ saṃgṛhitatvād eṣām abhāve tad-abhāvaḥ.

हेतु (with) cause फल effect आश्रय substratum; that which gives support आलम्बनैः object संगृहीतत्वात् because of being bound together एषाम् of these अभावे on the disappearance तद्-अभावः disappearance of them.

11. Being bound together as cause-effect, substratum-object, they (effects, i.e. *Vāsanās*) disappear on their (cause, i.e. *Avidyā*) disappearance.

If the *Vāsanās* form a continuous stream and no release from bondage is possible without their destruction how can Liberation be attained? The answer to this question was given in the theory of *Kleśas* which has been dealt with already in Section II. We saw that the cyclic progress of manifested life for the *Puruṣa* begins with the association of his consciousness with *Prakṛti* through the direct agency of *Avidyā*. *Avidyā* leads successively to *Asmitā*, *Rāga-Dveṣa* and *Abhiniveśa* and all the miseries of life in bondage.

If *Avidyā* is the ultimate cause of bondage and the whole process of the continuous generation of *Vāsanās* rests on this basis it follows logically that the only effective means of attaining freedom from bondage is to destroy *Avidyā*. All other means of ending the miseries and illusions of life which do not completely destroy *Avidyā* can, at best, be palliatives and cannot lead to the goal of *Yogic* endeavour—*Kaivalya*. How this *Avidyā* can be destroyed has been discussed very thoroughly and systematically in Section II and it is not necessary to deal with this question here.

१२. अतीतानागतं स्वरूपतोऽस्त्यध्वभेदाद्धर्माणाम् ।

Atītānāgataṃ svarūpato 'sty adhva-bhedād dharmāṇām.

अतीत the past अनागतं the future स्वरूपत: in reality; in its own form अस्ति exists अध्वभेदात् because of the difference of paths धर्माणाम् of properties.

12. The past and the future exist in their own (real) form. The difference of *Dharmas* or properties is on account of the difference of paths.

This is one of the most important and interesting *Sūtras* in Section IV because it throws light on a fundamental problem of philosophy. That there is a Reality underlying the phenomenal world in which we live our life is taken for granted in all schools of *Yoga*, the aim of *Yoga*, in fact, being the search for and discovery of this Reality. The question arises: 'Is this world of Reality absolutely independent of the phenomenal world in time and space which we contact with our mind or are the two worlds related to each other in some way?' According to the Great Teachers who have found the Truth the two worlds are related though it is difficult for the intellect to comprehend this relationship. If there is a relation existing between the two worlds we may further enquire whether the manifested worlds in time and space rigidly express a predetermined pattern of Divine Thought, just as a picture on a cinema screen is the result of a mechanical projection of the photographs in the film roll. Or does the procession of events in the phenomenal world merely conform to a Plan which exists in the Divine Mind in the same way as the construction of a building follows the plan of the architect? The first view will imply Determinism in its most rigid form while the second will leave some room for Free Will.

The *Sūtra* under discussion throws some light on this philosophical problem. It is composed of two separate parts, the second part amplifying the first. The statement 'the past and future exist in their own form' means obviously that the succession of phenomena which constitute the world process or any part of it are the expression, in terms of time, of some reality which exists in the subtler realms of consciousness beyond the range of the human intellect. This reality transcends time and yet expresses itself as time in the world process.

As this question of time will be dealt with thoroughly in connection with IV-33 let us pass on and proceed to consider the second part of the *Sūtra* with which we are immediately concerned at this stage. 'The difference of *Dharmas* is on account of the difference of paths.' This is apparently an abstruse statement which does not seem to make sense and the existing commentaries do not throw any light on it. Let us see whether it is not possible to get at the meaning of the author in the light of what has been said with regard to the nature of the past and future in the first part of the *Sūtra*.

If the succession of phenomena which we cognize with our mind is the expression of some reality and if this expression is not a mere mechanical projection implying Determinism in its rigid form then it follows logically that the fulfilment of this reality in terms of time and space must be possible along a number of paths any one of which may be actually followed as a result of all the forces working in the realm of Nature. The series of events which have taken place already and become the 'past' represent the path trodden by the Chariot of Time so far and have become fixed—part of the memory of Nature in the *Ākāśic* records. What about the events which are still in the womb of the 'future'? What shape are the events going to take in becoming the 'past' in their turn? As these events will not be the result of the working out of a rigid inexorable destiny but elastic adaptations to a Divine Pattern the path which they take must be at least to some extent indeterminate. There must be a certain amount of latitude for movement if there is freedom of choice and free will has any place in the scheme of things. Of course, there are forces working in the field which, to a certain extent, will determine the direction in which events will move. There is, for example, the pressure of evolutionary forces. There is the directing force of the Divine Plan and archetypes in every sphere of development. There is the tremendous pressure of the potential power of the *Saṃskāras* both in the realm of matter and mind. But within the limitations set by these different forces tending to mould the future there is, still, a certain freedom of movement which makes it possible for the future to develop along one of the many possible lines which open out from moment to moment. It is in this way, therefore, that in the world of the Relative, influenced by the Divine Pattern on the one hand and the momentum of the past on the other events move forward towards their final consummation.

Having understood the significance of the phrase 'difference of paths' let us now see how these different paths merely represent the emergence of different properties in the substratum, i.e. *Prakṛti*. The path taken by the course of events, if we analyse it carefully, is nothing else than a particular series of phenomena in a particular order, each element of this series, in its turn, being nothing more than a particular combination of properties or *Dharmas* which are all inherent in *Prakṛti*. If we represent, for the sake of illustration, these different properties by A, B, C, D, E, F, G, H, I, J, K, L, etc.

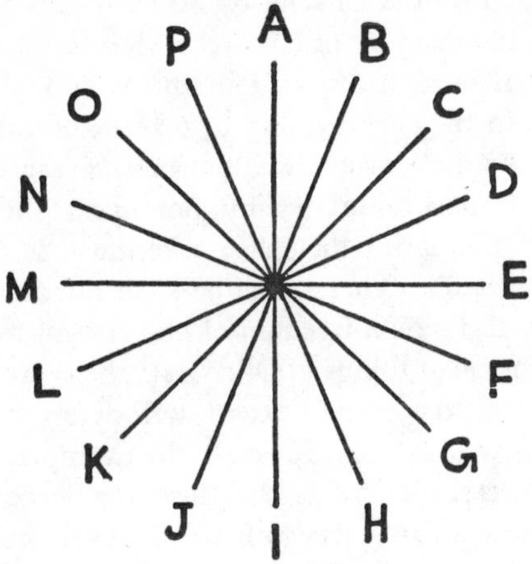

FIG. 13

then different courses of events may be represented by different series of phenomena in the following manner:

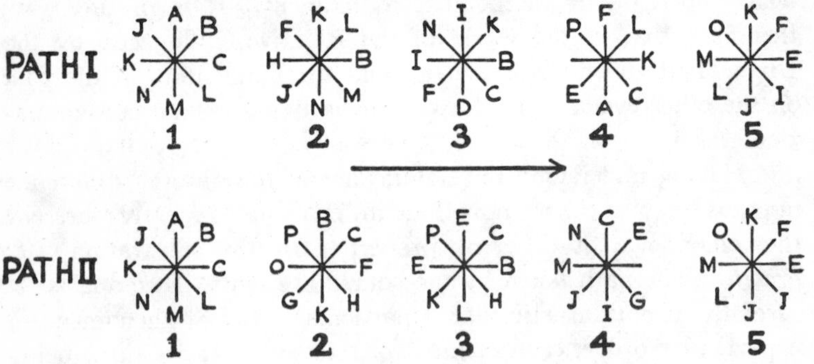

FIG. 14

It will be noted that each element of this phenomenon is nothing but a particular combination of *Dharmas* which have become manifest at a particular moment of time. It does not matter whether we consider the phenomena within a limited sphere like our Solar system or within the unlimited sphere of the Universe for they all take place within the realm of *Prakṛti*. It is thus possible, beginning with a particular situation, to arrive at another situation by two or more alternative paths.

These paths followed by the course of events in the phenomenal world are not of purely mechanical origin, as the materialists would have us believe. They, in some mysterious way, bring about the fulfilment of the Eternal as has been pointed out above. The lower phenomenal world does not exist for its own sake (being merely a law of mechanical necessity) but for the sake of fulfilling the Eternal. Its object is to bring about certain 'changes' in the higher spiritual worlds, these 'changes' being the very object of its existence. The use of the word 'changes' in connection with the Eternal is no doubt extremely incongruous but the student should understand that it is employed, for lack of a better term, to indicate that subtle and mysterious reaction which our life in the phenomenal world has on our eternal being. A specific instance will perhaps make the point clear. The unfoldment of the perfection which is latent in every human soul is the object of the reincarnations in the lower worlds through which it is made to pass. The different kinds of experiences through which the soul passes, life after life, stimulate gradually its spiritual nature and unfold the perfection which finds its consummation in *Kaivalya*. Now, the type and number of these experiences do not really matter as long as the objective is reached. A particular individual may go through a hundred lives of the most intense and painful experiences or he may take one thousand lives containing experiences of an entirely different nature to attain perfection. The path does not matter, it is the attainment of the goal which is important. The path lies in the world of phenomena which is unreal and illusory while the objective lies in the world of the Eternal which is Real.

It is this possibility of taking different paths that enables the *Yogi* to cut short the process of unfoldment in the phenomenal worlds and to attain perfection in the shortest possible time. He is not bound to go along the long and easy road of evolution which humanity as a whole is treading. He can step out of this broad road and take the short and difficult climb to the mountain top by following the path of *Yoga*. But if he is bent on breaking through the world of phenomena into the world of Reality he must first understand the nature of these phenomena and the manner in which they are perceived by the mind. That is why Patañjali has dealt with this question in IV-12.

१३. ते व्यक्तसूक्ष्माः गुणात्मानः ।

Te vyakta-sūkṣmāḥ guṇātmānaḥ.

ते they व्यक्त manifest सूक्ष्मा subtle; unmanifest गुणात्मानः of the nature of *Guṇas*.

13. They, whether manifest or unmanifest, are of the nature of *Guṇas*.

In the last *Sūtra* it was pointed out that all kinds of phenomena which are the object of perception by the mind are nothing but different combinations of *Dharmas* or properties which are inherent in *Prakṛti*. In this *Sūtra* the idea is carried one step further and it is pointed out that the *Dharmas* themselves are nothing but different combinations of the three primary *Guṇas*. This is a sweeping statement which is likely to startle anyone who is not familiar with the theory of *Guṇas* but to one who understands this theory it will appear as a perfectly logical conclusion which flows naturally from that theory. If the three *Guṇas* are the three fundamental principles of motion (inertia, mobility, vibration) and if motion of some kind or another lies at the basis of manifestation of all kinds of properties then these properties must be of the nature of *Guṇas*. Physical, chemical and other kinds of properties which modern Science has studied so far can be traced ultimately to motions and positions of different kinds and so the theory that properties are of the nature of *Guṇas* is in accord with the latest scientific developments as far as they go. But the statement in the *Sūtra* under discussion is of an all-embracing character and comprises not only physical properties which we can cognize with our physical senses but also subtle properties pertaining to the subtler worlds. Thoughts, emotions and in fact all kinds of phenomena involving *Dharmas* come within its scope.

The word *Sūkṣma* means not only properties related to the subtler planes but also those which are unmanifest or dormant. The only difference between manifest and dormant properties is that while the manifest properties are the result of particular combinations of *Guṇas in action* the dormant properties are those which exist potentially in *Prakṛti* in the form of theoretical combinations of *Guṇas* not yet materialized. Thousands of new compounds are being produced in the field of chemistry every year. Each of these represents a new combination of *Guṇas* which was latent so far and has only now become manifest. *Prakṛti* is like an organ having the potentiality for producing an innumerable number of notes. The manifest qualities are the notes which are struck and give their specific sound, the unmanifest qualities are the notes which are silent, lying in repose. But they are all there to emerge at any moment and play their part in the phenomena which are taking place everywhere, all the time.

The importance of the generalization contained in this *Sūtra* thus lies not only in the fact that it goes to the very bedrock in revealing the true nature of all kinds of phenomena but also in its extraordinary comprehensiveness. No generalization of modern Science can perhaps compare in its all-embracing nature with this doctrine of *Yogic* philosophy and as it is based upon a vision of the worlds of phenomena from the vantage-ground of Reality there is no doubt that the more Science advances into the realms of the unknown the more it will corroborate the *Yogic* doctrine.

१४. परिणामैकत्वाद्वस्तुतत्त्वम् ।

Pariṇāmaikatvād vastu-tattvam.

परिणाम transformation; change एकत्वात् on account of the uniqueness वस्तु of the object तत्त्वम् the essence; reality.

14. The essence of the object consists in the uniqueness of transformation (of the *Guṇas*).

What is the essential nature of any object or thing which is an object of mental perception? We can know of the existence and nature of anything only from the properties which it has at a particular moment. There is no other way. This 'bundle of properties' which in their totality constitute the thing must therefore be a unique combination of the three *Guṇas* since each property taken by itself is nothing more than a peculiar combination of the *Guṇas*. Anyone with some knowledge of modern Science can take up any physical object and break it up into its physical and chemical components—into molecules, atoms, electrons, etc. and these ultimately resolve into different kinds of forces and motions. Nothing material in the usual sense is left over if we take into consideration the fact that matter and energy are interconvertible. As far as we can see, it is all a play of different kinds of forces and motions of extraordinary variety and complexity. It is true we do not yet know exactly the nature of the nucleus of the atoms but from the trend of researches in this field it is very probable that this also will be found to be nothing more than a combination of different kinds of motions. So that, as far as it goes, modern Science corroborates the truth of the *Yogic* doctrine that every object which we perceive with our mind is merely a unique transformation of the three *Guṇas*. It should be noted that the clue to the meaning of the *Sūtra* lies in the word *Ekatvāt* which does not mean here 'oneness' but 'uniqueness'. Interpreted in this way the *Sūtra* fits in perfectly in the chain of reasoning adopted by Patañjali to explain the theory of mental perception.

१५. वस्तुसाम्ये चित्तभेदात् तयोर्विभक्तः पन्थाः ।

Vastu-sāmye citta-bhedāt tayor vibhaktaḥ panthāḥ.

वस्तुसाम्ये object being the same चित्तभेदात् because of there being difference of the mind तयोः of these two विभक्तः separate पन्थाः path; way of being.

15. The object being the same the difference in the two (the object and its cognition) are due to their (of the minds') separate path.

If each object is a unique transformation of the three *Guṇas* and has thus a definite identity of its own why then does it appear different to different minds? It is a matter of common experience that no two minds see the same thing alike. There is always a difference in cognition though the thing is the same. The reason for this difference, as pointed out in this *Sūtra*, lies in the fact that the minds which cognize the thing are in different conditions and thus naturally get different impressions from the same object. When one vibrating body strikes another vibrating body the result of the impact depends upon the condition of both the bodies at the time of the impact. The mental body which comes in contact with the object of perception is not a passive or static thing. It is vibrating in all sorts of ways and, therefore, must modify every impression received by its own rate of vibration. It is, therefore, not possible to obtain a true impression of the object as long as the mind itself is not free from its *Vṛttis*. The impression created will depend upon the condition of the receiving mind and as all minds are in different conditions, because they have followed different paths in their evolution, they must get different impressions from the same object. The student should keep in mind the distinction between the mental body which vibrates and the mind in which the *Vṛttis* are produced by these vibrations.

Is it possible to get a true impression of an object under any circumstances? Yes, when the mind has been freed from its *Vṛttis* and does not, in consequence, modify the impression made upon it by the object. When the *Vṛttis* have been eliminated the mind becomes one with the object (I-41), which is another way of saying that it receives an exact impression of the object without its own modifying influence. So it is only in *Samādhi*, when all the *Vṛttis* have been suppressed, that it is possible to know the object as it really is.

Even in our everyday life we find that the more a mind is influenced by different biases, prejudices and other disturbances the greater is the distortion produced in the impressions which are made upon it by men and things. A calm and dispassionate mind can alone see things correctly as far as this is possible under the limitations of ordinary life.

१६. न चैकचित्ततन्त्रं वस्तु तदप्रमाणकं तदा किं स्यात् ।

Na caika-citta-tantraṃ vastu tad-apramā-
ṇakaṃ tadā kiṃ syāt.

न not च and एक one चित्त mind तन्त्रम् dependent on वस्तु an object तत् that अप्रमाणकम् non-cognized; unwitnessed तदा then किम् what स्यात् would be; would happen to.

16. Nor is an object dependent on one mind. What would become of it when not cognized by that mind?

If each object of mental perception is a mere bundle of properties which produce different impressions upon different minds, then, mental perception may be considered as a purely subjective phenomenon and it may be argued that the object need not have an independent existence apart from the cognizing agent, i.e., the mind. This purely idealistic theory of philosophy is disposed of by the objection raised in this *Sūtra*. If the object of mental perception is only a product of the mind which perceives it and has no independent existence of its own, then, what becomes of the object when the mind ceases to perceive it? If we accept the purely idealistic theory that objects in the external world have no real existence of their own but are mere creations of the mind then we are led to the absurd conclusion that the external world appears and disappears with the appearance and disappearance of objects in the mind of each individual, and it becomes difficult to account for the uniformity of experiences of different people with regard to different things and the harmonious co-ordination of observations made by different individuals.

No useful purpose will be served by going further into the implications of this theory. It is enough to note that Patañjali does not accept it. The *Yogic* philosophy recognizes the existence of ' objects ' outside the mind. It is these objects which stimulate the mind in particular ways and produce impressions which are then perceived by the *Puruṣa*. It is true that the objects which produce the impressions are considered to be mere combinations of *Guṇas*. It is also true that the mind perceives not the objects themselves but the impressions made by them upon it. But still, there is something external to the mind which stimulates the mind to form images whatever its nature may be. It will be seen, therefore, that the theory of mental perception upon which the *Yogic* philosophy is based steers a middle course between pure idealism and pure realism and reconciles in a harmonious conception the essential features of both. The main postulates of the theory are given in the next few *Sūtras*.

१७. तदुपरागापेक्षित्वाच्चित्तस्य वस्तु ज्ञाताज्ञातम् ।

Tad-uparāgāpekṣitvāc cittasya vastu jñātājñātam.

तद्-उपराग the colouring thereby अपेक्षित्वात् because of needing चित्तस्य for the mind; by the mind वस्तु an object ज्ञात known अज्ञातम् unknown.

17. In consequence of the mind being coloured or not coloured by it, an object is known or unknown.

The first essential for the mind of an individual 'knowing' an object is that the object should affect or modify the mind in some way. The phrase actually used is 'colouring the mind'. The use of the word 'colouring' for 'modifying' is not merely a poetic way of stating a scientific fact. It is used with a definite purpose in view. The word 'modification' would merely imply a partial change in the mind while the idea which has to be conveyed is a change which may vary in intensity from a mere trace to a depth of any intensity. The knowledge of the object may be extremely superficial or very deep and all these progressively increasing degrees of understanding can best be conveyed by using the word 'colouring', the depth of the colour indicating the degree of assimilation of the object by the mind. Besides, it is only by the use of the word 'colouring' that the complete fusion of the object and the mind referred to in *Sūtra* I-41 can be properly understood.

Those who have ever tried to study a subject which is entirely new to them and much beyond their mental capacity will be able to form some idea regarding the necessity of an object 'colouring' the mind before it can be understood. The subject is not assimilated by the mind at all, simply refuses to sink into the mind as a dye sometimes refuses to stain a tissue. The mind must 'take in' the object to a certain extent at least if it is to 'know' it and the extent to which it assimilates the object determines the degree of knowledge. This 'colouring' of the mind by an external object is found on deeper analysis to be nothing more than the capacity of the mental vehicle to vibrate in response to the stimulus provided by the object. The more fully the vehicle can vibrate in this manner the greater is the knowledge of the object which the mind acquires. Herein comes the necessity of evolution of the vehicles in the earlier stages.

१८. सदा ज्ञाताश्चित्तवृत्तयस्तत्प्रभोः पुरुषस्यापरिणामित्वात् ।

Sadā jñātāś citta-vṛttayas tat-prabhoḥ
puruṣasyāpariṇāmitvāt.

सदा always ज्ञाताः (are) known चित्तवृत्तयः the modifications of the mind तत्-प्रभोः of its lord पुरुषस्य of the *Puruṣa* अपरिणामित्वात् on account of the changelessness or constancy.

18. The modifications of the mind are always known to its lord on account of the changelessness of the *Puruṣa*.

As soon as an object colours the mind the modification is at once witnessed by the *Puruṣa* and it is this witnessing by the *Puruṣa* which brings about the 'knowing' of the object. The use of the word 'witness' for the reaction of the *Puruṣa* to the modifications taking place in the mind is not appropriate but is resorted to in order to distinguish it from the simultaneous mental process which is generally called perception. All our words such as 'knowing', 'perceiving' are so closely identified with the activities of the mind that a new word is really needed to indicate this peculiar ultimate reaction of the *Puruṣa* to all mental processes. But, in the absence of such a word in the English language 'witnessing' will perhaps do for the present, provided we keep in mind its special significance. This 'witnessing' by the *Puruṣa* of the modification produced in the mind is the second indispensable condition of 'knowing' any object by the mind, the first being its 'colouring' by the object. Researches in psychology have shown that the mind is frequently modified by external objects even though it is not aware of them at the time, the proof of such modifications having taken place lying in the fact that such impressions can be recovered later from the mind by hypnotizing the person. So that, the 'witnessing' by the *Puruṣa* of the modifications produced in the mind is independent of the conscious activity of the mind. This is the significance of the word *Sadā* which means literally 'always' or 'ever'. What is meant to be conveyed in the *Sūtra* is that the *Puruṣa* is aware, in an unbroken manner, of all the changes which are taking place in the mind and it is not possible for any change to escape his notice. This is so because he is eternal. It is only a changeless, eternal consciousness which can provide such a constant and perfect background for the continuous and complex changes which are taking place in the mind. If the background itself is changeable there is bound to be confusion. You cannot project a cinema picture on a screen which itself is changing constantly.

Another point to note is that the *Puruṣa* should not only provide a constant background for the modifications of the mind but that his consciousness should be the ultimate background in order that he may be able to notice modifications in the mind at all its levels. When the *Yogi* passes into *Samādhi* and dives into the deeper levels of the mind he is not conscious of any break in his experiences. The new consciousness which emerges at each level seems to take in, understand and co-ordinate experiences of all the previous stages and, therefore, there must really be the same consciousness illuminating the *Citta* at all these different levels. It is not only our ordinary experiences at the level of the concrete mind of which this ultimate consciousness is constantly aware but also all the supra-mental experiences through which the *Yogi* passes in *Samādhi*.

The extraordinary comprehensiveness which characterizes consciousness of the *Puruṣa* in the ultimate background, is, of course, due to the fact that it is eternal, beyond time and space, and contains simultaneously within itself everything that can ever manifest in the realms of time and space. It is only white light which is a harmonious synthesis of all possible colours which can be used in the projection of a coloured film on a cinematographic screen. Coloured light which is incomplete cannot be used for such a purpose.

१९. न तत् स्वाभासं दृश्यत्वात् ।

Na tat svābhāsaṃ dṛśyatvāt.

न not तत् it स्वाभासम् self-illuminative दृश्यत्वात् because of its knowability or perceptibility.

19. Nor is it self-illuminative, for it is perceptible.

After stating in IV-18 that the *Puruṣa* is the sole eternal witness of all modifications in the mind at whatever level they may take place, Patañjali proceeds to substantiate this statement by a chain of reasoning developed in the next four *Sūtras*.

The first link in this chain is that the mind is not self-illuminative, i.e. capable of perceiving by its own power, because it is itself perceptible. It is not like the Sun which shines by its own light but like the moon which shines by the light of another heavenly body. The fact that the mind is perceptible follows from our ordinary experience of being able to watch its activities and modifications whenever we want to do so. It is true that when our attention is directed outwards we are not conscious of the changes which are taking place in our mind, but we can at any moment direct our attention inwards and observe these changes.

This fact of the mind being perceptible and performing its function of perception through the agency of some other power is brought home to the *Yogi* more vividly in *Samādhi* when he transcends different levels of the mind one after another. At each critical stage of this process of diving inwards towards the centre of his being, as he leaves one level of the mind for another, the perceiver seems to become the perceived. This continuous shifting of the boundary between the subjective and the objective proves to the *Yogi* that not only the lower concrete mind but even its subtlest grades are mere mechanisms of perception. The source of illuminating power of consciousness is somewhere else—in the *Puruṣa*.

२०. एकसमये चोभयानवधारणम् ।

Eka-samaye cobhayānavadhāraṇam.

एकसमये at the same time; simultaneously च and उभय both (opposite sides) अनवधारणम् absence of cognizing; non-comprehending.

20. Moreover, it is impossible for it to be of both ways (as perceiver and perceived) at the same time.

The fact that the mind is perceptible is a matter of experience. Now, if the mind is perceptible it cannot at the same time be the perceiver. The same thing cannot be the perceiver and the perceived. If the mind is perceptible it follows that there must be a power, of the nature of consciousness, which enables the mind to perform its functions of perception. Since the mind seems to perform its function of perception through the power of consciousness it cannot perceive consciousness itself, or to put it in other words, consciousness cannot be the object of perception by the mind. That is why it is impossible for us to know what consciousness is in itself as long as we are within the realms of the mind. As long as the cognitive aspect of consciousness acts through the medium of the mind it is turned outwards, as it were, and cognizes other things in the realm of the mind. It is only when it is released from the bondage of the mind and turns inwards upon itself that it can cognize itself, as explained in IV-22.

२१. चित्तान्तरदृश्ये बुद्धिबुद्धेरतिप्रसङ्गः स्मृतिसंकरश्च ।

Cittāntara-dṛśye buddhi-buddher atiprasaṅgaḥ smṛti-saṃkaraś ca.

चित्तान्तरदृश्ये in (one mind) being cognizable by another mind बुद्धिबुद्धेः cognition of cognitions अतिप्रसङ्गः superfluity of proving too much; *reductio ad absurdum* स्मृति of memories संकरः confusion च and.

21. If cognition of one mind by another (be postulated) we would have to assume cognition of cognitions and confusion of memories also.

Here a philosophical objection may be raised. Instead of postulating the existence of the one *Puruṣa* whose consciousness illuminates the mind at all its levels, we may suppose that each individual possesses a number of minds each subtler than the one which has been transcended. These different minds instead of being illuminated by one source of consciousness may be supposed to be independent of each other and the *Yogi* in *Samādhi* may be supposed to be merely passing into the realms of these different independent minds one after another. Such a supposition would dispense with the necessity of postulating the existence of the *Puruṣa* whose consciousness according to *Yogic* philosophy is the source of illumination for all the different grades of mind. But this hypothesis while doing away with the *Puruṣa* will lead us into all kinds of intellectual difficulties. For example, if we suppose that there are a number of independent minds, each mind perceiving those which are denser than itself and being perceived by those which are subtler, then there should be a corresponding number of *Buddhis*. According to the *Yogic* philosophy the mind is a mere instrument and the function of cognition which is a reflection of the cognitive aspect of Reality, *Citi*, is quite different from it though necessarily associated with it in all acts of mental perception. It follows, therefore, that if there are a number of independent minds then there must be a corresponding number of *Buddhis* also, for each mind must have its own separate *Buddhi* without which it cannot function. So, on the basis of this hypothesis, we would have not only a number of minds but also a corresponding number of *Buddhis* functioning simultaneously within the same individual which will mean cognition of cognition. The phrase *Atiprasaṅgaḥ* means not only 'too many' but also '*reductio ad absurdum*'. So both the meanings are applicable to the logical conclusion to which we are led from the original supposition. The absurdity lies in having to postulate the existence of a number of *Buddhic* functions where only one can exist. Just as the mind integrates the reports of the various sense-organs into one harmonized mental conception, so our *Buddhi* is supposed to integrate into one co-ordinated understanding the knowledge received through the different levels of the mind and it is impossible, therefore, to conceive that a number of *Buddhis* can function simultaneously within the same individual. It is possible to assume multiplicity of instruments for obtaining knowledge or experience but no multiplicity can be assumed with respect to the agency which co-ordinates and harmonizes all the knowledge gathered through different sources or instruments. This, by its very nature, must be one, otherwise there is bound to be chaos.

Besides this difficulty, another will be the confusion of memories. If there are a number of minds, each with its own set of memories, and there are also many independent *Buddhis*, the co-ordinating agency which integrates all these memories into one harmonious whole will be absent and the result must be chaos within our mind. The most remarkable fact with regard to our mind is the existence of perfect co-ordination and harmonization in the midst of the most complicated and multifarious mental phenomena and experiences. This is especially noticeable in the practice of *Yoga* when we dive into the deeper levels of the mind and traverse the subtler worlds with all their exquisitely fine and extraordinary experiences. It is the *Buddhic* principle within us which enables this co-ordination to be effected and the hypothesis of many independent minds which requires the elimination of this co-ordinating factor has therefore to be rejected.

२२. चितेरप्रतिसंक्रमायास्तदाकारापत्तौ स्वबुद्धिसंवेदनम् ।

Citer apratisaṃkramāyās tad-ākārāpattau
sva-buddhi-saṃvedanaṃ.

चितेः of the consciousness अप्रतिसंक्रमायाः (अ+प्रति+सं+क्रम) of such as does not pass from place to place तद्-आकार its form आपत्तौ: on the assumption (of) स्वबुद्धि self-cognition संवेदनम् knowing (of).

22. Knowledge of its own nature through self-cognition (is obtained) when consciousness assumes that form in which it does not pass from place to place.

If cognition takes place through the agency of the mind and in the subtlest cognitions pertaining to the deepest levels of the mind we can know only the mind thus illuminated by consciousness, the question naturally arises " How are we to know consciousness itself or that light which illuminates the mind at all its levels? " The answer to this important question is given in the *Sūtra* under discussion, but before we can understand its meanings it is necessary to consider carefully the various expressions used in it.

Citeḥ means ' of consciousness ' and is derived from *Citi* and not *Citta* which means the mind. *Apratisaṃkramāyāḥ* means ' not passing from one to another ', i.e. not passing from one level of *Citta* to another or from one vehicle to another. In *Samādhi* consciousness passes from one level of *Citta* to another and the phrase refers to the stage when this process stops or is brought to its limit. *Tad-ākārāpattau* means ' on the accomplishment or assumption of its own form '. Consciousness normally functions through the mind. This phrase refers to the condition in which it is freed from the limitations of the mind and is functioning in its own form. *Sva-buddhi* means *Buddhi* as it really is and not as it functions through the medium of the mind. We know only this function of perception as it appears in association with *Citta*. *Sva-buddhi* is the function of perception as it is when exercised upon itself. *Saṃvedanaṃ* means 'knowing of'. Knowing is really a function of consciousness but when exercised through the mind becomes knowing something outside or external to pure consciousness. The phrase *Sva-buddhi-saṃvedanaṃ* therefore means the knowledge which results when the faculty of *Buddhi* is turned upon itself. Normally, *Buddhi* functions through *Citta* and helps the mind to perceive and understand objects in its realm. But when it is freed from the association of *Citta* it automatically turns upon itself and illuminates its own nature, i.e. consciousness. It is because the power of illumination is inherent in it that it illuminates *Citta* when it functions through *Citta*. If a light is enclosed within a translucent globe it reveals the globe. If the globe is removed the light reveals itself. From the meanings and explanations of the different phrases given above the inner significance of the *Sūtra* should now be quite clear. *Buddhi*, as has been pointed out before, is that faculty which enables the mind to perceive and understand objects in the phenomenal worlds, the mind being inert and incapable of performing this function. As long as *Buddhi* is functioning through the medium of the mind it is not possible to know pure consciousness. It is only when it assumes that form in which all movement from one level of *Citta* to another has been eliminated that it reveals its real nature. As has been pointed out before, *Citta* or the mind has many levels corresponding to the different vehicles of consciousness and in *Samādhi* consciousness moves up and down from one level to another between the centre and periphery. In this kind of movement of consciousness there is no movement in space but only movement in different dimensions, the centre from which consciousness functions always remaining the same. When consciousness, in the state of *Samādhi*, has penetrated into the deepest level of *Citta* and then finally transcended even this level it is quite free from the limiting and obscuring action of *Citta* and it is only then that its true nature is realized. In this state the perceiver, perceived and perception all merge into one Self-illuminated Reality. So the answer to the question 'How are we to know consciousness itself?' is 'By diving in *Samādhi* into our consciousness until the mind in its subtlest form is transcended and the Reality hidden beneath it is revealed '.

From what has been said above it is apparent that we cannot understand the real nature of consciousness by applying the ordinary methods of modern psychology. What is known as consciousness in terms of modern psychology is only consciousness veiled by many layers of the mind, each of which increasingly obscures and modifies its nature as it infiltrates into the outermost physical mechanism, namely, the human brain. We thus observe consciousness in its ordinary manifestations through the physical brain under the greatest possible limitations and it is not possible to form any idea with regard to its true nature from these extremely partial and distorted manifestations. As well might a person who had always lived in a dungeon situated in a land where it was perpetually cloudy, try to form an idea regarding the light of the Sun from the gloom in which he lived. It will be seen, therefore, that not only is it impossible to know the true nature of consciousness by adopting the ordinary means available to the modern psychologist but also that the only effective means of doing so is to adopt the *Yogic* method. This is a subjective method, no doubt, and beyond the capacity of the ordinary man but it is the only method available. No amount of dissection of the brain and the nervous systems and study of human behaviour can unravel for us the mystery of consciousness itself. A great deal of research in this field of psychology is being carried on in very imposing laboratories in the West, a vast amount of so-called scientific data is being accumulated but all this effort is bound to prove futile from the very nature of the problem being tackled. The modern craze of submitting everything to physical examination may succeed with physical things but no physical instruments can ever be devised which will reveal the nature of consciousness which is of the nature of Spirit. All this waste of effort can be avoided and the whole field of modern psychology illuminated in the most effective manner if the facts of *Yogic* philosophy are properly understood and used in the study of psychological problems.

The student will have noticed that in the ideas set forth in the above pages no effort has been made to link up the facts of

Yogic philosophy with doctrines which are considered to be religious. But this does not mean that there is no relation between them. In fact, a religious man can see, if he studies the subject of *Yoga* with an open mind, that all the ideas of *Yogic* philosophy can be interpreted in religious terms, and the consciousness which the *Yogi* seeks to uncover within the folds of his mind is nothing but that Supreme Reality which is commonly referred to as God. God is recognized by every religion with any philosophical background to be a Mighty Being whose consciousness transcends the manifested Universe. He is considered to be hidden within every human heart. He is supposed to transcend the mind. Basically, these ideas are the same as those of *Yogic* philosophy. The main difference lies in the assertion by *Yogic* philosophy that this Supreme Reality or Consciousness is not merely a matter for speculation or even adoration but can be discovered by following a technique which is as definite and unfailing as the technique of any modern Science. *Yoga* thus imparts a tremendous significance to religion and places the whole problem of religious life and endeavour on an entirely new basis and it is difficult to understand how any religious man can reject its claims without giving them due consideration.

२३. द्रष्टृदृश्योपरक्तं चित्तं सर्वार्थम् ।

Draṣṭṛ-dṛśyoparaktaṃ cittaṃ sarvārtham.

द्रष्टृ the knower दृश्य and the knowable or known उपरक्तम् coloured (by) चित्तम् the mind सर्वार्थम् all-apprehending; all-including.

23. The mind coloured by the Knower (i.e., the *Puruṣa*) and the Known is all-apprehending.

This *Sūtra* apparently sums up what has been said about the *modus operandi* of mental perception in the previous *Sūtras*. Its real importance will, however, be seen only if we understand the significance of the phrase *Sarvārtham*. The mind, in order to know any object, has to be affected in two ways. Firstly, it must be modified or coloured, at least to some extent, by the object which is to be known, and secondly, it must be simultaneously illuminated by the consciousness of the *Puruṣa* which is eternally present in the ultimate background. Modified in this double manner the mind is capable of knowing everything in the phenomenal world, using the word 'knowing' in its most comprehensive sense. The significance of the word *Sarvārtham* which means literally 'all-including' or 'all-apprehending' lies in the fact that the word *Citta* does not stand merely for the medium through which the human intellect finds expression. It stands definitely for the all-inclusive medium through which phenomena of every kind, right from the physical to the *Ātmic* plane, are perceived. Even the thinnest veil of 'matter' which on the *Ātmic* plane obscures the consciousness of the *Puruṣa* and involves him in manifestation is associated with the finest grade of mind. *Citta* is thus co-extensive with *Prakṛti* and both are transcended simultaneously when *Puruṣa* attains Self-realization in *Kaivalya*.

२४. तदसंख्येयवासनाभिश्चित्रमपि परार्थं संहत्यकारित्वात् ।

Tad asaṃkhyeya-vāsanābhiś citram api
parārthaṃ saṃhatya-kāritvāt.

तद् that असंख्येय innumerable वासनाभिः by *Vāsanās* चित्रम् variegated अपि although परार्थम् for the sake of another संहत्यकारित्वात् by reason of acting in collaboration or association.

24. Though variegated by innumerable *Vāsanās* it (the mind) acts for another (*Puruṣa*) for it acts in association.

This *Sūtra* goes with the preceding one and should be studied along with it. Just as *Citta* is universal and embraces all vehicles through which the consciousness of the *Puruṣa* functions in the manifested worlds, in the same way *Vāsanā* is universal in its import and is associated with all the vehicles of consciousness and grades of *Citta*. The word *Vāsanā* is generally translated by the word desire but this is restricting its scope in the same manner as when we confine the meaning of the word *Citta* to that of the medium of the intellect. The clinging to the enjoyments of the lower worlds binds the soul to these worlds and produces all kinds of attachments and consequent suffering. Such clinging is generally known as desire or *Kāma*. But this clinging is not confined to the lower worlds. In its subtler forms it exists even in the higher worlds. In fact, wherever there is *Asmitā* or identification with a vehicle of consciousness there is clinging to the vehicle, however subtle this clinging may be and however spiritual may be the object of this clinging. If there were no clinging or attachment but perfect *Vairāgya* there would be no bondage but Liberation or *Kaivalya*. It is this clinging to the higher modes of existence which constitutes many of the 'fetters' which have to be broken on the path of Liberation.

It is only when *Vāsanā* is understood in this wider sense and not only in the sense of desires pertaining to the lower worlds that we can grasp the significance of the *Sūtra* under discussion. *Vāsanā* permeates life at all its levels including the highest. It has for its objectives things of the most varied nature, from the crudest physical indulgences to the most refined knowledge and bliss of the spiritual planes. But when we pursue these multifarious objectives—and the nature of the objects we seek continually changes as we evolve—what are we really seeking? Are we pursuing these objectives for their own sake? No! We are merely seeking the *Puruṣa* who is our real Self hidden beneath all these attractive objects of pursuit. It is for his sake that we are going through this long and tedious process of evolution. It is really not for the sake of these objects which promise to give us happiness that we pursue them but for the sake of someone else (*Parārthaṃ*) and that is the *Puruṣa*.

How do we know that it is the *Puruṣa* whom we are seeking in all these multifarious objectives? Because while the objectives keep changing all the time and never satisfy us he always remains in the background. He is the common factor in all our efforts to find happiness through ever-changing forms and, therefore, he must be the real object of our search. Simple reasoning, is it not?

He is thus not only the constant background of consciousness (IV-18) which illuminates the mind in all its activities but also the hidden drawing force of desire in all its forms and phases.

One important consequence of the *Puruṣa* being the ultimate goal amidst all the changing objectives which we pursue is that no condition of existence attained by the *Yogi*, however exalted it may be, can give him abiding peace. The Divine urge within him will, sooner or later, assert itself and make him dissatisfied with the condition he has attained, until he has found the *Puruṣa* in Self-realization. For the consciousness of the *Puruṣa* alone is Self-sufficient, Self-contained and Self-illuminated and until this is attained there can be no real security, no real freedom and no abiding peace.

२५. विशेषदर्शिन आत्मभावभावनाविनिवृत्तिः ।

Viśeṣa-darśina ātma-bhāva-bhāvanā-
vinivṛttiḥ.

विशेष the distinction दर्शिनः of him who sees आत्मभाव consciousness of the *Ātmic* plane भावना dwelling in or upon (in mind); reflection विनिवृत्तिः complete cessation (because of satisfaction). [Some editions read निवृत्तिः.]

25. The cessation (of desire) for dwelling in the consciousness of *Ātmā* for one who has seen the distinction.

When this fact is realized even the subtle *Vāsanā* which binds the *Yogi* to the transcendent bliss and spiritual illumination of the *Ātmic* plane ceases and he bends all his energies to tear down the last and the finest veil which hides the face of the Beloved. The distinction indicated by *Viśeṣa* has already been discussed in the previous *Sūtra*. It is the distinction between our true objective which is Self-realization and the innumerable and ever-changing objectives which we pursue in our search for happiness. The phrase *Ātma-Bhāva* is used for the exalted consciousness functioning on the *Ātmic* level—the last stage before *Kaivalya* is attained. The word *Bhāva* is a technical term used in *Yoga* for denoting the functioning of consciousness on the spiritual planes where perception is synthetic and all-inclusive and not of particular objects as on the lower planes. *Bhāvanā* is another technical term which means 'dwelling in mind upon' but used in conjunction with *Ātma-Bhāva* it will naturally mean living in and experiencing the transcendent knowledge and bliss of the *Ātmic* plane.

It may appear to the student that the renunciation of the attractions which bind the *Yogi* to the exalted condition of the *Ātmic* plane should be a comparatively easy matter considering the wisdom he has acquired and the *Vairāgya* he has developed. But, in judging of the effort required he should remember that the consciousness of this plane represents the acme of power, bliss and knowledge which is utterly beyond human comprehension and cannot be compared with anything with which we are familiar on the lower planes. Besides, the transcending of the *Ātmic* plane which he has now to attempt really means the destruction of his very individuality since the *Ātmā* is the very core of his separate existence in the realm of manifestation. It is true that a still higher and subtler kind of individuality emerges when the separate individual life of *Ātmā* is given up, but tremendous faith is needed for taking that final plunge into the void which now opens before him. And the basis of this faith is the realization that attachment to the transcendent consciousness of the *Ātmic* plane is still attachment to something which is not the Supreme Reality, which is still in the domain of *Citta* and *Vāsanā* and, therefore, subject to illusion, however subtle that illusion might be.

The desire for this transcendent bliss and knowledge which is inherent in the consciousness of the *Ātmic* plane destroys and eliminates the lower desires and brings the *Yogi* to the highest level of enlightenment which is possible within the realm of *Prakṛti*, but even this knowledge and bliss when they are acquired become, in their turn, the means of bondage and must be given up before the final objective is achieved. This is a fundamental law of life—the lower must be given up before the next higher can be gained.

२६. तदा हि विवेकनिम्नं कैवल्यप्राग्भारं चित्तम् ।

Tadā hi viveka-nimnaṃ kaivalya-
prāgbhāram cittam.

तदा then हि verily विवेकनिम्नं inclined towards discrimination कैवल्यप्राग्भारम् heading or gravitating towards *Kaivalya* चित्तम् the mind.

26. Then, verily, the mind is inclined towards discrimination and gravitating towards *Kaivalya*.

When the realization of the inadequacy of *Ātma-Bhāva* dawns upon the *Yogi* he determines to break this last fetter by renouncing the bliss and knowledge of the *Ātmic* plane. Thenceforward all his efforts are directed towards the attainment of *Kaivalya* by the constant exercise of that intense and penetrating discrimination which alone can pierce through the last veil of Illusion. This and the next three *Sūtras* throw some light on this last struggle of the soul to free itself completely from the bondage of matter before attaining *Kaivalya*.

It should be noted that the word used in this *Sūtra* for the agent which carries on this struggle is *Citta*. "The *Citta* is gravitating towards *Kaivalya* ". But how can *Citta*, which is sought to be transcended in the process, struggle to attain liberation from itself? It would be like a person trying to lift himself up by his boot-straps. The resolution of this paradox lies in the fact that it is not the mind really which is struggling to free the consciousness from the limitations in which it has got involved. Hidden behind the mind is the *Puruṣa*, who all along in the entire cycle of evolution is the real driving force behind the struggle to attain Self-realization. When the iron filings are attracted by a magnet it is the filings which appear to move but in reality it is the magnet which has induced magnetism in the filings and is the cause of the movement.

The weapons used in this last stage of the struggle for Liberation are *Viveka* and *Vairāgya*. The *Yogi* has obtained a glimpse of the Reality within him. He has to try and gain the awareness of Reality, again and again, through *Viveka* so that this awareness can be maintained without interruption (II-26). And, at the same time, he has to intensify his *Vairāgya* to such an extent that he passes into *Dharma-Megha-Samādhi* (IV-29). It is interesting to note that the weapons used in the last stage are the same as those used in the first stage. The *Yogi* enters the path of *Yoga* through *Viveka* and *Vairāgya* and he also leaves this path through *Viveka* and *Vairāgya*.

२७. तच्छिद्रेषु प्रत्ययान्तराणि संस्कारेभ्यः ।

Tac-chidreṣu pratyayāntarāṇi saṃskāre-bhyaḥ.

तच्छिद्रेषु in the breaks in it (discrimination) प्रत्ययान्तराणि other *Pratyayas* संस्कारेभ्यः from the force of impressions.

27. In the intervals arise other *Pratyayas* from the force of *Saṃskāras*.

This *Sūtra* describes the swaying, to and fro, of consciousness in the borderland which separates the Real from the unreal. The *Yogi* is trying to maintain his foothold in the world of Reality but he is thrown back again and again into the realm of Illusion, though this Illusion is of the subtlest kind. He cannot maintain steadily that condition of consciousness which is indicated by *Viveka Khyāti* and each relaxation in effort is followed instantly by the appearance of a *Pratyaya* which characterizes the functioning of consciousness through the medium of *Citta*. *Pratyaya*, as we have seen already, is a word used generally for the content of consciousness when it is functioning normally through a vehicle of any degree of subtlety. Emergence of a *Pratyaya*, therefore, means that the consciousness has temporarily receded from the Reality realized in *Nirbīja Samādhi* and is functioning at one or another level of *Citta*. It may be worthwhile pointing out here again that the word *Pratyaya* like *Citta* or *Vāsanā* is of universal import and is co-extensive with them. Wherever consciousness is functioning normally through any level of *Citta* in a vehicle there must be a content of consciousness which is called *Pratyaya* in *Yogic* terminology. It is only in *Asaṃprajñāta Samādhi* that there is no *Pratyaya* but this is so because consciousness is passing through a critical phase and is really hovering between two vehicles. Even on the highest level of *Citta* corresponding to the *Ātmic* plane there is a *Pratyaya* although it is impossible for us to visualize what it is like. When consciousness is thrown back into the *Ātmic* or any other lower vehicle owing to the relaxation of *Viveka*, *Pratyaya* of the corresponding plane emerges at once into the field of consciousness.

Why is the *Yogi's* consciousness thrown back into the vehicles which he has transcended and why do these *Pratyayas* appear, again and again, in this stage of his progress towards Self-realization? Because the *Saṃskāras* which he has brought over from his past are still present in his vehicles in a dormant condition and emerge into his consciousness as soon as there is relaxation of effort or a temporary interruption of *Viveka Khyāti*. As long as these 'seeds' are present merely in a dormant condition and have not been 'burnt' or rendered quite harmless by *Dharma-Megha-Samādhi* they must sprout into his consciousness as soon as a suitable opportunity presents itself.

२८. हानमेषां क्लेशवदुक्तम् ।

Hānam eṣāṃ kleśavad uktam.

हानम् removal एषाम् of these क्लेशवत् like that of the *Kleśas* or afflictions उक्तम् has been declared or described.

28. Their removal like that of *Kleśas*, as has been described.

The problem before the *Yogi* therefore is: How to prevent the emergence of these *Pratyayas* which have their source in the *Saṃskāras* brought over from the past? The activation of the *Saṃskāras* is to be prevented by the method which has been prescribed for the removal of *Kleśas* in Section II (10, 11 and 26). The reason for this should be obvious to the student if he has understood the nature of *Kleśas*, their relation to *Karmas* and the method of their removal as outlined in Section II. The *Karmas* or *Saṃskāras* which are rooted in *Kleśas* cannot become active if the *Kleśas* are quiescent. The *Kleśas* must remain quiescent in the absence of *Avidyā* from which they are all derived (II-4). *Avidyā* cannot manifest as long as the *Yogi* is able to keep undimmed his discriminative faculty and to manintain that awareness of Reality which is known as *Viveka Khyāti* (II-26). It follows logically, therefore, that the only way to prevent the dormant *Saṃskāras* from becoming active is to maintain undimmed *Viveka Khyāti* as indicated in II-26. The moment this is interrupted the door opens for the emergence of *Pratyayas* which are sought to be excluded completely at this stage. The chief effort of the *Yogi* in this last stage of his struggle to attain *Kaivalya* is thus to acquire the capacity to maintain undimmed and unbroken this high and penetrating state of discrimination which keeps the force of *Avidyā* in abeyance. Upon his capacity to maintain this condition indefinitely depends the possibility of his entering *Dharma-Megha-Samādhi* which burns the seeds of *Saṃskaras* and makes their re-activation impossible.

२९. प्रसंख्यानेऽप्यकुसीदस्य सर्वथा विवेकख्यातेर्धर्ममेघः समाधिः ।

Prasaṃkhyāne 'py akusīdasya sarvathā
viveka-khyater dharma-meghaḥ
samādhiḥ.

प्रसंख्याने in the knowledge of the highest meditation अपि even अकुसीदस्य of one who has no interest left सर्वथा in every way; by all means विवेकख्यातेः discrimination leading to awareness of Reality धर्ममेघः showering the *Dharmas*; relating to properties समाधिः trance.

29. In the case of one, who is able to maintain a constant state of *Vairāgya* even towards the most exalted state of enlightenment and to exercise the highest kind of discrimination, follows *Dharma-Megha-Samādhi*.

By the uninterrupted practice of *Viveka Khyāti* the *Yogi* keeps *Avidyā* at bay and prevents the emergence of *Pratyayas* in his exalted consciousness. To this is added the practice of that highest kind of mental renunciation which is known as *Para-Vairāgya*. In spite of the overpowering attraction of the high state of illumination and bliss which he has attained he renounces completely his attachment to it and maintains uninterruptedly this attitude of supreme non-attachment towards it. In fact, *Para-Vairāgya* which he is now practising is nothing new but is merely the culmination of the renunciation which he has been practising since his entry into the path of *Yoga*. Just as *Viveka Khyāti* has its beginnings in very simple forms of *Viveka* and is developed by prolonged and intensive practice during his progress, in the same way *Para-Vairāgya* develops from simple acts of renunciation and reaches its culmination in the renunciation of the bliss and illumination of the *Ātmic* plane. It should also be borne in mind that *Viveka* and *Vairāgya* are very closely related to each other and are really like two sides of the same coin. *Viveka*, by opening the eyes of the soul, brings about non-attachment to the objects which keep it in bondage and the non-attachment thus developed, in its turn, further clarifies the vision of the soul and enables it to see more deeply into the illusion of life. *Viveka* and *Vairāgya* thus strengthen and reinforce each other and form a kind of 'virtuous circle' which accelerates in an ever-increasing degree the progress of the *Yogi* towards Self-realization.

The combined practice of *Viveka Khyāti* and *Para-Vairāgya* when continued for a long time reaches, by a process of mutual reinforcement, a tremendous degree of intensity and culminates ultimately in *Dharma-Megha-Samādhi*, the highest kind of *Samādhi* which burns up the 'seeds' of *Saṃskāras* and unlocks the gates of the World of Reality in which the *Puruṣa* lives eternally. Why this *Samādhi* is called *Dharma-Megha-Samādhi* is not generally understood and the statements usually made are forced explanations which do not make sense. In most of these explanations the word *Dharma* is interpreted as virtue or merit and *Dharma-Megha* is taken to mean 'a cloud which showers virtues or merit' which, of course, explains nothing. The significance of the phrase *Dharma-Megha* will become clear if we assign to the word *Dharma* the meaning which it has in IV-12, namely that of property, characteristic or function. *Megha,* of course, is a technical term used in *Yogic* literature for the cloudy or misty condition through which consciousness passes in the critical state of *Asaṃprajñāta Samādhi* when there is nothing in the field of consciousness.

Now, *Nirbīja Samādhi* which is practised in this last stage which we are considering is a kind of *Asaṃprajñāta Samādhi* in which the consciousness of the *Yogi* is trying to free itself from the last veil of illusion to emerge into the Light of Reality itself. When this effort succeeds the consciousness of the *Yogi* leaves the world of manifestation in which *Guṇas* and their peculiar combinations, namely, *Dharmas,* operate and emerges into the world of Reality in which they no longer exist. His condition may be compared to the condition of a pilot in an aeroplane who comes out of a cloud bank into bright sunlight and begins to see everything clearly. *Dharma-Megha-Samādhi,* therefore, means the final *Samādhi* in which the *Yogi* shakes himself free from the world of *Dharmas* which obscure Reality like a cloud.

The passage through *Dharma-Megha-Samādhi* completes the evolutionary cycle of the individual and by destroying *Avidyā,* completely and for ever, brings about the end of *Saṃyoga* of *Puruṣa* and *Prakṛti* referred to in II-23. No more can *Avidyā* again obscure the vision of the *Puruṣa* who has attained full Self-realization. This process is irreversible and after reaching this stage it is not possible for the *Puruṣa* to fall again into the realm of *Māyā* from which he has obtained Liberation. Before this final goal was reached it was possible for the *Yogi* to fall even from a very high stage of enlightenment, but not after he has passed through *Dharma-Megha-Samādhi* and attained the Enlightenment of *Kaivalya.*

The next five *Sūtras* merely describe the results of passing through *Dharma-Megha-Samādhi* and attaining *Kaivalya.* It should be noted here that no effort is made to describe the experience of Reality. That would be futile for no one can imagine the transcendent glory of that consciousness into which the *Yogi* passes on attaining *Kaivalya.* Mystics have sometimes tried to convey in rapturous language the glorious visions of the higher planes which they have reached in *Samādhi.* These descriptions, though very inspiring, yet fail utterly to give to those who are still blind any idea of the beauty and grandeur of those planes. How can, then, anyone convey through the crude medium of language even a hint regarding that Supreme experience which the *Yogi* gains on attaining *Kaivalya* and Patañjali, knowing the futility of such a task, has not even attempted it. But he has given in a few *Sūtras* some of the results which accrue from the attainment of *Kaivalya.*

३०. ततः क्लेशकर्मनिवृत्तिः ।

Tataḥ kleśa-karma-nivṛttiḥ.

ततः thence क्लेश afflictions कर्म action and its reactions निवृत्तिः cessation; freedom from.

30. Then follows freedom from *Kleśas* and *Karmas*.

The first result of attaining *Kaivalya* is that the *Yogi* cannot thenceforward be bound by *Kleśas* and *Karmas*. The attainment of *Kaivalya* follows the destruction of *Kleśas* and *Karmas*. What the *Sūtra*, therefore, means is that the very potentiality for the re-emergence of these two instruments of bondage is destroyed. The *Jīvanmukta* cannot, after passing through *Dharma-Megha-Samādhi* and attaining *Kaivalya*, again fall into *Avidyā* and start generating *Karmas* which bind.

The relation of *Kleśas* and *Karmas* should always be borne in mind by the student, for on this is based the technique of attaining freedom from the binding action of *Karma*. *Kleśas* and *Karmas* are related to each other as cause and effect, as has been thoroughly explained under II-12 and no *Karma* can bind where there is no *Avidyā* but awareness of Reality. All action in this state is necessarily done in complete identification with the Divine Consciousness without the slightest identification with the individual ego. That is why no result accrues to the individual. The illusion of a separate life has been destroyed and no separate individual, in the ordinary sense, really exists under these conditions. It is true that according to the *Yogic* philosophy each *Puruṣa* is a separate individual but the separate individuality of each *Puruṣa* means merely that He is a separate centre of consciousness in the Supreme Reality and not that his consciousness is separated from that of other *Puruṣas* and pursues its separate individual ends as in the case of ordinary individuals blinded by illusion of a separate life. Separate individuality is perfectly compatible with the closest unification of consciousness, as every mystic or occultist who has experience of the higher spiritual consciousness definitely knows. In *Kaivalya* this paradoxical simultaneity of Individuality and Oneness reaches its utmost perfection.

३१. तदा सर्वावरणमलापेतस्य ज्ञानस्यानन्त्याज्ज्ञेयमल्पम् ।

Tadā sarvāvaraṇa-malāpetasya jñānasyā-
nantyāj jñeyam alpam.

तदा then सर्व all आवरण that which covers up, veils or distorts मल impurities अपेतस्य devoid of; from which is removed ज्ञानस्य of knowledge आनन्त्यात् because of the infinity of ज्ञेयम् the knowable अल्पम् but little.

31. Then, in consequence of the removal of all obscuration and impurities, that which can be known (through the mind) is but little in comparison with the infinity of knowledge (obtained in Enlightenment).

The second consequence of attaining *Kaivalya* is the sudden expansion of consciousness into the realm of infinite knowledge. When the last veil of illusion is removed in *Dharma-Megha-Samādhi* the Enlightenment which comes is of an entirely new kind. In the different stages of *Sabīja Samādhi* the knowledge which comes at each successive expansion of consciousness into a higher realm of *Citta* appears tremendously greater than in the preceding stage. But even the transcendent knowledge of the *Ātmic* plane which represents the highest reach of the mind in the realm of manifestation sinks into insignificance when compared with *Viveka-jaṃ-Jnānam* (III-55) which comes in the state of Enlightenment of *Kaivalya*. A million and a billion are increasingly tremendous magnitudes as compared with one, but they all sink into insignificance when compared with infinity as the following mathematical equations will show

$$\frac{1}{\infty} = 0 \qquad \frac{1,000,000}{\infty} = 0 \qquad \frac{1,000,000,000}{\infty} = 0$$

When we are in the realm of Infinity we are not in the realm of magnitudes at all. So the *Jīvanmukta* is not really in the realm of knowledge but has transcended knowledge and passed into the realm of pure consciousness. Knowledge is produced by the imposition of mental limitations on pure consciousness, and so even the highest kind of knowledge cannot be compared with the Enlightenment which comes when all these limitations are removed and the *Yogi* passes into the realm of pure consciousness. The relation of knowledge and Enlightenment is analogous to the relation of Time and Eternity. Eternity is not time of infinite extent but a state which transcends Time altogether. The two states do not belong to the same category.

It may be pointed out here that all the real mysteries of Life which we try to unravel by the help of the intellect are really rooted in the Eternal and are expressions in terms of Time and Space of realities which exist in their true form (*Svarūpa*) in the Eternal. That is why it is not possible to solve any real problem of Life as long as our consciousness is confined within the realm of the unreal, and much less so, while it is still confined within the narrow and cramping limitations of the intellect. The so-called intellectual solutions of our problems which academic philosophy seeks to provide are no solutions at all but merely statements of the same problems in different terms which really push back the problems to a deeper level. The only effective way to solve all these problems is to dive into our own consciousness by the help of the technique outlined in the *Yogic* philosophy and to free our consciousness from all limitations which obscure its Self-illumination. In the Light of the Eternal alone can all problems of Life be solved, because as said above, they are all rooted in the Eternal. To be more exact, the problems are not *solved* in the Light of the

Eternal consciousness, solution being a process characteristic of the illusion-bound intellect. They are *resolved.* They are no longer there, for they were shadows cast by the intellect in the realm of the unreal and naturally cannot exist in the domain of the Real.

It also follows from what has been said above that the Mystery of Life cannot be unravelled piecemeal. We cannot break up this Great Mystery into a number of component problems and then proceed to solve these problems, one by one, although this is what modern philosophy attempts to do. The resolution of the Mystery depends upon obtaining the synthetic vision of the Eternal and not upon putting together the separate and partial solutions obtained by the analytical processes of the intellect. It is a question of ' All or none '.

That is why the *Yogi* does not make any serious effort to solve the so-called problems of Life by the intellectual processes, knowing as he does that the best solution which he can get in this manner is not a real solution. Not that he despises the intellect, but he knows its inherent limitations and uses it only to transcend those limitations. He holds his soul in patience and bends all his energies in attaining the goal pointed out by the *Yogic* philosophy. This philosophy does not hold out any promise of solving the problems of Life but provides the key which unlocks the World of Reality in which all these problems are resolved and seen in their true nature and perspective.

३२. ततः कृतार्थानां परिणामक्रमसमाप्तिर्गुणानाम् ।

Tataḥ kṛtārthānāṃ pariṇāma-krama-
samāptir guṇānām.

ततः by that; therefore कृतार्थानां having fulfilled their object परिणाम of the changes क्रम process समाप्तिः the end गुणानाम् of the *Guṇas* or the three fundamental qualities.

32. The three *Guṇas* having fulfilled their object, the process of change (in the *Guṇas*) comes to an end.

In order to understand this *Sūtra* it is necessary to recall the theory of *Kleśas* discussed in Section II, especially II-23-24 which indicate the purpose and the means of bringing together *Puruṣa* and *Prakṛti*. That purpose having been fulfilled through the destruction of *Avidyā* and the attainment of *Kaivalya*, the compulsory association of *Purusa* and *Prakṛti* dissolves naturally and automatically and with this dissolution comes to an end the transformations of the *Guṇas*.

According to the *Yogic* philosophy the quiescent condition of *Prakṛti* which is known as *Sāmyāvasthā* is disturbed and the incessant transformations of the three *Guṇas* begin when *Puruṣa* and *Prakṛti* are brought together. These transformations continue as long as the association lasts and must come to an end when the association is dissolved, much in the same manner as the electric current stops when the magnetic field is removed in a dynamo. The subsidence of the disturbance in *Prakṛti* and the reversion of the *Guṇas* to the harmonized condition follows as a natural result of the dissociation of *Puruṣa* and *Prakṛti*.

What does this reversion of *Prakṛti* to the *Sāmyāvasthā* mean? Does it mean that *Puruṣa* and *Prakṛti* have reverted to their original state and the valuable fruits of the long evolutionary process are lost? No! The *Puruṣa* retains his Self-realization and *Prakṛti* retains the capacity to respond instantaneously to his consciousness and to serve as an instrument of his will through the efficient and sensitive vehicles which have been built up during the process of evolutionary development. But henceforth, the *Puruṣa* is not bound by the vehicles as he was before the attainment of *Kaivalya*. The vehicles on the different planes of manifestation may be retained or allowed to dissolve but they always remain in their potential form, to spring forth into activity whenever the *Puruṣa* wants to use them. He uses them as mere vehicles for his consciousness without any self-identification and, therefore, without gathering any new *Karmas* or *Saṃskāras*, and he is free to dissociate himself from them and retire into his Real form whenever he so wills. The association between *Puruṣa* and *Prakṛti* is now a completely free and perfect association involving no bondage or compulsion for the *Puruṣa*. He has destroyed *Avidyā* and there are no *Saṃskāras* to keep him bound to the world of manifestation as in the case of the ordinary *Jīvātmā*. The equilibrium of the *Guṇas* now evolved is so stable that they revert to it instantaneously and automatically the moment *Puruṣa* withdraws his consciousness into himself. Not only is it perfectly stable but it contains within it the potentiality of assuming instantaneously any combination that may be required for the expression of consciousness. The student should also read in this connection what has been said in dealing with II-18.

३३. क्षणप्रतियोगी परिणामापरान्तनिर्ग्राह्यः क्रमः ।

Kṣaṇa-pratiyogī pariṇāmāparānta-
nirgrāhyaḥ kramaḥ.

क्षण- moments प्रतियोगी corresponding परिणाम change अपरान्त (at) the final end निर्ग्राह्य: entirely apprehensible क्रम: process; succession.

33. The process, corresponding to moments which become apprehensible at the final end of transformation (of the *Guṇas*), is *Kramaḥ*.

This is one of the most important and interesting *Sūtras* in this Section because it throws some light on the nature of the manifested world and Time. In this *Sūtra* we have a remarkable illustration of the condensation in a few words of a whole theory of a scientific nature which would be dealt with in a volume by a modern writer.

Before we discuss the profound implications of this *Sūtra* it is necessary to explain the significance of some of the words which compose it. For these words stand for definite philosophical concepts and without a knowledge of their connotations it is not possible to appreciate the significance of the *Sūtra*. It is only with the help of such words which stand for a whole set of ideas and are pregnant with profound meanings that a *Sūtra* can be constructed.

Let us take the word *Kṣaṇa*. Literally it means a moment, but behind this simple meaning there is hidden a whole philosophy of Time which throws much light on our modern conception of Time. According to this philosophy, Time, contrary to our impression and belief, is not a continuous thing but discontinuous. Before the advent of modern Science matter was generally considered to be continuous, but investigations in the field of Chemistry showed that it was not continuous but discontinuous, being composed of discrete particles separated from one another by enormous empty spaces. In the same way investigations by *Yogic* methods showed that the apparently continuous series of changes which are taking place in the phenomenal world and by which we measure time, are not really continuous. The changes consist of a number of successive states which are quite distinct and separate from one another.

The mechanism for projecting a cinematographic picture on a screen provides an almost perfect illustration of this actual discontinuity hidden beneath apparent continuity. The following diagram will give some idea of the apparatus which is employed in projecting such a picture.

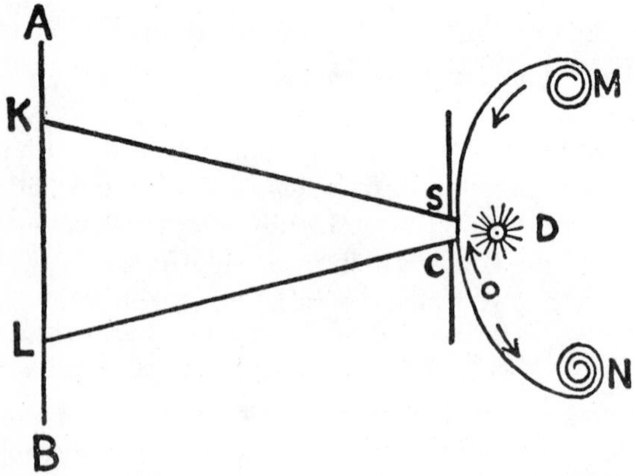

Fig. 15

AB is the screen. D is the source of light. O is an aperture which allows light from D to fall on the screen. This aperture opens and closes alternately and its movement is synchronized with the movement of the film. As the aperture opens, one of the series of pictures in the film comes opposite to it and a beam of light shooting through the picture projects it on the screen. The aperture then closes, the film moves, the next picture comes into place and is projected on the screen as before.

It will be seen, therefore, that the apparently continuous picture produced on the screen is really a series of separate images thrown on the screen in quick succession. The time interval between the successive images is less than one-tenth of a second and that is why we get the impression of a continuous picture.

According to *Yogic* philosophy the seemingly continuous phenomena which we cognize through the instrumentality of the mind are not really continuous and like the cinematographic picture on the screen consist of a series of discontinuous states. Each successive change in the phenomenal world which is separate and distinct produces a corresponding impression upon the mind but these impressions succeed one another with such rapidity that we get the impression of continuity. The interval of time corresponding to each of these successive states is called a *Kṣaṇa.* So *Kṣaṇa* may be called the smallest unit of time which cannot be broken up further.

The next word to be considered is *Kramaḥ.* We have seen just now that the impression of continuous phenomena in our mind is produced by a succession of discontinuous changes in *Prakṛti* around us. *Kramaḥ* stands for this process consisting of a relentless sucession of discontinuous changes underlying all kinds of phenomena. This process is ultimately based upon the unit of time, *Kṣaṇa,* as the projection of the cinematographic picture is based upon each opening and closing of aperture. As *Kṣaṇa* succeeds *Kṣaṇa* the whole manifested world passes from one distinct state to another distinct state, but the succession is so rapid that we are not conscious of the discontinuity.

It will be seen, therefore, that according to the *Yogic* philosophy not only is the whole basis of manifestation material—using the word material in its widest sense—but also that the changes which take place in *Prakṛti* and which produce all kinds of phenomena are essentially mechanical, that is, based on a hidden, essentially mechanical process. The whole manifested Universe and everything in it changes from moment to moment by a relentless law which is inherent in the very nature of manifestation.

If we have grasped the nature of the process indicated by the two words *Kṣaṇa* and *Kramaḥ* it should not be difficult to understand the meaning of the *Sūtra* under discussion. It means simply that the *Yogi* can become aware of the Ultimate Reality only when his consciousness is liberated from the limitations of this process which produces Time, by performing *Saṃyama* on this process as indicated in III-53. As long as his consciousness is involved in the process he cannot know his Real nature. It is only when he steps out of the world of the unreal into the Light of Reality that he realizes not only the true nature of Reality but also of the Relative world of Time and Space which he has left behind.

The thoughtful student may find in the profound idea adumbrated in this *Sūtra* the clue to the nature of Time and Energy and the Quantum Theory which has proved so helpful in the development of modern Science. It is not possible to go into these profound and fundamental problems here but the following two ideas should prove suggestive to the student who is interested in these subjects.

If the fundamental process underlying the phenomenal world is discontinuous then all apparently continuous processes which we can observe and measure must also be discontinuous. Take for example, the radiant energy which comes to us from the Sun. Does this energy flow to us continuously or does it come in discrete portions or quanta? If all the changes in the Solar system are discontinuous and the Solar system, as it were, comes into being and then disappears alternately from moment to moment, then the flow of energy from the Sun must be a discontinuous process. This conclusion which follows from the doctrines of the *Yogic* philosophy is in general accord with the basic idea underlying the Quantum Theory.

The two *Sūtras* III-53 and IV-33 also throw some light on the nature of Time. As the perception of phenomena is the result of the impressions produced in consciousness by a succession of mental images it is the number of mental images which will really determine the duration of the phenomenon which we call Time. There cannot thus be an absolute measure of Time. Time must be related to the number of images which pass through the mind. This idea will throw some light on the different measures of Time which are known to exist on the different planes of the Universe.

३४. पुरुषार्थशून्यानां गुणानां प्रतिप्रसवः कैवल्यं स्वरूपप्रतिष्ठा वा चितिशक्तेरिति ।

Puruṣārtha-śūnyānāṃ guṇānāṃ prati-prasavaḥ kaivalyaṃ svarūpa-pratiṣṭhā vā citi-śakter iti.

पुरुषार्थ aim of the *Puruṣa* शून्यानां devoid of गुणानां of the *Guṇas* or the three fundamental qualities प्रतिप्रसवः re-absorption; recession; re-mergence कैवल्यं Liberation स्वरूप (in) Real or own nature प्रतिष्ठा establishment वा or चितिशक्तेः of the power of pure Consciousness इति Finis.

34. *Kaivalya* is the state (of Enlightenment) following re-mergence of the *Guṇas* because of their becoming devoid of the object of the *Puruṣa*. In this state the *Puruṣa* is established in his Real nature which is pure Consciousness. Finis.

We now come to the last *Sūtra* which defines and sums up the ultimate state of Enlightenment which is called *Kaivalya*. The meaning of the *Sūtra* may be expressed simply in the following words: "*Kaivalya* is that state of Self-realization in which the *Puruṣa* gets established finally when the purpose of his long evolutionary unfoldment has been attained. In this state the *Guṇas*, having fulfilled their purpose, recede to a condition of equilibrium and therefore the power of pure Consciousness can function without any obscuration or limitation."

It should be noted that this is not a description of the content of Consciousness in the state of *Kaivalya*. As has been pointed out before, no one living in the world of the unreal can understand or describe the Reality of which the *Yogi* becomes aware on attaining *Kaivalya.* This *Sūtra* merely points out in a general way certain conditions which are present in *Kaivalya* and which serve to distinguish it from the exalted conditions of consciousness which precede it.

It is natural that vagueness should exist and a large number of misconceptions be prevalent about a state of consciousness and a goal of human achievement which is so utterly beyond human comprehension. But some of these misconceptions are so obvious that it would be worthwhile pointing them out before bringing this chapter to a close.

Does *Kaivalya* mean complete annihilation of the individuality and the merging of the *Yogi's* consciousness in the Divine Consciousness as implied by the well-known sentence 'the dewdrop slips into the Shining Sea'? In considering this important question which has been partly dealt with in II-18 we have to bear in mind that *Kaivalya* is the culmination of a tremendously long evolutionary process extending over innumerable lives and involving enormous periods of time. In the last phase of this evolutionary development which is brought about by the practice of *Yoga,* power, knowledge and bliss unfold from within the *Yogi's* consciousness by leaps and bounds and become so great towards the end that the human mind simply reels from its mere contemplation. At each stage of his progress the *Yogi* finds that the new consciousness which dawns within him is infinitely more vital and glorious than the preceding one and he seems to be progressively uncovering a tremendous Reality which is hidden within the deepest recesses of his own being. *Kaivalya* is attained by transcending the most transcendent state of consciousness which it is possible to attain within the realm of *Prakṛti.* Does it stand to reason that in the new consciousness which is attained his individuality is completely lost and the valuable fruits of evolution gathered at the cost of so much suffering and travail are washed away in one stroke?

It is reasonable to suppose that the experience of unity with the Divine Consciousness is so perfect and overwhelming that the *Yogi* seems to lose his own individuality for the time being but this does not necessarily mean that the individuality is dissolved and lost for ever in that glorious Reality. If the individuality is completely dissolved how do we then account for its reappearance in the lower worlds? For, it is an undoubted fact that these great Beings do return to the lower worlds after gaining Enlightenment. It is easy for the dewdrop to slip and be lost in the Shining Sea but it cannot be recovered from that Sea again. In the same way, if the individuality is merged and lost completely it cannot separate and manifest again. If it can do so, it simply means that a germ of individuality, however subtle it may be, still remains even in the perfect union of the *Jīvātmā* with *Paramātmā*. So let us not make the mistake of supposing that the long and tedious evolutionary development of a human being ends merely in his disappearance into a Reality from which there is no return and the hard earned fruits of evolution are lost both for him and others. Let us trust that the Almighty who has created this wonderful Universe and devised the Evolutionary Scheme has more intelligence than ourselves!

Then again, from the literal meaning of *Kaivalya* many people are led to imagine that it is a state of consciousness in which the *Puruṣa* is completely isolated from all others and lives alone in solitary grandeur like a man sitting on the peak of a mountain. Such a state, if it did exist, would be a horror and not the consummation of bliss. The idea of isolation implied in *Kaivalya* is to be interpreted in relation to *Prakṛti* from which the *Puruṣa* is isolated. This isolation frees him from all the limitations which are inherent in being involved in matter in a state of *Avidyā* but leads him, on the other hand, to the closest possible unification with Consciousness in all its manifestations. Complete isolation from *Prakṛti* means complete unification with Consciousness or Reality, because it is matter which divides the different units of consciousness, and in the world of Reality we are all one. The more we transcend matter and isolate our consciousness from it the greater becomes the degree of our union with *Parameśvara* and all the *Jīvātmās* who are centres in His Consciousness. And as *Ānanda* is inseparable from Love or the awareness of oneness we can see easily why this consciousness of *Kaivalya* which includes everyone in its vast embrace leads to the acme of Bliss.

The last question that might be dealt with in connection with IV-34 is whether *Kaivalya* represents the end of the journey.

Although a study of the *Yoga-Sūtras* might give the impression that *Kaivalya* is the final goal, those who have trodden the Path and passed further along it, as well as Occult tradition, declare with one voice that *Kaivalya* is only a stage in the unending unfoldment of consciousness. When the *Puruṣa* attains this stage of Self-realization he sees opening before him new vistas of achievement which are utterly beyond human imagination. As Lord Buddha said ' Veil upon veil shall lift, but still veil upon veil will be found behind.' The *Yoga-Sūtras* give the technique for achieving the final goal as far as human beings are concerned. What lies beyond is not only not our concern for the time being, but is totally beyond our comprehension and therefore cannot be the subject of study. The further mysteries which we have to unravel and the stages of the Path we have to tread are hidden within the still deeper recesses of our consciousness and will reveal themselves in due course when we are ready for them. Enough for us, for the time being, is the goal of achievement which is implied in *Kaivalya*.

INDEX

A

Abhiniveśa, 130, 150
Abhyāsa, 20, 21, 22
Ahiṃsā, 206, 237
Aliṅga, 114, 179
Ananta, 254
Antarāyāḥ, 70, 73, 84
Aparigraha, 206, 243
Apavarga, 171
Āsana, 205, 252
Asmitā, 130, 142, 387
Asteya, 206, 240
Ātmā, 269
Ātmabhāva, 426
Avidyā, 130, 138, 140, 196, 198, 200, 402

B

Bhoga, 171
Bhūtas, 171, 269
Brahmacarya, 206, 241
Buddhi, 269, 418, 420

C

Cetanā, pratyak, 71
Citta, 7, 85, 269, 275, 410, 412, 413, 414, 416, 417, 418, 423, 424, 428
Citta, means for making steady, 85, 87, 88, 89, 90, 91, 93
Citta, nirmāṇa, 387, 389, 390

D

Dhāraṇā, 205, 267, 275, 291
Dharma, 403, 408
Dharmī, 303
Dhyāna, 205, 278, 291
Draṣṭā, 10, 11, 169, 185, 198, 423
Dṛśyam, 169, 171, 188, 423
Duḥkha, 82, 148, 161, 168
Dvaṃdva, 256
Dveṣa, 130, 148

G

Guṇas, 171, 179, 408, 409, 437, 443

I

Indriyas, 171, 269, 271

Īśvara, 56, 59, 61
Īśvara-praṇidhāna, 54, 127, 220, 250
Īśvara, vācaka of, 62

K

Kaivalya, 198, 365, 372, 428, 443
Karmas, 160, 391
Karmāśaya, 157, 390
Kleśas, 157, 159, 430, 434
Kleśas, attenuation of, 129
Kleśas, nature of, 130
Kleśas, philosophy of (synopsis), 137
Kleśas, reduction of, 152
Kleśas, suppression of, 155
Krama, 305, 368, 437, 439
Kṣaṇa, 368, 439

L

Liṅga, stage of guṇas, 179

M

Mahā-vratam, 218
Mantra, 377

N

Nidrā, 13, 18, 91
Nirodha, 6, 122
Nirodha Pariṇāma, 292
Niyama, 205, 220

P

Pariṇāma, 305, 307, 383, 437, 439
Pariṇāma, dharma-lakṣaṅa, 300
Pariṇāma, ekāgratā, 298
Pariṇāma, nirodha, 292, 296
Pariṇāma, samādhi, 297
Prajñā, 34, 117, 119, 287
Prakṛti, 188, 189, 191, 383
Prakṛtilaya, 44
Pramāṇa, 13, 16
Praṇava, 62
Praṇava, japa of, 68, 70
Prāṇāyāma, 87, 205, 258, 264, 265, 266, 267
Pratyāhāra, 205, 268, 271
Puruṣa, 56, 185, 188, 191, 337, 372, 414, 424, 434

R

Rāga, 130, 147

S

Samādhi, 205, 250, 280, 291, 377
Samādhi, aspects of, 32
Samādhi, asaṃprajñāta, 41
Samādhi, dharma-megha, 431
Samādhi, nirbīja, 122, 292
Samādhi, nirvicāra, 112, 115, 117, 119
Samādhi, nirvitarka, 109
Samādhi, sabīja, 114, 121
Samādhi, saṃprajñāta, 31
Samādhi, savicāra, 112
Samādhi, savitarka, 101
Saṃskāra, 316, 396
Saṃtoṣa, 220, 247
Saṃyama, 286, 287
Sattva, 336, 363, 372
Satya, 206, 239
Śauca, 220, 245, 246
Siddhas, 333
Siddhis, 307, 343, 377
Siddhi, kaivalya, 365
Siddhi, knowledge of past and future, 307
Siddhi, knowledge of sounds uttered, 314
Siddhi, knowledge of previous birth, 316
Siddhi, knowledge of another's mind, 317
Siddhi, knowledge of time of death, 320
Siddhi, knowledge of the small, the hidden and the distant, 324
Siddhi, knowledge of the solar system, 326
Siddhi, knowledge of the arrangement of stars, 328
Siddhi, knowledge of ˬhe movements of stars, 329
Siddhi, knowledge of the organization of the body, 330
Siddhi, knowledge of Puruṣa, 337
Siddhi, mastery of indriyas, 359
Siddhi, mastery of omnipotence and omniscience, 363
Siddhi, mastery of pañca-bhutas, 351, 357
Siddhi, mastery of Pradhāna, 361
Siddhi, power of disappearance, 318, 319
Siddhi, power of entering another's body, 343
Siddhi, power of immovability, 332
Siddhi, power of increasing gastric fire, 346
Siddhi, power of increasing strength, 323
Siddhi, power of inhibiting hunger and thirst, 331
Siddhi, power of intuition (pratibhā), 334, 341
Siddhi, power of knowing the nature of mind, 335
Siddhi, power of levitation, 345
Siddhi, power of Maha-Videhā, 349
Siddhi, power of passage through space, 348
Siddhi, power of seeing Perfected Beings, 333
Siddhi, power of strengthening qualities, 322
Siddhi, power of superphysical hearing, 347
Smṛti, 13, 19, 109, 396, 418
Sukha, 85, 147, 247
Sūtra, method of exposition, 3
Svādhyāya, 127, 220, 250

T

Tanmātras, 269
Tapas, 127, 220, 248, 377

V

Vairāgya, 20, 25, 30
Vāsanā, 394, 400, 402, 424
Videha, 44
Vikalpa, 13, 17
Vikṣepa, 73
Vikṣepa, elimination of, 85, 87, 88, 89 90, 91, 93
Vikṣepa, symptoms of, 82
Viparyaya, 13, 17
Vitarka, 230, 232
Vivekajaṃ jñānam, 368, 369, 370
Viveka-khyātiḥ, 200, 202, 431
Vṛtti, 8, 12

Y

Yama, 205, 206
Yoga, definition of, 6
Yoga, kriyā, 127
Yogi, bhava-pratyaya, 44
Yogi, his mastery, 94
Yogi, upāya-pratyaya, 47

QUEST BOOKS

are published by The Theosophical Society in America, a branch of a world organization dedicated to the promotion of brotherhood and the encouragement of the study of religion, philosophy, and science, to the end that man may better understand himself and his place in the universe. The Society stands for complete freedom of individual search and belief. Quest Books are offered as a contribution to man's search for truth.